Index to emergency topics

OXFORD MEDICAL PUBLICATIONS

Oxford Handbook of
Respiratory Medicine

Oxford Handbooks

Oxford Handbook of
Respiratory Medicine

Stephen Chapman
Specialist Registrar, Respiratory Medicine,
Oxford Rotation

Grace Robinson
Specialist Registrar, Respiratory Medicine,
Oxford Rotation

John Stradling
Professor of Respiratory Medicine,
University of Oxford

Sophie West
Specialist Registrar, Respiratory Medicine,
Oxford Rotation

OXFORD
UNIVERSITY PRESS

OXFORD
UNIVERSITY PRESS

Great Clarendon Street, Oxford OX2 6DP

Oxford University Press is a department of the University of Oxford.
It furthers the University's objective of excellence in research, scholarship,
and education by publishing worldwide in

Oxford New York

Auckland Cape Town Dar es Salaam Hong Kong Karachi
Kuala Lumpur Madrid Melbourne Mexico City Nairobi
New Delhi Shanghai Taipei Toronto

With offices in

Argentina Austria Brazil Chile Czech Republic France Greece
Guatemala Hungary Italy Japan Poland Portugal Singapore
South Korea Switzerland Thailand Turkey Ukraine Vietnam

Oxford is a registered trade mark of Oxford University Press
in the UK and in certain other countries

Published in the United States
by Oxford University Press Inc., New York

A catalogue record for this title is available from the British Library

Library of Congress Cataloging in Publication Data

Oxford handbook of respiratory medicine / Stephen Chapman ... [et al.].
Includes bibliographical references and index.
    1. Respiratory organs–Diseases–Handbooks, manuals, etc. [DNLM: 1. Respiratory
Tract Diseases–diagnosis–Handbooks.   2. Respiratory Tract Diseases–therapy–
Handbooks. WF 39 O98 2005] I. Title: Handbook of respiratory medicine.
II. Chapman, Stephen.
RC732.O97 2005   616.2'00475–dc22   2005006671

Typeset by Newgen Imaging Systems (P) Ltd., Chennai, India
Printed in Italy
on acid-free paper by Legoprint S.p.A

ISBN   0–19–852977–5 (flexicover)   978–0–19–852977–4 (flexicover)

10 9 8 7 6 5 4 3 2 1

Preface

This *Handbook of Respiratory Medicine* has been written largely by specialist registrars, for specialist registrars. Three of the four authors, Stephen Chapman, Grace Robinson, and Sophie West, are specialist registrars on the Oxford rotation and John Stradling is Professor of Respiratory Medicine in Oxford. It is in a format that the authors would like to have had when they started their specialist registrar training. However, we hope that any health worker or student with an interest in respiratory medicine will find this text a rapid and useful reference source.

The layout of the book tries to fulfil the requirement to be able to look up a topic quickly when the clinical need arises, but also to provide a bit more insight into the more difficult areas. Therefore the chapters are of necessity different in style and reflect the authors' own views on how to best approach and understand an area.

The handbook is divided into five sections: clinical presentations and approaches to symptoms and problems; the clinical conditions themselves; supportive information; procedures; and useful appendices (also on the inside covers), containing more technical and reference information.

We hope you find it helpful. Feedback on errors and omissions would be much appreciated. Please post your comments via the OUP website: *www.oup.com/uk/medicine/handbooks*.

Stephen Chapman
Grace Robinson
John Stradling
Sophie West
June 2005

Acknowledgements

We would like to offer our grateful thanks to the following friends and colleagues for their reviewing and advice on various sections of this book.

Dr Nicholas Bates, Dr Lesley Bennett, Dr Rachel Bennett, Dr Malcolm Benson, Dr Penny Bradbury, Mrs Debbie Buttar, Dr James Calvert, Dr Jane Collier, Dr Graham Collins, Dr Chris Conlon, Dr Chris Davies, Dr Helen Davies, Dr Rob Davies, Dr Thearina de Beer, Mrs Joan Douglass, Dr Rachael Evans, Dr Fergus Gleeson, Dr Maxine Hardinge, Dr Ling Pei Ho, Dr Andrew Jeffreys, Dr Nick Maskell, Dr Phil Mason, Dr Kim McAnaulty, Dr Fiona McCann, Dr Sarah Menzies, Dr Annabel Nickol, Dr Jayne Norcliffe, Dr Jeremy Parr, Ms Gerry Pengelly, Mrs Lisa Priestley, Dr Naj Rahman, Dr Catherine Richardson, Mrs Jo Riley, Dr Peter Sebire, Dr Mark Slade, Dr S Rolf Smith, Dr Catherine Swales, Dr Denis Talbot, Dr David Taylor, Dr Catherine Thomas, Dr Estée Török, Dr David Waine, Dr Chris Wathen, Dr John Wiggins, and Dr Eleanor Wood.

Contents

Part 2 **Clinical conditions**

Part 3 **Supportive care**

Part 4 **Practical procedures**

Appendices

Abbreviations

A–a	alveolar to arterial gradient
ABG	arterial blood gas
ABPA	allergic bronchopulmonary aspergillosis
ACE	angiotensin-converting enzyme
ADH	antidiuretic hormone
AFB	acid-fast bacillus
AFP	alpha-fetoprotein
AIA	aspirin-induced asthma
AIDS	acquired immune deficiency syndrome
AIP	acute interstitial pneumonia
ANA	antinuclear antibody
ANCA	antinuclear cytoplasmic antibody
ANP	atrial natriuretic peptide
APTT	activated partial thromboplastin time
ARDS	acute respiratory distress syndrome
ATRA	all-trans retinoic acid
ATS	American Thoracic Society
AVM	arteriovenous malformation
BAL	bronchoalveolar lavage
BCG	bacille Calmette–Guérin
bd	twice a day
BHR	bronchial hyperreactivity or hyperresponsiveness
BIPAP	bi-level positive airways pressure
BMI	body mass index (kg/metres^2)
BOOP	bronchiolitis obliterans organizing pneumonia
BP	blood pressure
BPD	bronchopulmonary dysplasia
BSAC	British Subaqua Club
BTS	British Thoracic Society
CABG	coronary artery bypass graft
CAP	community-acquired pneumonia
CCF	congestive cardiac failure
CF	cystic fibrosis
CFA	cryptogenic fibrosing alveolitis
CFT	complement fixation test
CFTR	cystic fibrosis transmembrane conductance regulator

CHART	continuous hyperfractionated accelerated radiotherapy
CI	contraindication
CLL	chronic lymphocytic leukaemia
CMV	cytomegalovirus
CNS	central nervous system
CO	carbon monoxide
CO_2	carbon dioxide
COHb	carboxyhaemoglobin
COP	cryptogenic organizing pneumonia
COPD	chronic obstructive pulmonary disease
CPAP	continuous positive airway pressure
CRP	C-reactive protein
CSA	central sleep apnoea
CSF	cerebrospinal fluid
CT	computerized tomography
CTPA	computerized tomographic pulmonary angiogram
CVA	cardiovascular accident
CVD	cardiovascular disease
CXR	chest radiograph
DIC	disseminated intravascular coagulation
DIP	desquamative interstitial pneumonitis
dsDNA	double-stranded DNA
DVLA	Department of Vehicle Licensing Authority
DVT	deep vein thrombosis
ECG	electrocardiogram
Echo	echocardiogram
ECOG	Eastern Cooperative Oncology Group
EEG	electroencephalogram
EGFR	epidermal growth factor receptor
EIA	enzyme immunoassay
ELCAP	Early Lung Cancer Action Project
ELISA	enzyme-linked immunosorbent assay
EMG	electromyogram
ENT	ear, nose, and throat
EOG	electrooculogram
EPAP	expiratory positive airways pressure
ERS	European Respiratory Society
ESR	erythrocyte sedimentation rate
ESS	Epworth sleepiness scale/score
FBC	full blood count

FEV_1	forced expiratory volume in 1 second
FiO_2	fractional inspired oxygen
FNA	fine needle aspirate
FOB	fibre optic bronchoscopy
FRC	functional residual capacity
FVC	forced vital capacity
g	gram
GBM	glomerular basement membrane
GI	gastrointestinal
GORD	gastro-oesophageal reflux disease
GU	genitourinary
H2	histamine receptors, type 2
HAART	highly active antiretroviral therapy
HACE	high altitude cerebral oedema
HAPE	high altitude pulmonary oedema
Hb	haemoglobin
HCG	human chorionic gonadotrophin
HCO_3^-	bicarbonate
HHT	hereditary haemorrhagic telangiectasia
HIV	human immunodeficiency virus
HLA	human leucocyte antigen
HP	hypersensitivity pneumonitis
HRCT	high resolution computerized tomography
HSV	herpes simplex virus
ICU	intensive care unit
IFA	indirect immuno fluorescence assay
IgE	immunoglobulin E
IgG	immunoglobulin G
IgM	immunoglobulin M
IIP	idiopathic interstitial pneumonia
ILD	interstitial lung disease
IM	intramuscular
INR	international normalized ratio
IPAP	inspiratory positive airways pressure
IPF	idiopathic pulmonary fibrosis
ITU	intensive therapy unit
IV	intravenous
IVC	inferior vena cava
JVP	jugular venous pressure
kCO	carbon monoxide transfer factor

l	litre
LAM	lymphangioleiomyomatosis
LCH	Langerhans' cell histiocytosis
LDH	lactate dehydrogenase
LFTs	liver function tests
LIP	lymphoid interstitial pneumonia
LOS	lower oesophageal sphincter
LTOT	long-term oxygen therapy
LVRS	lung volume reduction surgery
M, C & S	microscopy, culture, and sensitivity
MDI	metered dose inhaler
MDR-TB	multidrug-resistant TB
MDT	multidisciplinary team
mg	milligrams
MGUS	monoclonal gammopathy of uncertain significance
MI	myocardial infarction
min	minute
MRI	magnetic resonance imaging
MRSA	methicillin (or multiply) resistant *Staphylococcus aureus*
MTB	mycobacterium tuberculosis
ng	nanograms
NIPPV	non-invasive positive pressure ventilation
NIV	non-invasive ventilation
NNRTI	non-nucleoside reverse transcription inhibitor
NO	nitric oxide
NO_2	nitrogen dioxide
non-REM	non-rapid eye movement sleep
nREM	non-rapid eye movement sleep
NSAID	non-steroidal anti-inflammatory drug
NSIP	non-specific interstitial pneumonia
NTM	non-tuberculous mycobacteria
OCP	oral contraceptive pill
od	once a day
OSA	obstructive sleep apnoea
OSAHS	obstructive sleep apnoea/hypopnoea syndrome
OSAS	obstructive sleep apnoea syndrome
$PaCO_2$	arterial carbon dioxide tension
PAF	platelet-activating factor
PaO_2	arterial oxygen tension
PAP	pulmonary artery pressure

PAS	para-aminosalicylic acid
PC_{20}	provocative concentration (of histamine or methacholine) causing a 20% fall in FEV_1
PCO_2	carbon dioxide tension
PCP	*pneumocystis carinii* (now *jiroveci*) pneumonia
PCR	polymerase chain reaction
PE	pulmonary embolus
PEEP	positive end expiratory pressure
PEFR	peak expiratory flow rate
PEG	percutaneous endoscopic gastrostomy
PFTs	pulmonary function test
PHLS	Public Health Laboratory Service
PHT	pulmonary hypertension
PO	orally/by mouth
PO_2	oxygen tension
PPH	primary pulmonary hypertension
prn	as required
PSA	prostate-specific antigen
PSB	protected specimen brush
PSG	polysomnography
PT	prothrombin time
PTH	parathyroid hormone
qds	four times a day
RADS	reactive airways dysfunction syndrome
RAST	radioallergosorbent test
RBBB	right bundle branch block
RB-ILD	respiratory bronchiolitis-associated interstitial lung disease
RCP	Royal College of Physicians
RCT	randomized controlled trial
REM	rapid eye movement sleep
RNP	ribonuclear protein
RSV	respiratory syncytial virus
RT-PCR	reverse transcriptase polymerase chain reaction
RV	residual volume
RVH	right ventricular hypertrophy
SaO_2	arterial oxygen saturation
SARS	severe acquired respiratory syndrome
SBE	subacute bacterial endocarditis
SCL-70	scleroderma antibody (to topoisomerase 1)
SCUBA	self-contained underwater breathing apparatus

SE	side-effect
SLE	systemic lupus erythematosus
SO_2	sulphur dioxide
SOB	shortness of breath
SVC	superior vena cava
SVCO	superior vena caval obstruction
TB	tuberculosis
TBB	transbronchial biopsy
tds	three times a day
Th2	T-helper 2 cell
TIA	transient ischaemic attack
TLC	total lung capacity
TLCO	total lung carbon monoxide transfer factor
TNF	tumour necrosis factor
TSH	thyroid-stimulating hormone
U & E	urea and electrolytes
UIP	usual interstitial pneumonia
UK	United Kingdom
URT	upper respiratory tract
URTI	upper respiratory tract infection
USS	ultrasound scan
V/Q	ventilation/perfusion ratio
VAP	ventilator acquired pneumonia
VATS	video-assisted thoracoscopic surgery
VC	vital capacity
VTE	venous thromboembolism
WBC	white blood cell count
WCC	white cell count
WHO	World Health Organisation
ZN	Ziehl–Neelson
βHCG	beta human chorionic gonadotrophin
μg	micrograms

Part 1

Clinical presentations— approaches to problems

Breathlessness

Clinical assessment and causes

Physiological mechanisms of breathlessness

Dyspnoea refers to the abnormal and uncomfortable awareness of breathing. Its physiological mechanisms are poorly understood; possible afferent sources for the sensation include receptors in respiratory muscles, juxtacapillary (J) receptors (sense interstitial fluid), and chemo-receptors (sensing $\uparrow CO_2$ and $\downarrow O_2$).

Clinical assessment

All patients need a full history and examination. Key points in the assessment are:

- Duration and onset of breathlessness. The box opposite groups the causes of breathlessness by speed of onset, although in practice some variability and overlap exists. Patients often underestimate the duration of symptoms—inquiring about exercise tolerance over a period of time is a useful way of assessing duration and progression
- Severity of breathlessness. Assess the level of handicap and disability by asking about effects on lifestyle, work, and daily activities
- Exacerbating factors. Ask about rest and exertion, nocturnal symptoms, and body position. The timing of nocturnal breathlessness may provide clues to the likely cause: left ventricular failure causes breathlessness after a few hours of sleep, and resolves after about 45 minutes; asthma tends to occur later in the night; laryngeal inspiratory stridor causes noisy breathlessness of very short duration (<1 min); and Cheyne–Stokes apnoeas result in breathlessness that is recurrent and clears each time in less than 30 sec. Orthopnoea is suggestive of left ventricular failure or diaphragm paralysis, although it is also common in many chronic lung diseases. Breathlessness during swimming is characteristic of bilateral diaphragm paralysis. Trepopnoea refers to breathlessness when lying on one side as a result of ipsilateral pulmonary disease
- Associated symptoms, such as cough, haemoptysis, chest pain, wheeze, stridor, fever, loss of appetite and weight, ankle swelling, and voice change. Wheeze may occur with pulmonary oedema, pulmonary embolism, bronchiolitis, and anaphylaxis, in addition to asthma and COPD
- Personal and family history of chest disease
- Lifetime employment, hobbies, pets, travel, smoking, illicit drug use, medications
- Examination of the cardiovascular and respiratory systems. Observe the pattern and rate of breathing. Assess for signs of respiratory distress. Look for paradoxical abdominal movement if the history suggests diaphragmatic paralysis. A useful bedside test is to exercise the patient (e.g. by stepping on and off a 15 to 20 cm block) until their breathlessness occurs, and then measure oximetry immediately on stopping when the finger is still; a fall in oxygen saturation is expected with organic causes of dyspnoea.

Investigations

Initial investigations typically include resting oximetry, peak flow and spirometry, CXR and ECG. Further tests depend on clinical suspicion; options include full PFTs with measurement of lung volumes lying and standing, gas transfer and flow-volume loop, bronchial hyperresponsiveness or reversibility testing, maximal mouth or inspiratory sniff pressures, ABGs (with measurement of A–a gradient, see page 718), exercise oximetry, ventilation-perfusion scanning and CTPA, HRCT, blood tests (full blood count and TSH), echo, exercise ECG, and cardiac catheterization.

Causes of breathlessness grouped by speed of onset

Instantaneous
- Pneumothorax
- Pulmonary embolism.

Acute (minutes–hours)
- Airways disease (asthma, exacerbation of COPD, upper airways obstruction)
- Parenchymal disease (pneumonia, pulmonary oedema, pulmonary haemorrhage, acute hypersensitivity pneumonitis)
- Pulmonary vascular disease (pulmonary embolism)
- Cardiac disease (e.g. acute myocardial infarction, arrhythmia, valvular disease, tamponade, aortic dissection)
- Metabolic acidosis
- Hyperventilation syndrome.

Subacute (days)
- Many of the above, plus:
  - Pleural effusion
  - Lobar collapse
  - Acute interstitial pneumonia
  - Superior vena cava obstruction
  - Pulmonary vasculitis.

Chronic (months–years)
- Some of the above, plus:
  - Obstructive airways disease (COPD, asthma)
  - Diffuse parenchymal disease (including usual interstitial pneumonia, sarcoidosis, bronchiectasis, lymphangitis carcinomatosis)
  - Pulmonary vascular disease (chronic thromboembolic disease, primary pulmonary hypertension, veno-occlusive disease)
  - Hypoventilation (chest wall deformity, neuromuscular weakness, obesity)
  - Anaemia
  - Thyrotoxicosis.

Specific situations

Causes of breathlessness with a normal CXR

- Airways disease (asthma, upper airways obstruction, bronchiolitis)
- Pulmonary vascular disease (pulmonary embolism, primary pulmonary hypertension, intrapulmonary shunt)
- Early parenchymal disease (e.g. sarcoid, interstitial pneumonias, infection—viral, PCP)
- Cardiac disease (e.g. angina, arrhythmia, valvular disease, intracardiac shunt)
- Neuromuscular weakness
- Metabolic acidosis
- Anaemia
- Thyrotoxicosis
- Hyperventilation syndrome (page 535).

Causes of episodic/intermittent breathlessness

- Asthma
- Pulmonary oedema
- Angina
- Pulmonary embolism
- Hypersensitivity pneumonitis
- Vasculitis
- Hyperventilation syndrome.

Distinguishing cardiac and respiratory causes of breathlessness

This can be difficult. Resting ECG is useful—in practice, a cardiac cause of breathlessness is unlikely in the setting of a completely normal ECG. Exercise ECG, echo, and cardiac catheterization may be required. Measurement of B-type natriuretic peptide (BNP) is a recent development that may be of value in the diagnosis of cardiac failure; in patients presenting as an emergency with breathlessness, a serum BNP level <50 ng/l makes cardiac failure very unlikely. Cardiac and respiratory diseases can of course coexist.

Further information

Rapid measurement of B-type natriuretic peptide in the emergency diagnosis of heart failure. Maisel AS, Krishnaswamy P et al. N Engl J Med 2002; **347**: 161–7

Chronic cough and normal CXR

Aetiology, clinical assessment, and treatment

Cough is a frequent symptom of many respiratory diseases and is often associated with underlying lung pathology and an abnormal CXR.

Cough can occur in otherwise healthy people and is often a self-limiting symptom. Persistent chronic coughing can be a socially disabling and distressing symptom, for which help is often sought. **Cough syncope** is loss of consciousness following violent coughing, a Valsalva type manoeuvre, which impairs venous return to the heart and provokes bradycardia and vasodilatation (similar to an ordinary faint).

- Patients with a normal CXR and persistent cough are often grouped under the heading 'chronic cough'
- **Chronic cough = cough lasting more than 8 weeks**
- It can sometimes be difficult to diagnose the underlying cause
- Investigation is warranted, but successful response to therapeutic trials may aid determination of the underlying cause. Centres vary in their approach to this
- Specialist cough clinics suggest they achieve diagnosis and effective treatment in over 80% of patients referred with chronic cough.

Aetiology In practice, over 90% of cases of chronic cough with a normal CXR are caused by one or more of:
- Cough variant asthma or eosinophilic bronchitis
- Gastro-oesophageal reflux disease
- Postnasal drip, due to perennial or allergic rhinitis, vasomotor rhinitis, or chronic sinusitis.

In clinic: full history History can be unhelpful. Cough is most commonly due to asthma, reflux, or postnasal drip, but unfortunately there may be no specific symptoms to suggest these diagnoses.
- Duration of cough
- When it tends to occur—nights or early morning, after exertion, on exposure to dust, pollen or cold air (asthma), after meals or on sitting or bending over (GORD), nocturnal (postnasal drip and asthma)
- Non-productive or productive and, if so, how much sputum and colour
- Haemoptysis
- Fever
- Associated symptoms
  - Shortness of breath
  - Wheeze
  - Throat clearing
  - Sensation of postnasal drip
  - Chest pain
  - Ankle swelling
  - Orthopnoea/paroxysmal nocturnal dyspnoea
  - Dyspepsia
- Previous respiratory disease, such as childhood asthma, eczema, or hay fever
- History of sinus disease or perennial rhinitis

- History of severe respiratory infections, such as whooping cough, that may have caused bronchiectasis
- Known cardiac disease or valvular heart disease
- Drug history ?ACE inhibitor
- Occupation ?workplace irritants
- Pets/birds
- Smoker
- Use of recreational drugs.

Examination can also be unhelpful, as it is usually normal. Look for signs of underlying lung disease, or other medical conditions, such as heart failure, neurological disease (particularly bulbar involvement).

Investigations

Initially

- **Spirometry** may indicate restrictive or obstructive defect. Performance of spirometry may provoke cough and bronchospasm
- **Methacholine provocation test** (page 701) provides the best positive predictive value for cough due to asthma. A lack of response suggests cough variant asthma is extremely unlikely. PC_{20} is normal in eosinophilic bronchitis
- **Serial peak flow recordings** Twice daily for two weeks. Greater than 20% diurnal variation suggests asthma. Can be normal in cough variant asthma
- **Induced sputum examination**, if available, for eosinophil counts, to suggest either asthma or eosinophilic bronchitis. Usually a research tool.

Later

- **Consider chest HRCT** if any features suggestive of lung cancer or interstitial lung disease, as a small proportion may present with a normal CXR (central tumour)
- **Consider ENT examination** if predominantly upper respiratory tract disease, resistant to treatment. Consider sinus CT
- **Consider bronchoscopy** if foreign body possible, or history suggestive of malignancy, small carcinoid, endobronchial disease. Perform after CT to help guide bronchoscopist
- **Consider oesophageal pH monitoring**.

Treatment The initial treatment of patients with a chronic cough is determined by what the most likely underlying cause is, based on the history and investigations. The key is to give any drug treatment at a high enough dose, and for a long enough time (such as 3 months), to be effective.

Causes of cough (with or without CXR abnormality)

Respiratory
- Infection: viral upper and lower respiratory tract infections, bacterial pneumonia, TB, pertussis
- Chronic bronchitis
- Obstructive airways disease: COPD, asthma
- Cough variant asthma
- Eosinophilic bronchitis
- Obstructive sleep apnoea (nocturnal only)
- Lung cancer
- Bronchiectasis, cystic fibrosis
- Interstitial lung disease
- Airway irritants: smoking, dusts and fumes, acute smoke inhalation
- Airway foreign body.

Mediastinal
- External compression of trachea by enlarged lymph nodes (e.g. lymphoma, TB)
- Mediastinal tumours/cysts/masses.

Cardiac
- Left ventricular failure
- Left atrial enlargement (e.g. severe mitral stenosis).

ENT
- Acute or chronic sinusitis
- Postnasal drip due to perennial, allergic, or vasomotor rhinitis.

GI
- GORD
- Oesophageal dysmotility, stricture, or pharyngeal pouch causing repeated aspiration
- Oesophago-bronchial fistula.

CNS
- Neurological disease affecting swallowing causing repeated aspiration, such as stroke, multiple sclerosis, motor neurone disease, or Parkinson's disease.

Drugs
- ACE inhibitors
- Some inhaler preparations can cause cough.

Other
- Idiopathic
- Ear wax (vagal nerve stimulation)
- Psychogenic.

Causes of chronic cough: asthma, GORD

Asthma or 'cough variant asthma', 'cough predominant asthma'. This represents one end of the asthma spectrum, with airway inflammation, but may have minimal bronchoconstriction. There is not always a typical asthma history, but ask about wheeze, atopy, hay fever, or childhood asthma or eczema. Cough is typically worse after exercise, in cold air, or in the mornings.

Spirometry may be normal, without evidence of airflow obstruction. There may be typical asthmatic diurnal peak flow variation of >20%, or peak flows may be stable.

Methacholine challenge should be positive. If negative, other causes of cough should be sought.

Treatment should be for at least 2 months, with high-dose inhaled steroids. Response may take days or weeks. Bronchodilators may make little difference. If inhaled steroid therapy has been tried unsuccessfully, ensure inhaler technique is optimal and a high dose has been used. Alternatively prescribe a two-week course of oral prednisolone 40 mg/day and assess response. If the cough improves, high-dose inhaled steroids should be continued and slowly reduced after about 2 months.

Eosinophilic bronchitis Airway eosinophilia, rarely with peripheral blood eosinophilia, causing heightened cough reflex, but no bronchial hyper-responsiveness/wheeze or peak flow variation. Diagnosis based on negative asthma investigations and induced sputum eosinophilia. Improves with inhaled corticosteroids, usually after 2–3 weeks. Sputum eosinophil count also reduces with treatment.

Gastro-oesophageal reflux disease (GORD) Cough may be related to distal reflux at the lower oesophageal sphincter (LOS), or due to micro-aspiration of acid into the trachea. There may be associated oesophageal dysmotility. LOS reflux is often longstanding and is associated with a productive or non-productive daytime cough and minimal nocturnal symptoms. It is worse after meals and when sitting down, due to increased intraabdominal pressure being transmitted to the LOS. Micro-aspiration is associated with more prominent symptoms of reflux or dyspepsia, although these are not always present. Patients may have an intermittent hoarse voice, dysphonia, and sore throat.

Laryngoscopy may reveal posterior vocal cord inflammation, but this is not a reliable sign.

A trial of treatment for both is recommended. This is with a high-dose proton pump inhibitor for at least 3 months, although longer treatment may be required to control cough. H2 receptor blockers are also effective and pro-kinetics like metoclopramide may help. Other reflux avoidance measures should be carried out: avoiding caffeine, wearing loose fitting clothes, sleeping with an empty stomach (avoid eating <4 hours before bed), sleeping propped up.

Investigation, if required, due to treatment failure or diagnostic uncertainty, is with 24-hour ambulatory pH monitoring, which determines the presence of reflux events. These may not necessarily be responsible for the cough, so it is not a very specific or sensitive test. Oesophageal manometry can be used to measure the LOS pressure and oesophageal contractions after swallowing to determine the presence of oesophageal dysmotility.

Causes of chronic cough: rhinitis, post-infectious, ACE inhibitors

Rhinitis, sinusitis, and postnasal drip Rhinitis is defined as sneezing, nasal discharge, or blockage for more than an hour on most days for either a limited part of the year (seasonal) or all year (perennial). Furthermore, rhinitis may be allergic (e.g. hayfever), non-allergic, or infective. The associated nasal inflammation may irritate cough receptors directly or produce a postnasal drip. These secretions may pool at the back of the throat, requiring frequent throat clearing, or drip directly into the trachea, initiating cough. A history of facial pain and purulent nasal discharge may suggest sinusitis, which can also predispose to postnasal drip. Symptoms of cough may occur on lying, but can be constant, regardless of position.

Sinusitis is an infection of the paranasal sinuses, which may complicate an URTI and is frequently caused by *Haemophilus influenzae* or *Streptococcus pneumoniae*. It causes frontal headache and facial pain. Chronic sinusitis may require further investigation with CXR or CT, which shows mucosal thickening and air-fluid levels. May need surgery.

ENT examination may reveal swollen turbinates, nasal discharge, or nasal polyps. CT of the sinuses may show mucosal thickening and fluid levels.

Treatment Nasal preparations should be taken by kneeling with the top of the head on the floor ('Mecca' position), or lying supine with the head tipped over the end of the bed.

- **Non-allergic rhinitis** Trials suggest the best results are with an initial 3 weeks of nasal decongestants with first-generation antihistamines (which have helpful anticholinergic properties) and pseudoephedrine. Alternatives are nasal ipratropium bromide or xylometazoline. This is then followed by 3 months of high-dose nasal steroids, which are ineffective when used as first-line treatment. Second-generation antihistamines (i.e. non-sedating) are of no use in non-allergic rhinitis
- **Allergic rhinitis** Second-generation antihistamine and high-dose nasal steroids for 3 months at least
- **Vasomotor rhinitis** Nasal ipratropium bromide for 3 months
- **Chronic sinusitis** Treat as for non-allergic rhinitis, but include 2 weeks of antibiotics active against *H. influenzae*, such as doxycycline or co-amoxiclav.

Post-infectious Respiratory tract infections, especially if viral in nature, can cause a cough. This may take weeks or months to resolve spontaneously, although most settle within 8 weeks. The cough is related to a heightened cough reflex. Associated laryngospasm can occur, which is a sudden hoarseness, with associated stridulous inspiratory efforts and a sensation of being unable to breathe.

Treatment with anti-tussives, such as codeine linctus, may ease the symptoms. Inhaled steroids have been tried, but there is no trial evidence that these work.

ACE inhibitor cough occurs with any ACE inhibitor and is related to bradykinin not being broken down by angiotensin-converting enzyme, and accumulating in the lung. Occurs in 10% of people on ACE inhibitors; more frequent in women. Can occur 3–6 months after starting the drug. Cough usually settles within a week of stopping the drug, but may take months. Avoid all ACE inhibitors thereafter and may need change to change to an angiotensin receptor antagonist.

Further information

Review Series on Cough. A Morice, J Kastelik. *Thorax* 2003: **58**; 901–5 and GA Fontana and M Pistolesi, *Thorax* 2003; **58**: 1092–5

Eosinophilic bronchitis: clinical features, management and pathogenesis. Birring SS *et al*. *Am J Respir Med* 2003; **2**: 169–73

The diagnosis and treatment of cough. Irwin RS and Madison JM. *NEJM* 2000; **343**: 1715–21

Chest pain

The majority of patients with chest pain referred to the respiratory team have either acute pleuritic pain or persistent, well-localized pain. Cardiac pain rarely presents in this manner, although it should be considered in exertional pain or in the presence of risk factors for ischaemic heart disease. Within the respiratory system, pain may arise from the parietal pleura, major airways, chest wall, diaphragm, and mediastinum; the lung parenchyma and visceral pleura are insensitive to pain. Processes involving the upper parietal pleura cause a pain localized to that part of the chest. The lower parietal pleura and outer region of diaphragmatic pleura are innervated by the lower six intercostal nerves, and pain here may be referred to the abdomen. The central region of the diaphragm is supplied by the phrenic nerve (C3, 4 and 5), and pain may be referred to the ipsilateral shoulder tip. Tracheobronchitis tends to be associated with retrosternal pain.

Acute pleuritic chest pain

- Pleuritic pain is sharp, well-localized, worse on coughing and inspiration, and the subsequent limitation of inspiration often leads to a degree of breathlessness
- Causes of acute pleuritic chest pain include:
  - Pulmonary infarction (following embolism)
  - Pneumonia
  - Pneumothorax
  - Pericarditis
  - Pleural infection (empyema, tuberculous)
  - Autoimmune disease (e.g. systemic lupus erythematosus, rheumatoid arthritis)
  - Musculoskeletal
  - Fractured rib
- In addition, consider atypical presentations of serious conditions such as myocardial infarction, aortic dissection, oesophageal rupture, and pancreatitis. Consider angioinvasive fungi such as aspergillus as a cause of chest pain in the immunocompromised
- Diagnosis is typically based on 'pattern recognition' of clinical features followed by selected investigations. Initial investigations typically include CXR, ECG, ABGs, serum inflammatory markers, and D-dimers. Further investigations may include V/Q scanning or CT pulmonary angiography, pleural aspiration, and measurement of serum autoantibodies
- Pulmonary embolism (page 407) commonly presents with pleuritic pain, and exclusion of this diagnosis is the usual reason for referral. Assess risk factors for thromboembolic disease. Normal oxygen saturations and PaO_2 in the 'normal' range do not exclude the diagnosis; calculate the A–a gradient (page 718). The presence of a pleural rub is a non-specific sign that occurs with pleural inflammation of any cause
- In young adults, pneumococcal pneumonia may present with acute onset pleuritic chest pain, although systemic symptoms such as fever usually predate the pain by hours

- The pain from pericarditis is pleuritic but central, and relieved on leaning forward; there may also be a pericardial rub, characteristic ECG features, and a small pericardial effusion on echo
- Musculoskeletal pain may occur as a result of cervical disc disease, arthritis of the shoulder or spine, a fractured rib, or costochondritis (Tietze's syndrome), which often follows a viral infection
- The presence of chest wall tenderness does not invariably indicate a benign, musculoskeletal cause; tenderness may be seen in malignant chest wall infiltration and sometimes following pulmonary infarction
- Other features besides pleurisy that may suggest a diagnosis of systemic lupus erythematosus include rash, photosensitivity, oral ulcers, arthritis, pericarditis, renal or neurological disease, cytopenia, positive ANA, and dsDNA.

Chronic chest pain

- Persistent chest pain that is well-localized is typically caused by chest wall or pleural disease. Causes include:
  - Malignant pleural disease or chest wall infiltration
  - Benign musculoskeletal pain
  - Pleural infection (empyema, tuberculous)
  - Benign asbestos pleural disease
  - Autoimmune disease (e.g. systemic lupus erythematosus, rheumatoid arthritis)
  - Recurrent pulmonary infarction (emboli, vasculitis)
- Pain from malignant chest wall infiltration is often 'boring' in character, and may disturb sleep; it is frequently not related to respiration. Causes include primary lung cancer, secondary pleural malignancy, mesothelioma, and rib or sternal involvement from malignancy (including myeloma and leukaemia)
- Chronic thromboembolic disease tends to present with breathlessness; when chest pain occurs, it is usually episodic rather than persistent
- As with acute pleuritic pain, investigations are directed by initial clinical suspicion. Consider CT chest, bone scan, serum autoantibodies, full blood count and film, serum electrophoresis. CXR may appear normal in malignant chest wall disease.

Haemoptysis

Clinical assessment and causes

Haemoptysis is a common and non-specific feature of many lung diseases. It can be a sign of significant underlying lung disease. In up to one-third of cases, no cause will be found. An early assessment of the likely underlying cause needs to be made and investigated accordingly.

Diagnostic approach to haemoptysis Small volume haemoptysis is a commonly encountered problem in the out-patient department. It can be safely and efficiently investigated as an out-patient. Massive haemoptysis is usually encountered in the accident and emergency department or in a patient already on the ward, with known underlying lung disease. The approaches to small volume and massive haemoptysis are different.

History

- Past history of lung disease?
- Document volume of blood and whether old (altered) or fresh
- Time course (intermittent, constant)
- Definitely from the airway and not from the nose or mouth or haematemesis? (though haemoptysis may easily be swallowed, and then vomited)
- Presence of systemic features—associated infection, symptoms consistent with underlying malignancy?

Examination May be normal or show signs of underlying lung disease, e.g. bronchiectasis, bronchial carcinoma, or symptoms of circulatory collapse.

In practice the usual differential diagnosis lies between:

- Malignancy
- Bronchiectasis
- Tuberculosis/infection
- PE.

Causes of haemoptysis

Common

- Bronchial tumour (benign, e.g. carcinoid or malignant). Haemoptysis is a common presenting feature of bronchogenic malignancy, indicating endobronchial disease, which may be visible endoscopically
- Bronchiectasis. Small volume haemoptysis is a common feature of bronchiectasis, particularly during exacerbations. It can be a cause of massive haemoptysis, from dilated and abnormal bronchial artery branches that form around bronchiectatic cavities
- Active tuberculosis. Haemoptysis occurs in cavitating and non-cavitating disease, active disease and inactive disease (bronchiectatic cavity, e.g. containing mycetoma)
- Pneumonia (especially pneumococcal)
- Pulmonary thromboembolic disease
- Vasculitides/alveolar haemorrhage syndromes, e.g. Wegener's granulomatosis, SLE, Goodpasture's syndrome
- Warfarin with any of the above.

Rare
- Lung abscess
- Mycetoma
- Fungal/viral/parasitic infections
- Fat embolism
- Arteriovenous malformation e.g. in hereditary haemorrhagic telangiectasia (HHT) (see page 565)
- Severe PHT (see page 391)
- Mitral stenosis (rare)
- Congenital heart disease
- Aortic aneurysm
- Aspergillus—invasive fungal disease (intracavity mycetoma) can be a cause of massive haemoptysis
- Coagulopathy including disseminated intravascular coagulation
- Endometriosis
- Pulmonary haemosiderosis
- Iatrogenic, e.g. lung biopsy, bronchoscopy.

Investigations

The investigation of haemoptysis can often be carried out as an out-patient, but patients with significant bleeding or likely serious underlying cause should be admitted if there are concerns.

NB Beware of the apparently small bleed, which is a sentinel/herald bleed for massive bleeding. This is fortunately rare.

Out-patient investigations and management

First-line investigations

- *Blood tests* FBC, clotting, group and save. Autoantibodies—ANCA, anti-GBM, ANA (if vasculitis suspected)
- *Sputum cytology* and M, C, & S and AFB if infection suspected
- *CXR* may show mass lesion, bronchiectasis, consolidation, or an AVM
- *CT chest* should be done prior to bronchoscopy, as prior knowledge of the site of abnormality leads to increased pick up rates at bronchoscopy. Similarly, a definitive diagnosis, e.g. AVM, may be made from the CT, obviating the need for further investigations. This depends on local resources, CT may miss an upper airway abnormality, but bronchoscopy should not
- *Bronchoscopy* to visualize airways and localize the site of bleeding. May also be therapeutic, for example if a bleeding tumour can be injected with vasoconstricting agent or catheter inserted for tamponade (see massive haemoptysis)
- *Transbronchial biopsies*—if vasculitis suspected.

Second-line investigations

Usually done if first-line investigations fail to demonstrate a cause
- *CTPA* to exclude PE
- *Bronchial angiogram* Diagnostic and therapeutic. Rare for the actual bleeding site to be identified; more often the bleeding site is assumed from visualizing a mesh of dilated and tortuous vessels, e.g. around a bronchiectatic cavity. Usually done during an episode of bleeding, to maximize the chance of identifying the site of bleeding
- *Bronchial artery embolization*—therapeutic approach to embolize the bleeding artery, usually with coils or glue (specialist centre only)
- *ENT review* The source of the bleeding may be the upper airway
- *Echocardiogram* Moderate/severe PHT can cause haemoptysis, especially in a patient on anticoagulants.

Cryptogenic haemoptysis In around one-third of cases, despite appropriate investigations as above, no cause for the haemoptysis can be found. This has a good prognosis. Often the haemoptysis will settle without treatment and will become less worrying to the patient over time, especially as investigations have failed to determine the cause.

Management of massive haemoptysis

Massive haemoptysis (100–600 ml blood in 24 hours) is a life-threatening emergency, with a mortality of up to 80%.

Massive haemoptysis is extremely distressing for the patient, relatives, and medical staff, but is fortunately rare. Investigations will follow treatment, which may be difficult, and is often unsuccessful. In some cases, active treatment may be inappropriate, and palliative treatment with oxygen and diamorphine may be warranted.

- Airway protection and ventilation

Protection of the non-bleeding lung is vital to maintain adequate gas exchange. This may involve lying on the bleeding side (to prevent blood flowing into the unaffected lung), or intubation with a double lumen tube.

If intubation is not needed, or not appropriate, give high flow oxygen.

- Cardiovascular support
  - Large bore/central intravenous access
  - Clotting factors, group and save
  - Fluid resuscitation ± transfusion
  - Reverse anticoagulants
  - Inotropes
- Nebulized adrenaline (5–10 ml of 1 in 10,000)
- Oral tranexamic acid (500 mg tds, not if in severe renal failure)
- CXR ± Chest CT (depending on stability of patient)
- Early bronchoscopy—diagnostic and therapeutic
- Rigid bronchoscopy (with general anaesthesia) is preferable. May allow localization of the site of bleeding, balloon tamponade with a Fogarty catheter
- Bronchial artery embolization—therapeutic approach to embolize bleeding artery, usually with coils or glue (specialist centre only)
- Surgery—resection of bleeding lobe (if all other measure have failed).

Unexplained respiratory failure

Causes

Definition Respiratory failure is conventionally divided into type I (hypoxia only, $PaO_2 < 8$ kPa) and type II (hypoxia and hypercapnia, $PaCO_2 > 6$ kPa): they are conceptually quite different. Type I is an increased alveolar-to-arterial (A–a) gradient with no impairment of ventilation. The number of causes is of course vast, including most of respiratory medicine, and requires the usual 'history, examination, and investigations'.

A more difficult, less common, clinical scenario, is an unexplained rise in $PaCO_2$ (>6 kPa, type II), with no obvious cause following a standard assessment. This may occur in the out-patient, ward, A&E, or ICU setting.

Pathophysiology A rise in $PaCO_2$ can be due to V/Q mismatch with inadequate compensatory hyperventilation, e.g. overwhelming asthma, when there will also be a large A–a gradient indicating this increased V/Q mismatch. However, it can also be due to inadequate ventilatory drive, or primary ventilatory pump failure, where the A–a gradient will usually be normal. The list below contains mainly the causes that might not have been suspected from the initial assessment, but for completeness also includes more obvious causes. The conditions with asterisks are the ones most commonly discovered when the cause is not immediately obvious.

Failure of drive
Brainstem abnormality
- Polio and post-polio syndrome* (exact mechanism unclear)
- Brainstem stroke
- Arnold–Chiari malformation—herniation of cerebellum into foramen magnum compressing the brainstem
- Syringobulbia—expansion of a fluid compartment in the middle of the spinal cord extending up into the medulla (can be associated with Arnold–Chiari malformation)
- Encephalitis
- Brainstem tumour.

Suppression
- Sedative drugs*
- Metabolic alkalosis (hypokalaemic alkalosis, diuretic-induced).

Pump failure
Neurological (particularly if diaphragm involved)
- Myopathies
  - Acid maltase deficiency (Pompe's), diaphragm paralysis commonly occurs early on*
  - Duchenne muscular dystrophy
  - Myotonic dystrophy
  - Several other very rare myopathies
- Neuropathy
  - Motor neurone disease (MND) can affect diaphragm early on*
  - Bilateral diaphragm paralysis, e.g. bilateral neuralgic amyotrophy, trauma*
  - Guillain–Barré*

- Spinal muscular atrophy
- High cord transection
- Neuromuscular junction abnormalities
  - Myasthenia gravis*
  - Eaton–Lambert syndrome
  - Anti-choline esterase poisoning
- Mixed
  - Post ITU ('critical care neuropathy'), post muscle relaxant drugs*
- *Chest wall*
  - Obesity*
  - Scoliosis*
  - Post thoracoplasty (usually 'three stage', many ribs caved in starting from the top down—done for tuberculosis pre effective chemotherapy)
  - Flail chest
  - Pneumothorax/large effusion
  - Severe ankylosing spondilitis
- *Airways obstruction/mixed*
  - Unrecognized COPD/severe asthma*
  - Obstructive sleep apnoea and associated COPD/obesity/muscle weakness.*

Clinical presentation

Slow onset

In several of the above conditions, e.g. acid maltase deficiency, MND, and scoliosis, the onset of ventilatory failure can be insidious and include:

- General fatigue
- Headaches on awakening
- Morning confusion
- Morning cyanosis
- Dyspnoea in the swimming pool (diaphragm paralysis)
- Swallowing difficulties (MND)
- Ankle oedema (fluid retention, cor pulmonale, from the hypoxia).

Rapid onset

Sometimes the significance of these symptoms is missed and a relatively trivial respiratory tract infection tips the balance and the patient goes into severe ventilatory failure with coma. These individuals will end up ventilated on ICU and may be difficult to wean, or present again a few weeks after discharge.

Clinical assessment and management

History, examination, and investigations

History A more carefully taken history, particularly for symptoms of a subtle weakness prior to presentation, episode of shoulder pain (neuralgic amyotrophy), past history of polio, orthopnoea (diaphragm weakness), drug history, may be helpful. Often this is not available as the patient may present unconscious.

Examination A thorough examination, particularly neurological, may reveal clues, such as fasciculation, diaphragm weakness (inward drawing of abdomen on inspiration/sniffing: *masked* if on positive pressure ventilation), myotonia, as well as rarer signs seen in some of the conditions listed previously.

Blood gases taken breathing air (following >20 minutes off extra O_2)
- Degree of CO_2 retention
- Presence of a base excess indicating chronicity of CO_2 retention
- Calculate A–a gradient to detect any V/Q mismatch (page 718)
- In pure hypoventilation there should be no significant A–a gradient (<2 kPa), unless there is associated basal atelectasis from poor lung expansion and/or obesity.

Pulmonary function tests (page 705)
- Presence of unexpected severe airways obstruction
- Reduction in vital capacity (neurological or chest wall)
- Further fall of VC on lying down—indicative of diaphragm paralysis
- The supine VC is most predictive of ventilatory failure, <1 litre indicates a high chance of this being the cause of the failure
- Mouth pressures, sniff pressures, or trans-diaphragmatic pressures; not much more helpful than VC, lying and standing.

Specific tests—for some of the conditions listed above such as:
- EMG studies—MND, myotonia
- MRI—gadolinium enhanced: Arnold–Chiari, brainstem lesion, syrinx
- CPK—some myopathies
- Sleep study—REM hypoxia, obstructive sleep apnoea
- Muscle biopsy—acid maltase deficiency (glycogen-containing vacuoles and low enzyme levels).

Management Management of the underlying condition, if available, is paramount. In the situation of irreversibility, the decision will need to be taken as to whether non-invasive ventilation is appropriate. Page 600.

Lying down and sleeping with the ***whole bed tipped head up*** by about 20° greatly improves ventilation in the presence of bilateral diaphragm paralysis. Just elevating the top half of the bed and leaving the abdomen and legs horizontal does not work. The abdominal contents have to descend into the pelvis to effectively 'offload' the diaphragm. This posture will also improve the ability to wean from assisted ventilation.

Pleural effusion

Clinical assessment

Pleural effusion is a common presentation of a wide range of different diseases.

Commonest causes in UK and USA (in order): cardiac failure, pneumonia, malignancy, pulmonary embolism.

Priority is to make a diagnosis and relieve symptoms with minimum number of invasive procedures. The majority of patients do not require a chest drain and can be managed as out-patients. Procedures such as therapeutic thoracentesis may be performed readily on a day unit. Consider admission and chest drain insertion for:

- Patients with malignant effusions who are candidates for pleurodesis
- Empyema or parapneumonic effusion with purulent fluid or a pleural fluid pH < 7.2 (the majority of these effusions are unlikely to resolve without drainage and antibiotics)
- Patients who are unwell with an acute massive effusion.

Key steps in the management of the patient with a pleural effusion (see also abbreviated algorithm in following section):

1. **History, examination, CXR** (PA and lateral).

2. **Does the patient have heart failure?** If so, this should be treated, with no need for pleural tap unless atypical features (such as very asymmetrical bilateral effusions, unilateral effusion, chest pain, or fever) or fails to respond within 3 days (75% of cardiac failure effusions resolve following 48 hours of diuresis).

3. **Thoracentesis** (= 'pleural tap', or pleural fluid aspiration) may be diagnostic and/or therapeutic, depending on the volume of fluid removed. See page 676 for procedure details. Following diagnostic tap:
   - Note pleural fluid *appearance*
   - Send sample in sterile pot to biochemistry for measurement of *protein* and *LDH*
   - Send a fresh, 20 ml sample in sterile pot to *cytology* for examination for malignant cells and differential cell count
   - Send samples in sterile pot and blood culture bottles to *microbiology* for Gram stain and microscopy, culture, and AFB stain and culture
   - Process non-purulent, heparinized samples in arterial blood gas analyser for **pH**
   - Consider measurement of cholesterol and triglycerides, haematocrit, glucose, and amylase, depending on the clinical circumstances.

If the patient is breathless they may benefit from removal of a larger volume of fluid (therapeutic tap, page 677).

4. **Is the pleural effusion a transudate or exudate?** Helpful in narrowing the differential diagnosis. In patients with a normal serum protein, pleural fluid protein <30 g/l = transudate and protein >30 g/l = exudate. In borderline cases (protein 25–35 g/l), or

in patients with abnormal serum protein, apply Light's criteria—effusion is exudative if it meets one of following criteria:

Pleural fluid protein/serum protein ratio > 0.5

Pleural fluid LDH/serum LDH ratio > 0.6

Pleural fluid LDH > two-thirds the upper limit of normal serum LDH

These criteria are very sensitive in the diagnosis of exudative effusions, although may occasionally falsely identify transudates as being exudates, e.g. patients with partially treated heart failure on diuretics may be misidentified as exudates.

5. **Further investigations** if the diagnosis remains unclear:
   • CT chest with pleural contrast (ideally scan prior to complete fluid drainage, to improve images of pleural surfaces; useful in distinguishing benign and malignant pleural disease, page 300).
   • Repeat pleural fluid cytology
   • Further pleural fluid analysis, e.g. cholesterol, triglyceride, haematocrit, glucose, amylase, fungal stains
   • Pleural tissue biopsy for histology and TB culture (ultrasound- or CT-guided, closed Abrams', or thoracoscopic biopsy; image-guided biopsies are superior to Abrams' for malignant disease; use Abrams' biopsy only in cases when tuberculosis is suspected; thoracoscopy is 'gold-standard', biopsies have sensitivity of 90% for malignancy, and allow therapeutic talc pleurodesis at the same time)
   • Reconsider pulmonary embolism and tuberculosis
   • Consider thoracoscopy if persistent undiagnosed pleural effusion.

Bronchoscopy has no role in investigating undiagnosed effusions unless the patient has haemoptysis or a CXR/CT pulmonary abnormality. Pleural fluid may compress the airways and limit bronchoscopic views, and so if bronchoscopy is indicated it is best performed following drainage of the effusion.

Further information

Pleural effusions: the workup and treatment. Holm KA and Antony VB. *J Respir Dis* 2001; **22**: 211–9

Pleural effusion. Light RW. *NEJM* 2002; **346**: 1971–7

BTS Guidelines for the investigation of a unilateral pleural effusion in adults. Maskell NA, Butland RJA. *Thorax* 2003; **58** (suppl. II) ii8–17

Diagnostic algorithm for the patient with a pleural effusion

1. **History, examination, CXR.**

2. **Does the patient have heart failure,** with no atypical features (such as asymmetrical bilateral effusions, unilateral effusion, normal heart size on CXR, chest pain, fever)?

No | Yes

Diuresis

Effusions persist

3. **Thoracentesis** (diagnostic ± therapeutic).
   Pleural fluid analysis: appearance, protein, LDH, cytology, microbiology, pH (± cholesterol, triglyceride, haematocrit, glucose, amylase).

4. **Is the pleural effusion a transudate or exudate?**

Exudate | Transudate

Treat cause

Effusion persists

5. **Further investigations** if diagnosis remains unclear:
   - CT chest with contrast to enhance pleura
   - Repeat pleural fluid cytology
   - Further pleural fluid analysis, e.g. cholesterol, triglyceride, haematocrit, glucose, amylase, fungal stains
   - Pleural tissue biopsy for histology and TB culture (ultrasound- or CT-guided, closed Abrams', or thoracoscopic biopsy)
   - Reconsider pulmonary embolism and tuberculosis
   - Consider thoracoscopy if persistent undiagnosed pleural effusion.

Transudative pleural effusions

Mechanisms involve either increased hydrostatic pressure or reduced osmotic pressure (due to hypoalbuminaemia) in the microvascular circulation.

Differential diagnosis

Cause	Notes
Common	
Left ventricular failure	Investigate further if atypical features (very asymmetrical bilateral effusion, unilateral effusion, chest pain, fever); frequently complicated by pulmonary embolism (up to one-fifth of cases at autopsy)
Cirrhotic liver disease ('hepatic hydrothorax')	Ascites often but not invariably present; majority right-sided; remove ascites and treat hypoalbuminaemia (page 514)
Pulmonary embolism	10–20% are transudates (page 314)
Peritoneal dialysis	Pleural fluid analysis resembles dialysis fluid, with protein <1 g/dl and glucose >300 mg/dl
Nephrotic syndrome	Usually bilateral; consider secondary pulmonary embolism if atypical features
Atelectasis	Common on ITU or post-operatively; usually small effusion, may be bilateral; rarely needs investigation
Less common	
Constrictive pericarditis	May be unilateral or bilateral
Hypothyroidism	May be transudate or exudate; pleural effusions occur most commonly in association with ascites, pericardial effusion, and cardiac failure, although may be an isolated finding
Meigs' syndrome	Unilateral (often right-sided) or bilateral pleural effusions and ascites; occur in women with ovarian or other pelvic tumours; resolve following removal of tumour
Urinothorax	Effusion ipsilateral to obstructed kidney with retroperitoneal urine leak, resolves after treatment of obstruction; pleural fluid smells of urine, pH usually low; pleural fluid creatinine > serum creatinine is diagnostic
Malignancy	Up to 5% are transudates

Treatment of transudative effusions is directed at the underlying cause; consider further investigation if fails to respond.

Exudative pleural effusions

Mechanisms involve an increase in capillary permeability and impaired pleural fluid resorption.

Differential diagnosis

Cause	Notes and page references
Common	
Parapneumonic effusion	Occurs in 40% of bacterial pneumonias; commonest exudative effusion in young patients (page 306)
Malignancy	Commonest exudative effusion in patients > 60 years (page 302)
Pulmonary embolism	80–90% are exudates (page 314)
Rheumatoid arthritis	Typically low pleural fluid glucose, often <1.6 mmol/l (page 314)
Mesothelioma	Pleural fluid cytological analysis has low sensitivity (page 324)
Less common	
Empyema	Pleural fluid pH < 7.2; clinical features of infection, e.g. fever, sweats (page 306)
Tuberculosis	Typically lymphocytic effusion; pleural fluid AFB smear positive in 10% of cases, culture positive in 25%, Abrams' biopsy histology sensitivity 90% (page 312)
Other infections	Very rare; include viral, parasitic, rickettsial, and fungal (e.g. aspergillus, histoplasma, coccidioidomycosis)
Hepatic, splenic or subphrenic abscess	
Oesophageal rupture	Initially sterile exudate, followed by empyema; pH < 7.2, raised salivary amylase, often history of vomiting
Pancreatitis	Pleural fluid pancreatic amylase may be raised
SLE	Lupus erythematosus cells in fluid are diagnostic; may respond quickly to prednisolone
Other autoimmune diseases	Churg–Strauss syndrome (intensely eosinophilic fluid), Sjögren's syndrome, scleroderma, dermatomyositis, Wegener's granulomatosis
Sarcoidosis	Effusions are uncommon
Post-cardiac injury syndrome (Dressler's syndrome)	Pleural effusions common; may be blood-stained
Post-coronary artery bypass surgery	(page 315)
Radiotherapy	May cause small, unilateral effusions up to 6 months after treatment
Uraemia	Effusions frequently resolve after starting dialysis
Chylothorax	Presence of chylomicrons or pleural fluid triglyceride level >110 mg/dl (page 40)

Benign asbestos-related pleural effusion	(page 320)
Drug-induced	Drugs include amiodarone, bromocriptine, methotrexate, phenytoin, and nitrofurantoin; see www.pneumotox.com for full list; effusions usually resolve following discontinuation of drug
Other, rare causes	Include yellow nail syndrome, cryptogenic organizing pneumonia, amyloidosis, familial Mediterranean fever

Treatment of exudates involves treatment of the underlying cause, as well as measures to improve breathlessness and remove pleural fluid, e.g. therapeutic thoracentesis (page 677), intercostal drainage (page 685), and pleurodesis (page 692).

Pleural fluid analysis 1

'Routine' pleural fluid analysis comprises assessment of:
- Pleural fluid appearance
- Biochemistry (protein and LDH)
- Cytology (for malignant cells and differential cell count; ideally fresh 20 ml sample)
- Microbiology (Gram stain and microscopy, culture, and AFB stain and culture; inoculation of blood culture bottles with pleural fluid may increase yield)
- pH.

Although considered routine, some of these investigations may be unnecessary and even misleading, depending on the clinical picture (e.g. microbiological analysis on patients suspected as having transudates).

Additional pleural fluid investigations such as measurement of cholesterol and triglycerides, haematocrit, glucose, and amylase may be helpful in certain clinical circumstances.

Appearance

Appearance	Possible causes
Bloody	Trauma, malignancy, pulmonary infarction, pneumonia, post-cardiac injury syndrome, pneumothorax, benign asbestos-related pleural effusion, aortic dissection/rupture; defined as haemothorax if pleural fluid haematocrit >50% of peripheral blood haematocrit (page 314)
Turbid or milky	Empyema, chylothorax, pseudochylothorax (clear supernatant after centrifuging favours empyema; cloudy after centrifuging suggests chylothorax or pseudochylothorax, page 40)
Putrid odour	Anaerobic empyema
Viscous	Mesothelioma
Food particles	Oesophageal rupture
Urine odour	Urinothorax
Black	Aspergillus infection
Brown, 'anchovy sauce'	Amoebic liver abscess draining into pleural space

Differential cell count

Predominant cell type	Possible causes
Neutrophils	Any acute effusion, e.g. parapneumonic, pulmonary embolus
Mononuclear cells	Any chronic effusion, e.g. malignancy, tuberculosis
Lymphocytes	Tuberculosis, especially if over 80%; other causes include malignancy, sarcoidosis, lymphoma, rheumatoid pleurisy, post-CABG
Eosinophils	Often unhelpful; associations include air or blood in pleural space (haemothorax, pulmonary infarct, pneumothorax, previous tap), malignancy, infection (parapneumonic, tuberculous, fungal, parasitic), drug- and asbestos-induced effusions, Churg–Strauss syndrome or idiopathic
Mesothelial cells	Predominate in transudates; variable numbers in exudates, typically suppressed in inflammatory conditions, e.g. tuberculosis
Lupus erythematosus cells	Diagnostic of systemic lupus erythematosus

Pleural fluid analysis 2

Pleural fluid pH and glucose Pleural fluid pH may be measured using an arterial blood pH analyser. The sample should be appropriately heparinized, e.g. aspirate a few ml of pleural fluid into a pre-heparinized blood gas syringe. Frankly purulent samples should not be analysed—it is unnecessary, and might damage the machine.

Normal pleural fluid pH is about 7.6. An abnormally low pH (<7.3) suggests pleural inflammation and is often associated with a low pleural fluid glucose (<3.3 mmol/l or pleural fluid/serum glucose ratio <0.5). The mechanism probably involves increased neutrophil phagocytosis and bacterial or tumour cell breakdown, resulting in the accumulation of lactate and carbon dioxide.

Causes of low pH and low glucose effusions:
- Parapneumonic effusion and empyema (pH < 7.2 indication for drainage of pleural space, as unlikely to resolve spontaneously)
- Rheumatoid pleuritis (glucose < 1.7 mmol/l in 66% and < 2.8 mmol/l in 80% of cases)
- Malignant pleural effusion (associated with advanced disease and poor survival, higher sensitivity of pleural fluid cytological analysis, and failure of pleurodesis)
- Tuberculous pleural effusion
- Oesophageal rupture
- Lupus pleuritis.

Urinothorax is the only transudative effusion that can cause a pH < 7.3. An abnormally high (alkaline) pH may rarely occur in the setting of *Proteus* pleural infection.

Pleural fluid triglyceride and cholesterol Measure in turbid or milky effusions or where chylothorax is suspected.

Chylothorax occurs following disruption of the thoracic duct, and pleural fluid may appear turbid, milky, serous, or blood-stained. The presence of pleural fluid chylomicrons or a pleural fluid triglyceride level >110 mg/dl confirm the diagnosis. Causes of chylothorax:
- Malignancy (particularly lymphoma)
- Trauma
- Following thoracotomy
- Pulmonary lymphangioleiomyomatosis.

Pseudochylothorax occurs due to cholesterol crystal deposition in chronic effusions, most commonly due to rheumatoid pleurisy or tuberculosis, and may cause a milky effusion; raised pleural fluid cholesterol (> 200 mg/dl) and cholesterol crystals at microscopy distinguish it from chylothorax.

Pleural fluid amylase Abnormal if pleural fluid amylase > upper normal limit for serum amylase, or if amylase pleural fluid/serum ratio > 1.0. Causes include:

- Pleural malignancy and oesophageal rupture (both associated with raised *salivary* amylase)
- Pancreatic disease (acute and chronic pancreatitis, pancreatic pseudocyst; associated with raised *pancreatic* amylase).

NB May be normal early in the course of acute pancreatitis or oesophageal rupture.

Diffuse lung disease

Causes

Diffuse lung disease is common and its diagnosis is frequently challenging. This chapter describes a diagnostic approach based on clinical features, imaging, and other investigations; more detailed descriptions of the diseases themselves are presented later in the book. The term 'diffuse lung disease' is used here to describe any widespread pulmonary disease process. Patients typically present with breathlessness and bilateral CXR shadowing. The rate of onset and severity of breathlessness are extremely variable, however, and presentations range from an asymptomatic patient with longstanding radiological changes to an acute onset of breathlessness over days leading rapidly to respiratory failure and death.

Anatomy of diffuse lung disease

An understanding of lung anatomy is helpful when considering the causes of diffuse lung disease and their appearance on HRCT. Many diffuse lung diseases primarily affect the interstitium ('interstitial lung disease', also described as 'diffuse parenchymal lung disease'), a poorly defined term that refers to the connective tissue fibrous framework of the lung. Centrally, connective tissue surrounds bronchovascular bundles (each consisting of a bronchus and its accompanying pulmonary artery) that originate at the hila. Peripherally, these connective tissue sheaths are in continuity with fibrous interlobular septa that organize the lung into units called 'secondary pulmonary lobules', polyhedral structures with approximately 2 cm sides. Interlobular septa, which define and separate secondary pulmonary lobules, contain lymphatics and venules. A secondary pulmonary lobule contains around 5–12 acini and is supplied at its centre by a bronchiole and pulmonary arteriole.

The term 'interstitial lung disease' is confusing because many primarily interstitial processes also involve the airways, vasculature, and alveolar airspaces. Disease processes that primarily affect the airways (e.g. bronchiectasis), vessels (e.g. vasculitis), or airspaces (e.g. pneumonia) may also present with diffuse CXR shadowing and so are included in this chapter.

Causes

There are several hundred causes of diffuse lung disease, and it is useful to divide these into groups based on their rate of onset and aetiology/disease mechanism (see table opposite).

Further information

Picture of secondary pulmonary lobule
www.vh.org/adult/provider/radiology/DiffuseLung/AnatImages/2LobuleRadiograph Schema.html

British Thoracic Society. BTS guidelines on the diagnosis, assessment and treatment of diffuse parenchymal lung disease in adults. *Thorax* 1999; **54** (suppl. 1): S1–30

Causes of diffuse lung disease

Disease onset	Cause/ mechanism	Examples (common conditions in bold)
Acute (days– weeks)	Infection	**Bacterial** (pneumococcal, staphylococcal, Gram-negative, anaerobic, TB), viral (influenza, parainfluenza, adeno, RSV, measles, varicella, hanta), atypical, fungal (aspergillosis, histoplasmosis, PCP)
	Miscellaneous	**Adult respiratory distress syndrome,** acute interstitial pneumonia (AIP), acute hypersensitivity pneumonitis
Acute or chronic	Drugs	Immunosuppressants (methotrexate, azathioprine, cyclophosphamide); treatment of connective tissue disease (gold, penicillamine, sulfasalazine); cytotoxics (chlorambucil, melphalan, busulfan, lomustine, carmustine, bleomycin, mitomycin); antibiotics (nitrofurantoin, cephalosporins); anti-arrhythmics (amiodarone); illicit (cocaine inhalation, heroin, methadone, IV talc)
	Toxins	Radiotherapy, high concentration oxygen, paraquat
	Vasculitis/alveolar haemorrhage	Wegener's granulomatosis, Churg–Strauss syndrome, Goodpasture's syndrome, SLE, microscopic polyangiitis, idiopathic haemosiderosis
	Pulmonary venous hypertension	**Cardiogenic pulmonary oedema,** pulmonary venoocclusive disease
	Miscellaneous	**Sarcoidosis,** cryptogenic organizing pneumonia (COP), eosinophilic pneumonia, lipoid pneumonia
Chronic (months– years)	Idiopathic interstitial pneumonias	**Usual interstitial pneumonia (UIP),** non-specific interstitial pneumonia (NSIP), desquamative interstitial pneumonia (DIP), lymphocytic interstitial pneumonia (LIP), respiratory bronchiolitis-associated interstitial lung disease (RB-ILD)
	Inhalational Inorganic	**Asbestosis,** coal workers' pneumoconiosis, silicosis, metals, e.g. cobalt, aluminium
	Organic	Hypersensitivity pneumonitis, e.g. bird fanciers' lung, farmers' lung
	Connective tissue disease	**Rheumatoid arthritis,** SLE, scleroderma, poly- and dermato-myositis, ankylosing spondylitis, Sjögren's syndrome, Behçet's disease
	Malignancy	Lymphangitis carcinomatosa, bronchoalveolar cell carcinoma, pulmonary lymphoma
	Miscellaneous	**Bronchiectasis,** Langerhans' cell histiocytosis, amyloidosis, lymphangioleiomyomatosis, alveolar proteinosis, microlithiasis

Clinical assessment and imaging

History Clinical features may provide useful clues to the underlying diagnosis. Key points in the history are:

Presenting symptoms

- Breathlessness is the most common symptom, and its rate of onset may be useful diagnostically (see table on preceding page)
- Causes of truly *episodic* breathlessness/diffuse CXR shadowing include eosinophilic pneumonia, vasculitis, Churg–Strauss syndrome, hypersensitivity pneumonitis, cryptogenic organizing pneumonia, allergic bronchopulmonary aspergillosis, and pulmonary oedema
- Cough may occur, although its diagnostic value is uncertain; it may be a prominent symptom in lymphangitis carcinomatosis, hypersensitivity pneumonitis, cryptogenic organizing pneumonia, sarcoid, and eosinophilic pneumonia. Chronic production of purulent sputum suggests bronchiectasis. Bronchorrhoea (production of large volumes of sputum) may occur with bronchoalveolar cell carcinoma. Haemoptysis suggests alveolar haemorrhage, malignancy, or pulmonary venous hypertension
- Wheeze may occur in asthma associated with eosinophilic pneumonia or Churg–Strauss syndrome
- Weight loss and fever are non-specific symptoms associated with many diffuse lung diseases.

Other medical conditions e.g. malignancy, connective tissue disease, HIV infection, other immunosuppression. Ask about old CXRs, which may be helpful in assessing disease duration.

Drugs

- See table on preceding page for common drug causes of diffuse lung disease
- Delays of months or even years may occur between starting the drug and developing lung involvement
- Illicit drug abuse (crack cocaine or heroin—pulmonary oedema, eosinophilic pneumonitis, diffuse alveolar haemorrhage, interstitial pneumonia; intravenous drug use—IV talcosis, septic emboli)
- Oily nose drops (lipoid pneumonia).

Occupation, lifestyle, hobbies, and pets

- May involve inhalation of inorganic or organic dusts. Document lifelong employment history, including probable exposure levels, use of protective equipment, and names of employers
- Inorganic dusts associated with development of diffuse lung disease include asbestos, silica, cobalt, beryllium, aluminium, isocyanates, copper sulphate, iron, tin, barium, and antimony
- Hypersensitivity pneumonitis may result from inhalation of organic dusts such as *Thermoactinomycetes* in mouldy hay (farmers' lung), avian proteins or feathers (bird fanciers' lung), mushroom compost, mouldy cheese, cork or sugar cane, and isocyanates
- Risk factors for immunocompromise (opportunistic infection, LIP, lymphoma)

- Smoking history (Langerhans' cell histiocytosis, respiratory bronchiolitis-associated interstitial lung disease, desquamative interstitial pneumonia, and Goodpasture's syndrome are more common in smokers).

Evidence of extrapulmonary disease Manifestations of connective tissue disease, vasculitis, sarcoidosis, e.g. arthralgia, skin rash, ocular symptoms, muscular pain and weakness, Raynaud's, nasal/sinus disease, haematuria. Infertility in males (immotile cilia syndrome, cystic fibrosis).

Travel Tuberculosis, pulmonary eosinophilia from parasites (tropics), histoplasmosis (north and central United States, parts of South America and Africa), hydatid disease (Middle East, Australasia, Mediterranean).

Family history α_1-antitrypsin deficiency, rare familial forms of UIP and sarcoidosis.

Examination

- Cyanosis and signs of cor pulmonale in severe disease
- Clubbing (usual interstitial pneumonitis, asbestosis, bronchiectasis)
- Basal crackles (usual interstitial pneumonitis, asbestosis, connective tissue disease, pulmonary oedema, lymphangitis, drugs); crackles in bronchiectasis are characteristically coarse
- Absence of crackles despite a significant CXR abnormality may be suggestive of sarcoidosis, pneumoconiosis, hypersensitivity pneumonitis, or Langerhans' cell histiocytosis
- Squeaks suggest the presence of bronchiolitis
- Skin, joint, and eye disease (connective tissue disease, sarcoidosis, vasculitis).

Imaging

CXR is an essential test and is diagnostic in at least 50% of cases. Up to 10% of patients with biopsy-proven diffuse lung disease have a normal CXR, however. Previous CXRs are helpful in assessing disease duration and progression.

High-resolution CT (HRCT) chest is more sensitive and specific than CXR for diagnosing diffuse lung disease (see following page and Appendix 4). HRCT is often in itself diagnostic, and should always precede biopsy in the investigation of diffuse lung disease. HRCT also enables assessment of disease extent, and optimal biopsy site if required. HRCT appearance correlates to some extent with disease activity in the interstitial pneumonias: a predominantly 'ground-glass' appearance may signify a steroid-responsive, inflammatory state, whereas reticulation and honeycombing are often associated with fibrosis, poor response to treatment, and a worse prognosis.

HRCT diagnosis

HRCT (and to a limited extent CXR) appearances can be classified according to the pattern and distribution of disease, and the presence of additional features (see also Appendix 4):

1. Imaging pattern

Reticular (or linear) pattern Causes include:
- Interstitial pulmonary oedema
- Usual interstitial pneumonitis (UIP; reticular shadowing is typically patchy, subpleural, and basal; other features include loss of architecture of secondary pulmonary lobules, honeycombing, ground-glass change, traction bronchiectasis)
- Asbestosis (similar features to UIP, often with pleural plaques)
- Connective tissue disease-associated fibrosis (similar features to UIP)
- Chronic hypersensitivity pneumonitis (often associated with regions of ground-glass change, air-trapping on expiration, and centrilobular micronodules)
- Drug-induced fibrosis
- Sarcoidosis.

Nodular pattern consists of numerous discrete, round opacities 0.1–1 cm in diameter.
- Interstitial processes result in nodularity within interlobular septa, around bronchovascular bundles, and subpleurally (e.g. sarcoidosis, which may demonstrate associated perihilar reticular shadowing and lymphadenopathy)
- Airspace diseases may lead to affected acini becoming visible as nodules (e.g. hypersensitivity pneumonitis, miliary TB, COP, malignancy).

Ground-glass change is an increase in lung density through which pulmonary vasculature is still visible (compare the lung density with that of air within the bronchi). May occur as a result of airspace or interstitial disease, and may be patchy or diffuse. Causes include:
- Pulmonary oedema or haemorrhage, ARDS
- Hypersensitivity pneumonitis
- Drugs
- Certain idiopathic interstitial pneumonias (NSIP, RB-ILD, DIP, AIP)
- PCP
- Sarcoidosis
- Bronchoalveolar cell carcinoma
- Alveolar proteinosis.

Ground-glass appearance may be artefactual, the increased density resulting from breath-holding during expiration. It may also be confused with 'mosaic perfusion', where densities vary in different regions of the lung as a result of variable perfusion, e.g. in chronic thromboembolic disease, small airways disease.

Consolidation (or airspace shadowing) is an increase in attenuation characterized by air bronchograms (air-filled bronchi superimposed against opacified alveoli) and the loss of visibility of adjacent vessels. It occurs as

disease processes infiltrate and fill alveolar airspaces, for example, with water, blood, pus, malignant cells, or fibrous tissue. Causes include:
- Pneumonia
- Pulmonary oedema or haemorrhage, ARDS
- Drugs
- Cryptogenic organizing pneumonia (COP)
- Bronchoalveolar cell carcinoma, lymphoma
- Other rare conditions (e.g. eosinophilic pneumonia, alveolar proteinosis).

Cystic change refers to well-defined air spaces with a thin wall. Causes include:
- Langerhans' cell histiocytosis (bizarrely shaped cysts and nodules, apical predominance)
- Usual interstitial pneumonitis (subpleural honeycombing)
- PCP
- Lymphocytic interstitial pneumonia
- Septic emboli
- Lymphangioleiomyomatosis (thin-walled cysts, otherwise normal lung)
- Centrilobular emphysema may simulate cystic disease, but there is absence of a well-defined wall.

Interlobular septal thickening occurs as a result of processes affecting the lymphatics or venules within interlobular septa, such as:
- Pulmonary oedema (smooth thickening)
- Lymphangitis carcinomatosis (irregular, nodular thickening of interlobular septa and bronchovascular bundles, no architectural distortion)
- Sarcoidosis
- Usual interstitial pneumonitis.

2. Imaging distribution
- Upper zone: silicosis, pneumoconiosis, chronic sarcoidosis, hypersensitivity pneumonitis, ankylosing spondylitis, tuberculosis, Langerhans' cell histiocytosis
- Lower zone: UIP, connective tissue diseases, asbestosis
- Mid-zone: sarcoidosis, pulmonary oedema, *Pneumocystis carinii* pneumonia
- Peripheral: UIP, eosinophilic pneumonia, drugs (amiodarone), COP
- Sharp borders: radiation pneumonitis.

3. Additional imaging features
- Lymphadenopathy: sarcoidosis, lymphoma, malignancy, infection, silicosis, berylliosis, LIP
- Pleural effusion/involvement: pulmonary oedema, connective tissue diseases, infection, malignancy, asbestosis, drugs, LAM.

Further information
Diagnostic approach to the patient with diffuse lung disease. Ryu JH et al. Mayo Clin Proc 2002; **77**: 1221–7

Further investigations

Urine and blood tests Consider the following investigations:
- Urine dipstick and microscopy for detection of renal disease associated with vasculitis/connective tissue disease
- ESR, CRP, full blood count (look specifically at the eosinophil count), renal and liver function, calcium (increased in >10% of patients with sarcoidosis)
- Autoantibodies (including anti-Jo-1, occurs with myositis-associated interstitial pneumonia; positive rheumatoid factor or ANA may occur in infection, malignancy, and UIP as well as in connective tissue disease)
- ANCA (vasculitis), anti-GBM (Goodpasture's syndrome)
- Serum precipitins (to antigens in hypersensitivity pneumonitis; poor specificity)
- Serum ACE levels may be increased in sarcoidosis, but this is a non-specific and relatively insensitive test and is unhelpful diagnostically.

Sputum
- Cytology may be diagnostic in bronchoalveolar cell carcinoma
- Induced sputum may be useful in the diagnosis of PCP and TB.

Pulmonary function tests
- Useful in assessing severity of disease and response to treatment, but often unhelpful diagnostically
- Typically show restrictive pattern with reduced vital capacity and transfer factor. Normal values do not exclude mild, early lung disease
- Obstructive pattern rare, but may be seen in sarcoidosis, Langerhans' cell histiocytosis, and lymphangioleiomyomatosis; may see mixed picture if coexisting COPD
- Transfer factor may be increased transiently (days) in alveolar haemorrhage. Reduced transfer factor with preserved lung volumes in scleroderma is suggestive of pulmonary vascular disease (such as pulmonary arterial hypertension or vasculitis)
- Disease progression and response to treatment are best assessed by serial measurements of vital capacity and transfer factor
- Check oxygen saturation and consider ABGs. A fall in oxygen saturation on simple exercise may be performed in the clinic setting, and is a useful clue to underlying lung disease in patients with normal saturation and lung function at rest and an unremarkable CXR.

Cardiac investigations
- *ECG* Conduction abnormality in sarcoidosis; cardiogenic pulmonary oedema is unusual in the presence of a completely normal ECG
- *Echocardiography* Assess left ventricular and valvular function if cardiac pulmonary oedema suspected, and measure pulmonary arterial pressure in scleroderma and suspected pulmonary veno-occlusive disease.

Bronchoalveolar lavage
- Most useful in diagnosis of opportunistic infection (bacterial or fungal pneumonia, tuberculosis, PCP), malignancy, alveolar proteinosis, eosinophilic pneumonia, and alveolar haemorrhage
- BAL differential cell counts usually unhelpful diagnostically.

Lung biopsy

Which patients need a lung biopsy?

In cases of uncertain aetiology, despite clinical assessment and HRCT, lung biopsies often provide a definitive diagnosis. Ideally they should be taken before treatment is started. The decision to biopsy varies amongst clinicians, and should take into account the individual patient's clinical condition and wishes, and the likely benefit of a definitive diagnosis in terms of predicting treatment response and prognosis. Some take a pragmatic approach when a diagnosis (or group of diagnoses with the same treatment) is likely but not biopsy-proven, and treat empirically. In some cases, the patient may be too unwell for biopsy and require empirical treatment. Biopsy of end-stage fibrosis is unhelpful in eliciting an underlying aetiology.

Biopsy techniques

Transbronchial biopsy provides small samples, but relatively high diagnostic yield in diseases with a 'centrilobular' distribution, e.g. sarcoidosis, hypersensitivity pneumonitis, malignancy, infection (fungi, tuberculosis), and cryptogenic organizing pneumonia. Take 4–6 samples. Additional blind endobronchial biopsies may be diagnostic in sarcoidosis.

Open lung biopsy via thoracotomy or video-assisted thoracoscopic (VATS) biopsy provide larger samples than TBB, and have diagnostic yields of at least 90%. Both require general anaesthesia. VATS probably has a lower morbidity, and is generally preferred in stable patients; open biopsy is required in ventilator-dependent patients.

Open or VATS biopsy (rather than TBB) is required for diagnosis of idiopathic interstitial pneumonias, vasculitis, lymphoma, lymphangioleiomyomatosis, and Langerhans' cell histiocytosis.

Percutaneous image-guided biopsy may be useful in the diagnosis of well-localized and dense peripheral infiltrates. A cutting needle biopsy technique is best and, if the lesion(s) abuts the pleural surface, pneumothorax is uncommon.

Diffuse alveolar haemorrhage

Bleeding within the lungs can be from the bronchial circulation, such as when a lung cancer erodes a bronchial vessel, or from the pulmonary circulation.

Bleeding into the alveoli is often a feature of a small vessel vasculitis of the lungs. This blood tends to remain in the lungs and is not expectorated.

Patients with diffuse alveolar haemorrhage may have a background history of vasculitis over the preceding weeks to months. They can present with slowly progressive dyspnoea with possible haemoptysis, or be acutely unwell with hypoxia. They may require ventilatory support.

Presentation Abrupt onset haemoptysis is the most common symptom, although this is not present in one-third of cases. Also cough, dyspnoea, low-grade fever, weight loss, arthralgia, myalgia.

Examination May be non-specific, or they may have signs of underlying vasculitis with skin rashes, nail fold infarcts, digital gangrene. Episcleritis, corneal ulceration, epistaxis, nasal crusting, or deafness may be present. Patients may be breathless. Haematuria and proteinuria on urine dip.

Investigations
- May be hypoxic—check SaO_2 ± ABG
- May have falling haemoglobin
- CXR showing bilateral alveolar infiltrates—difficult to distinguish from pulmonary oedema or infection
- Consider chest HRCT
- Raised kCO as increased intra-alveolar haemoglobin available to combine with carbon monoxide. Abnormal if raised by more than 30%. If breathless at rest, they will not be able to perform this test as it requires breath-holding of an air, carbon monoxide, and helium mixture for 10 seconds. This test can be used to monitor disease progress
- BAL shows bloodstained lavage, which becomes sequentially more so with each washing. Cytology shows haemosiderin-laden macrophages
- Renal involvement: blood and/or protein in the urine, raised urea and creatinine
- Send blood for urgent ANA, ANCA, anti-GBM, dsDNA, and rheumatoid factor
- Consider biopsy of lung, kidney, or other affected site if well enough to make a tissue diagnosis.

Management
- Admit to hospital
- Support with intravenous fluids, blood transfusion, and oxygen if necessary
- Closely monitor, paying particular attention to oxygen saturations and keeping them above 92% with oxygen therapy. May need respiratory support with intubation and ventilation or CPAP. Monitor haemoglobin with further transfusion if necessary. Monitor urine output and renal function
- Treatment with plasma exchange, high dose steroids and cyclophosphamide, and dialysis if required.

Key questions

- Is this isolated lung disease?
- Is there accompanying renal disease?
- Are there other features of an underlying disease?—ENT, joints etc.

Causes of alveolar haemorrhage, first three are the commonest

	See page
Goodpasture's disease	508
Wegener's granulomatosis	504
SLE	492
Rheumatoid arthritis	490
Microscopic polyangiitis	507
Progressive systemic sclerosis	496
Mixed connective tissue disease	
Polyarteritis nodosa	
Behçet's disease	
Essential mixed cryglobulinaemia	
Tumour-related vasculitis	
Endocarditis-related vasculitis	
Idiopathic rapidly progressive glomerulonephritis	
D-penicillamine induced	
Cocaine	
Idiopathic pulmonary haemosiderosis	
Chemicals: trimellitic anhydride	
lymphangiography	
Leptospirosis	
Isolated pauci-immune pulmonary capillaritis	
Coagulopathy, such as disseminated intravascular coagulation	

Pulmonary infiltrates in the immunocompromised host (non-HIV)

Clinical assessment

Respiratory disease is a significant cause of morbidity and mortality in the immunocompromised, and its diagnosis and management are challenging. In the UK this is encountered most commonly in the setting of immunocompromise secondary to cytotoxic chemotherapy, haematological malignancy, immunosuppression post-transplant (particularly renal and bone marrow), prolonged corticosteroid use, and AIDS (page 65).

Most pulmonary diseases present in a similar manner in the setting of immunocompromise, with fever, dyspnoea, dry cough, chest pain, and often hypoxia. This non-specific clinical presentation, combined with the large number of possible causes, makes reaching a precise diagnosis difficult; the diagnosis remains unclear in up to 10% of cases even at autopsy. There is limited evidence to demonstrate that obtaining a definitive diagnosis leads to an overall improvement in mortality, although, in subgroups such as patients with respiratory infection, early identification and treatment of pathogens has been shown to improve outcome.

Causes of pulmonary infiltrates in the non-HIV-infected immunocompromised are presented on page 62, and treatment on page 64. Specific conditions are described separately (e.g. invasive aspergillosis page 264; PCP page 270).

Key steps in the management of these patients are:

Clinical assessment In the *history*, the underlying cause of immunocompromise and the timing and location of respiratory disease onset may provide clues to the diagnosis. Different types of pathogen are associated, to a certain extent, with community- or hospital-acquired infection, although considerable overlap exists and this distinction is often of limited clinical use. *Staphylococcus aureus* (including MRSA), *Pseudomonas aeruginosa,* and other Gram-negative bacteria, and fungi such as *Aspergillus* and *Candida* are particularly associated with hospital-acquired infection.

The rate of disease onset may also suggest possible causes:
- **Acute onset** (< 24 hours) Bacterial pneumonia, viral pneumonitis (e.g. CMV), pulmonary oedema or haemorrhage, pulmonary emboli, ARDS
- **Subacute onset** (days) Fungi (e.g. *Pneumocystis*, *Aspergillus*), bacteria (e.g. *Nocardia, Legionella*), viral (e.g. CMV), drug-induced pneumonitis
- **Chronic onset** (weeks) Malignancy, mycobacteria, fungi.

Chest **examination** may suggest the extent of pulmonary involvement, although this can be misleading and there are often no abnormal signs (e.g. PCP). Assess fluid status; pulmonary oedema is common following transplantation. Extrapulmonary involvement may be helpful in suggesting a pathogen, e.g. cutaneous lesions (herpes simplex and varicella-zoster; necrotic lesions from *Pseudomonas* and other Gram-negative bacteria, mycobacteria, and fungi; subcutaneous abscesses in *Staphylococcus aureus* and *Nocardia*), central nervous system involvement (*Pseudomonas, Aspergillus, Cryptococcus, Nocardia*, mycobacteria, *Streptococcus pneumoniae, Haemophilus influenzae*, varicella-zoster).

Initial investigations

- *CXR* appearance is very variable; may be normal or show consolidation, nodular infiltrate, or diffuse shadowing. CXR is of limited diagnostic value, as appearances are non-specific and atypical presentations are common; the 'first-choice' diagnosis based on CXR is correct in only a third of cases. CXR may however be helpful in monitoring disease progression and response to treatment
- *Blood and pleural fluid* (if available) sampling for microscopy and culture. Consider viral serology (e.g. CMV following transplantation), urinary legionella antigen
- *Sputum examination* is often of little diagnostic value in immunocompromised patients, with the possible exceptions of invasive aspergillosis and tuberculosis. Send sputum for acid-fast stain and mycobacterial culture, fungal stain, and culture. Induced sputum has a low yield for PCP in non-HIV patients
- *The degree of* **hypoxia** is often not appreciated; measure oxygen saturations and consider ABGs. Severe hypoxia tends to be more commonly associated with infection due to bacteria, viruses or *Pneumocystis* than with mycobacteria or fungi.

Is immediate antibiotic treatment required? Immediate, empirical treatment with broad-spectrum antibiotics prior to further investigation should be considered, depending on the nature of immunological defect and local hospital policy. In general, neutropenic patients with fever or pulmonary infiltrates are at significant risk of developing overwhelming sepsis, and should receive prompt antibiotic cover, irrespective of the CXR appearance. More invasive diagnostic procedures can then be reserved for patients who deteriorate or fail to improve within a period of observation (e.g. 2–3 days). In non-neutropenic patients, depending on the clinical circumstances, it is often possible to withhold treatment until definitive investigations have taken place.

Further investigations

More invasive diagnostic techniques are usually required for a definitive diagnosis:

CT chest
- Specific indications not yet defined. Probably not needed in typical cases of bacterial pneumonia or PCP
- Useful in identifying the location and extent of pulmonary disease and aiding invasive sampling procedures
- Often detects pulmonary disease in the presence of a normal CXR— consider if respiratory symptoms but normal CXR
- May be diagnostic, e.g. pulmonary embolism (CTPA); lymphangitis carcinomatosis; invasive aspergillosis ('halo' and 'air crescent' signs).

Bronchoscopy with bronchoalveolar lavage
- First-line investigation, consider early in management. Diagnostic in about 60% of patients overall, up to 70% of patients with infection; results in change to treatment in around 50% of cases overall. Complications are rare
- Useful in the diagnosis of bacterial pneumonia, PCP (sensitivity 80–90%), cytomegalovirus (sensitivity 85–90%), aspergillosis (sensitivity 50%), tuberculosis, malignant disease, diffuse alveolar haemorrhage, and alveolar proteinosis
- BAL fluid analysis: routine microscopy and culture for bacteria; additional stains and culture for fungi, mycobacteria, *Nocardia*; silver or immunofluorescence stain for *Pneumocystis*; cytology, including flow cytometry for malignant cells; viral serology; haemosiderin-laden macrophages if alveolar haemorrhage suspected
- Consider additional tests on BAL fluid, such as *Cryptococcus* antigen detection or CMV PCR. *Aspergillus* antigen detection or PCR and *Toxoplasma gondii* PCR are less well validated
- Transbronchial biopsy has a slightly higher sensitivity than BAL for the diagnosis of infection, but carries a risk of bleeding and pneumothorax, which can be serious complications in this patient group; it is not usually performed at initial bronchoscopy, although may be considered, e.g. if lymphangitis is suspected.

Lung biopsy Consider as a second-line investigation if BAL is non-diagnostic. Options include:
- *Repeat bronchoscopy with transbronchial lung biopsy* is useful in the diagnosis of malignancy, mycobacteria, fungi, organizing pneumonia, and drug-induced lung disease
- *VATS or open lung biopsy* has a greater diagnostic yield than TBB although it is unclear if this can be directly translated into an improved survival. Results in change to treatment in <50% of patients, and complications may be serious
- *Percutaneous image-guided fine-needle aspiration or biopsy* for investigation of peripheral nodules.

Further information

Pulmonary infiltrates in the non-HIV-infected immunocompromised patient. Shorr AF *et al. Chest* 2004; **125**: 260–71

Causes

Infectious causes (*>75% of cases*) Infection is the commonest cause of respiratory disease in the immunocompromised. The nature of immunological defect may provide clues to the likely infectious agent (table opposite), although considerable overlap exists and this should serve only as a guide. The pattern of infection will be further modified by prophylactic treatment, e.g. CMV and PCP prophylaxis post-transplantation.

Non-infectious causes (*<25% of cases*) Often present with similar, if not identical, clinical and radiological features to infection, and signs such as fever do not reliably differentiate between them. Non-infectious causes include:

- *Pulmonary oedema* Particularly following renal or bone marrow transplant
- *ARDS* e.g. secondary to sepsis or drugs such as cytarabine, gemcitabine, or 'engraftment syndrome' following bone marrow transplantation
- *Drug-induced disease* Causes include all-trans retinoic acid (ATRA), anti-thymocyte globulin, azathioprine, bleomycin, busulfan, carmustine, chlorambucil, cyclophosphamide, cytosine arabinoside, hydroxyurea, liposomal amphotericin B, melphalan, mitomycin, methotrexate, sirolimus
- *Respiratory involvement from the underlying disease* e.g. lymphoma, leukaemic infiltration, lymphangitis carcinomatosis, connective tissue disease, leucostasis with very high leucocyte counts in leukaemia
- *Diffuse alveolar haemorrhage* Relatively common complication of leukaemia; haemoptysis often absent; diverse CXR appearances; underlying infection common
- *Pulmonary embolism* Often complicated by secondary infection; clinical and radiological features may be confused with invasive aspergillosis
- *Radiation-induced pulmonary disease* Pneumonitis and cryptogenic organizing pneumonia (COP)
- *'Idiopathic pneumonia syndrome'* following bone marrow transplantation (breathlessness with hypoxia and diffuse CXR infiltrate, diagnosis of exclusion, high mortality)
- *Chronic graft-versus-host disease* following allogeneic bone marrow transplantation (dry cough, obstructive lung disease, rarely necrotizing bronchiolitis obliterans)
- *Post-transplant lymphoproliferative disease*
- *Pulmonary alveolar proteinosis* (page 544).

Multiple disease processes About a third of patients are thought to have two or more disease processes accounting for their respiratory involvement. Co-infection with multiple pathogens is common, and secondary infection with a different infectious agent (commonly *Aspergillus* or Gram-negative bacteria such as *Pseudomonas*) may complicate either a primary respiratory infection or a non-infectious process such as pulmonary embolism. Secondary infection is associated with a poor prognosis, and should be considered particularly in patients who deteriorate after an initial response to treatment, and in patients who are neutropenic.

Infectious causes of pulmonary infiltrates based on underlying immunological defect and clinical condition

Clinical conditions	Immunological defect	Infectious agent
Leukaemia Cytotoxic treatment Aplastic anaemia Rare genetic conditions	Neutropenia or impaired neutrophil function	Bacteria (Pseudomonas aeruginosa, Staphylococcus aureus, Escherichia coli, Klebsiella, Haemophilus influenzae, Nocardia) Fungi (Aspergillus—page 260, Candida, Mucormycosis)
Post-transplantation Cytotoxic treatment High-dose steroids Lymphoma AIDS (page 65) Renal impairment Rare genetic conditions	Impaired T-lymphocyte function	Fungi (PCP, Cryptococcus neoformans, Candida, Histoplasma, Coccidioides, Blastomyces)—pages 274–9 Viruses (Cytomegalovirus, herpes simplex, varicella-zoster)—pages 218, 220 Bacteria (Mycobacteria, Listeria, Legionella, Nocardia) Parasites (Toxoplasma gondii)
Myeloma Acute and chronic lymphocytic leukaemia Lymphoma Common variable immuno-deficiency Rare genetic conditions	Hypogammaglobulinaemia or impaired B-lymphocyte function	Encapsulated bacteria (Streptococcus pneumoniae, Haemophilus influenzae)
Genetic conditions (e.g. complement component deficiency, mannose-binding lectin deficiency)	Impaired complement activation	Streptococcus pneumoniae

Treatment

Antimicrobials Depending on the clinical circumstances, antimicrobials may need to be started prior to definitive investigations (see above), although blood cultures should always precede antibiotic treatment. Choice of antimicrobial depends on the underlying condition and local hospital policy.

- In general, most neutropenic patients are treated with broad-spectrum antibiotics providing both Gram-positive and Gram-negative cover, e.g. piperacillin (4.5 g IV qds) and netilmicin (5 mg/kg od by IV infusion, may need higher dose initially); antifungals are considered if slow response to treatment or subsequent deterioration. Consider vancomycin if MRSA is a possibility
- Treatment for CMV and PCP is associated with significant side-effects, and ideally should be based on a definitive diagnosis. In unwell patients who are strongly suspected to have PCP, treatment (page 272) can be started immediately, as BAL *Pneumocystis jiroveci* stains remain positive for up to two weeks
- Antituberculous treatment should only rarely be administered in the absence of a microbiological diagnosis.

Diuretics Fluid overload and pulmonary oedema are common following renal and bone-marrow transplantation, and typical clinical and radiological signs may be disguised; consider a trial of diuretics.

Steroids Despite a lack of randomized, controlled trials, prednisolone (1–2 mg/kg/day PO, or up to 2 g methylprednisolone IV) is often considered in the treatment of drug- or radiation-induced lung disease, diffuse alveolar haemorrhage, and idiopathic pneumonia syndrome following bone marrow transplantation. Ideally exclude underlying infection prior to starting steroids. Prednisolone (40–80 mg daily PO) is recommended for the treatment of PCP in patients with respiratory failure.

Supportive treatment Administer oxygen to maintain saturations >95%. Respiratory failure in immunocompromised patients is associated with a poor outcome: mortality following intubation and mechanical ventilation ranges 60–100%. Early, intermittent use of non-invasive ventilation in immunocompromised patients with pulmonary infiltrates and hypoxia (defined as breathlessness, respiratory rate >30/min and PaO_2/FiO_2 ratio <200) has been shown to reduce the need for intubation and improve mortality. Before NIV is commenced, a decision regarding suitability for intubation and mechanical ventilation should be made.

Surgery Surgical wedge resection or lobectomy may be considered in the treatment of invasive aspergillosis, either acutely for lesions adjacent to pulmonary vessels that are judged to have a significant risk of massive haemoptysis, or at a later date for residual lesions at risk of reactivation with further chemotherapy.

Further information
Non-invasive ventilation in immunosuppressed patients with pulmonary infiltrates, fever, and acute respiratory failure. Hilbert G et al. NEJM 2001; **344**: 481–7

Pulmonary infiltrates in the immunocompromised host (HIV)

Clinical assessment

Widespread use of highly active antiretroviral therapy (HAART) and antimicrobial prophylaxis in HIV has resulted in a longer survival as well as changes in the nature of respiratory involvement. Respiratory disease remains common in the setting of HIV, and patients should be managed in consultation with a HIV-specialist.

Causes of respiratory disease in the HIV-infected patient are listed on page 69. Specific conditions are described separately (e.g. PCP page 270, TB page 227). Key steps in management are:

Clinical assessment

- As with other causes of immunocompromise, clinical features of respiratory disease in HIV-infected patients are non-specific: breathlessness, cough, fever, weight loss, and fatigue are common, although chest symptoms are not always present
- Ask about treatment and compliance with HAART and PCP prophylaxis
- Source of HIV infection may be relevant: Kaposi's sarcoma occurs particularly in homosexual men and in African men and women; tuberculosis and bacterial pneumonia are more common in IV drug users
- Travel history may be useful: infection with 'endemic mycoses' (e.g. histoplasmosis, blastomycosis, coccidioidomycosis) is well-recognized in the USA but rare in the UK
- Careful examination may provide clues to the respiratory condition. Pulmonary Kaposi's sarcoma is unusual in the absence of disease elsewhere; palatal Kaposi's sarcoma in particular is predictive of pulmonary involvement. Extrapulmonary mycobacterial disease is common, and may involve the liver, lymph nodes, pericardium, and meninges.

Investigations

CXR

- CXR changes are relatively non-specific
- PCP classically appears as bilateral perihilar infiltrates that progress to alveolar shadowing; more unusual patterns include small, nodular infiltrates or focal consolidation. CXR is normal in 10% of cases. Pneumothorax is suggestive of PCP
- Appearances of bacterial pneumonia are often atypical, e.g. diffuse bilateral infiltrates mimicking PCP
- Pleural effusion or hilar/mediastinal lymphadenopathy are unusual in PCP, and are more suggestive of mycobacterial infection or Kaposi's sarcoma. CXR cavitation is unusual in tuberculosis occurring late in the course of HIV.

CD4 count Useful in narrowing the differential diagnosis. Bacterial infection, including tuberculosis, occurs at any stage of disease, although infection is more severe at lower CD4 counts; PCP and atypical presentations of tuberculosis occur most commonly at CD4 $< 200 \times 10^6$/l; non-tuberculous mycobacteria, Kaposi's sarcoma, and lymphoma occur late in the disease (CD4 $< 50 \times 10^6$/l).

Blood cultures should be taken prior to antimicrobial treatment. Bacteraemia is relatively common with bacterial pneumonia in HIV, particularly with *S. pneumoniae* infection. Bacteraemic tuberculosis may occur in advanced disease.

Other blood tests Raised inflammatory markers are a non-specific finding.

Sputum Induced sputum may assist the diagnosis of PCP and mycobacterial disease. Induced sputum has a sensitivity of about 60% for the diagnosis of PCP. Tuberculosis is more likely to be smear-negative in the setting of HIV, as cavitation in these patients is less common. Induced sputum should ideally be obtained in a negative-pressure room.

Other cultures Consider sampling urine, stool, lymph node, or bone marrow in suspected mycobacterial disease, as extrapulmonary disease is common.

CT chest is useful in looking for evidence of respiratory disease in patients with symptoms but a normal CXR, and may be helpful in directing invasive diagnostic procedures. CT is also of benefit in the diagnosis and staging of Kaposi's sarcoma and lymphoma.

Further investigations and treatment

Bronchoscopy and BAL

- Bronchoscopy and BAL are safe and frequently diagnostic in this patient group, and should be considered early in management, particularly in the presence of a diffuse CXR abnormality or following non-diagnostic induced sputum analysis. BAL should also be considered in patients with a localized CXR abnormality that has not responded to a trial of broad-spectrum antibiotics
- BAL fluid analysis: routine microscopy and culture for bacteria; additional stains and culture for fungi, mycobacteria, *Nocardia*; silver or immunofluorescence stain for *Pneumocystis*; cytology, including flow cytometry for malignant cells; viral serology. Consider additional tests such as *Cryptococcus* antigen detection or CMV PCR
- Both *Nocardia* and *Rhodococcus equi* stain weakly acid-fast, and may be confused with mycobacteria
- Kaposi's sarcoma appears as 'raised bruises' in the trachea or bronchi on bronchoscopy; routine biopsy is not recommended, as diagnostic yield is low and significant haemorrhage may occur.

Lung biopsy If bronchoscopy and BAL are non-diagnostic, consider repeat bronchoscopy with TBB or surgical lung biopsy. TBB has a greater sensitivity than BAL, but potentially serious complications such as pneumothorax or haemorrhage are significantly more common.

Treatment

- Consider broad spectrum antibiotics and empirical treatment for PCP (high-dose co-trimoxazole, and steroids if the patient is in respiratory failure—page 272). BAL *Pneumocystis* stains remain positive for up to two weeks despite treatment, and so empirical treatment for PCP should not be delayed if the patient is unwell and this diagnosis is suspected
- Further antimicrobial treatment can be directed at specific pathogens isolated from BAL or biopsy. CMV is commonly isolated from BAL fluid, but rarely, if ever, causes lung disease in the setting of HIV and the value of antiviral treatment in such cases is unknown
- Supportive therapy with oxygen; consider NIV. ITU admission for invasive ventilation may be required. PCP is the commonest cause of respiratory failure requiring ITU admission in HIV-positive patients. Mortality from PCP requiring mechanical ventilation is about 60%, although it may be significantly higher in patients with low CD4-counts
- Steroids may be effective in the treatment of non-specific interstitial pneumonitis and lymphocytic interstitial pneumonitis.

Causes of respiratory disease in HIV infection *(commoner causes in bold)*

Infectious

Bacteria
- **Streptococcus pneumoniae**
- **Haemophilus influenzae**
- **Staphylococcus aureus**
- **Gram-negative bacteria, especially Pseudomonas**
- Nocardia
- Rhodococcus equi.

Mycobacteria
- **Mycobacterium tuberculosis**
- **Mycobacterium avium-intracellulare**
- Mycobacterium kansasii.

Viruses
- Influenza
- Parainfluenza
- Respiratory syncytial virus
- Herpes simplex
- Adenovirus.

Fungi
- **Pneumocystis jiroveci**
- Aspergillus spp
- Cryptococcus neoformans
- Endemic mycoses.

Parasites
- Strongyloides stercoralis (hyperinfection syndrome—rare).

Non-infectious
- **Kaposi's sarcoma**
- Lymphoma
- Drug-induced lung disease
- Non-specific interstitial pneumonitis
- Lymphocytic interstitial pneumonitis
- Cardiogenic pulmonary oedema
- Increased risk of lung cancer.

The respiratory sleep patient

History

The problem Sleep apnoea and related problems are now a common reason for referral to many respiratory units. This is due to a much better recognition of the syndromes and the increasing prevalence of obesity in the general population. Most respiratory units with sleep services are seeing patients primarily for possible obstructive sleep apnoea (OSA) and therefore most patients tend to be sleepy, and referrals for insomnia are not usually encouraged.

Patients arrive at a respiratory sleep unit for several different reasons; they are commonly:
- Concerns that the patient may have sleep apnoea, with or without a full house of symptoms
- Loud snoring, with the patient or spouse seeking advice about noise reduction
- Referrals from the ENT department who may be considering offering surgery for snoring, and wish to exclude OSA first
- Excessive daytime sleepiness, diagnosis unclear, might just be OSA, might be narcolepsy, etc.
- Other nocturnal symptoms such as sleep walking, panic arousals, etc.

Thus in sleep out-patients the issues revolve around making the correct diagnosis of the excessive daytime sleepiness or nocturnal symptoms (and referring on if appropriate), offering simple advice for snoring, or putting the patient through the nasal continuous positive airway pressure (CPAP) induction programme.

Some units perform a sleep study first on the basis of an appropriate referral letter; others see the patient first and then book a sleep study if indicated. For the purposes of this account it is assumed that the patient is seen first.

History A clear history of the exact presenting complaint is obviously necessary, concentrating on the following points when OSA is suspected (a full discussion is available in the section on OSA, page 332).
- Sleepiness: how severe, what does it interfere with, over how long has it been coming on, and does it reduce quality of life? The Epworth sleepiness scale is useful to assess this (see page 75). This is scored out of 24; 0–9 is considered normal and >9 excessively sleepy. It is only a guide
- Important to differentiate sleepiness (tendency to nod off, due to inadequate sleep) from tiredness (feelings of exhaustion due to many causes, often without a tendency to nod off)
- Snoring and apnoeas. Best assessed from a witness: how loud, continuous, intermittent, and are there recognized 'stopping breathing' or choking episodes during sleep?
- Other OSA symptoms, such as nocturia and restless sleep
- History of weight and neck size changes over the last 5 to 10 years (recent weight gains common)
- History of nasal or other ENT surgery (particularly previous palate surgery, which increases discomfort of CPAP)

- Previous medical history (certain risk factors such as mandibular surgery, hypothyroidism, acromegaly, etc.)
- Previous cardiovascular/cerebrovascular history and hypertension history (may influence decision to treat)
- Alcohol and smoking history
- Occupation and shift working
- Driving issues, such as sleepiness while driving and 'near misses' or actual sleep-related accidents
- Does the patient drive for a living and what kind of vehicle?

If OSA seems unlikely, then other causes of sleepiness need to be considered, concentrating on the commonest.

Alternative diagnoses for excessive daytime sleepiness

- Depression, often missed
- Lifestyle issues—alcohol, late night working, shift work, caffeine abuse, family circumstances, etc.
- Drugs—some of the anti-hypertensives (e.g. β blockers) and psychoactive drugs (e.g. antidepressants and anxiolytics) can provoke sleepiness
- Narcolepsy—e.g. cataplexy (sudden loss of muscle tone in response to excitement or anticipation), sleep paralysis (frightening paralysis on wakening for a few seconds or minutes), and prolific vivid dreaming, often at sleep onset
- Periodic limb movements during sleep (associated with restless legs during the day, especially in renal failure)
- Post severe head injury or cranial irradiation (hypothalamic damage)
- Post-infectious (e.g. Epstein–Barr virus)
- Idiopathic (sometimes hereditary)
- Certain neurological disorders such as myotonic dystrophy, Parkinson's, and previous stroke
- Simply being at the sleepier end of the normal spectrum
- The symptom may really be tiredness, such as in 'ME' or insomnia, when the ESS is usually low
- Blind insomnia/sleepiness—circadian problem when 24 hour cycle not linked with the real world through light and melatonin production.

Examination and investigations

Examination of these patients is often relatively unhelpful.

In OSA the main features are:
- The neck circumference (best measure of the obesity contribution to the cause of OSA, >17 in) and BMI
- Examination of the oropharynx (usually crowded with boggy mucosa, with perhaps large tonsils)
- Assessment of teeth (crowding suggests small mandible, and mandibular advancement devices require sound teeth)
- Nasal patency (how easy will nasal CPAP be?).

Also:
- Assessment of respiratory function, signs of cor pulmonale, FEV_1/VC ratio and SaO_2 (COPD increases likelihood of being in type II respiratory failure, so-called 'overlap syndrome')
- Blood pressure (may influence decision to treat OSA)
- Evidence of endocrine abnormalities: hypothyroidism, acromegaly, Cushing's, diabetes.

It may also be appropriate to look for:
- Evidence of a neuromuscular disorder, including a previous stroke
- Evidence of heart failure (central sleep apnoea, or Cheyne–Stokes respiration, which can produce overnight oximetry traces similar to those of OSA).

Clinic tests to perform

- Blood gas estimation if respiratory failure suspected (these OSA patients require more urgent treatment)
- Thyroid function (hypothyroidism not always clinically obvious) plus other hormones if indicated
- Routine haematology and biochemistry (prevalence of type II diabetes will be high in this overweight population)
- Some would recommend a fuller cardiovascular risk assessment including cholesterol, fasting triglycerides, glucose, and folate since these patients are often in a high risk group (10 year cardiovascular event risk typically about 35%).

Other scenarios If it is known already that the patient has OSA, then the clinic appointment will revolve around a joint decision between the doctor and the patient as to whether a trial of treatment is indicated (usually nasal CPAP). This will depend mainly on the severity of symptoms, versus the perceived inconvenience of the treatment. Weight loss is important but rarely achievable, and, of course, other treatable causes of OSA must not be missed (e.g. hypothyroidism, tonsillar hypertrophy) simply because nasal CPAP is available.

If the patient has come via ENT, and is being considered for pharyngeal surgery, then the respiratory physician's role is to dissuade the patient from this route as the objective success rate is poor, and the hazards significant. The presence of significant OSA is a contraindication to surgery.

All other approaches to snoring, such as the use of mandibular advancement devices, should be considered first, and pharyngeal surgery regarded as the last resort of the totally desperate.

EPWORTH SLEEPINESS SCALE

Name:..Hospital number .... Date:......................

Your age (Yrs)....................Your sex (Male = M / Female = F).....................

- How likely are you to doze off or fall asleep in the situations described in the box below, in contrast to feeling just tired?
- This refers to your usual way of life in recent times.
- Even if you haven't done some of these things recently try to work out how they would have affected you.
- Use the following scale to choose the <u>most appropriate number</u> for each situation:-

0 = would <u>never</u> doze   2 = <u>Moderate</u> chance of dozing
1 = <u>Slight</u> chance of dozing   3 = <u>High</u> chance of dozing

Situation	Chance of dozing
Sitting and reading	☐
Watching TV	☐
Sitting, inactive in a public place (e.g. a theatre or a meeting)	☐
As a passenger in a car for an hour without a break	☐
Lying down to rest in the afternoon when circumstances permit	☐
Sitting and talking to someone	☐
Sitting quietly after a lunch without alcohol	☐
In a car, while stopped for a few minutes in the traffic	☐
Thank you for your cooperation Total score =	☐

The breathless, pregnant patient

Causes

Normal physiological changes of pregnancy

- Elevated serum progesterone levels stimulate respiratory drive and lead to an increased tidal volume and raised minute ventilation, with only a modest increase in oxygen consumption. The subsequent fall in maternal pCO_2 facilitates fetal CO_2 transfer across the placenta; any cause of maternal hypercapnia leads quickly to fetal respiratory acidosis. Respiratory rate is unaffected by pregnancy. Elevation of the diaphragm occurs due to the enlarging uterus, leading to a reduced functional residual capacity, although diaphragm function is normal and vital capacity is unaffected. Peak flow and FEV_1 are unaffected by pregnancy
- Increased cardiac output occurs due to an increase in heart rate (by about 15/min) and stroke volume; peripheral resistance falls. Blood pressure is reduced in the first and second trimesters by 10–20 mmHg, but is normal at term. Peripheral pulses tend to be increased in volume. Dependent oedema is common. Third heart sound and ejection systolic murmurs are commonly heard. May hear venous hums in the neck
- Raised levels of coagulation factors and impaired fibrinolysis, combined with venous stasis, result in a 5-fold increased risk of venous thromboembolism
- Upper airway oedema, particularly in the setting of pre-eclampsia, may predispose to upper airways obstruction during sleep, but rarely frank obstructive sleep apnoea. OSA tends to occur in obese women, and may be associated with impaired fetal growth and pre-eclampsia. Snoring in pregnancy is a poor predictor of OSA.

Causes of breathlessness in pregnancy

Causes are listed in the box opposite. In general, breathlessness may be due to:

- Normal physiological changes of pregnancy. Up to 75% of pregnant women experience a degree of breathlessness, perhaps as a result of the increase in ventilation. Tachypnoea is a useful sign, as it is abnormal in pregnancy and suggests an underlying disease process
- New disease process. Pulmonary embolism is the commonest and is a major cause of maternal death. Other, rare but serious causes include amniotic fluid embolism and ARDS
- Exacerbation of chronic respiratory or cardiac disease. Asthma is the commonest. Unsuspected underlying disease may present for the first time in pregnancy, e.g. structural heart disease such as mitral stenosis; lymphangioleiomyomatosis. Pulmonary hypertension is associated with a particularly poor prognosis during pregnancy. Patients with interstitial lung disease and vital capacity <1 l should also consider avoiding pregnancy. In patients with cystic fibrosis, the presence of pulmonary hypertension or FEV_1 < 50% predicted are associated with a poor outcome.

Causes of breathlessness in pregnancy

Pulmonary
- Exacerbation of pre-existing lung disease, e.g. asthma (page 106), cystic fibrosis, lymphangioleiomyomatosis
- Pneumonia (page 176)
  - Bacterial: usual organisms, including tuberculosis (page 242) and aspiration (page 198)
  - Viral: particularly varicella, influenza (pages 220, 216)
  - Fungal: particularly coccidioidomycosis (page 278)
- Aspiration pneumonitis
- Pulmonary metastases from choriocarcinoma (very rare).

Pleural
- Pneumothorax (page 287), particularly during labour
- Small, asymptomatic effusions postpartum
- Ovarian hyperstimulation syndrome (very rare).

Vascular
- Pulmonary embolism (page 420)
- Amniotic fluid embolism (page 422)
- Air embolism (page 422)
- Pulmonary hypertension (page 391).

Cardiogenic pulmonary oedema
- Exacerbation of pre-existing cardiac disease, e.g. mitral stenosis
- Peripartum cardiomyopathy.

Non-cardiogenic pulmonary oedema
- Iatrogenic fluid overload
- Tocolytic therapy (β-agonists used to inhibit uterine contractions in preterm labour)
- ARDS due to pre-eclampsia, sepsis, massive haemorrhage, amniotic fluid embolism.

Other
- Anaemia
- Oesophageal rupture
- Hemidiaphragm rupture.

Investigations

Liaise with your obstetrics team, as well as paediatricians and anaesthetists if delivery is approaching. Management of specific conditions is discussed in the individual disease chapters in Part 2.

The following investigations may be affected by the pregnancy itself:

- **ABGs.** Normal maternal $pO_2 > 13.3$ kPa and pCO_2 3.7–4.3 kPa. A compensatory fall in serum bicarbonate (to 18–22 mmol/l) occurs, resulting in an average pH of 7.44. During the third trimester, perform ABGs in an upright position, as pO_2 may be 2.0 kPa lower when supine. A–a gradient is unaffected during pregnancy, except when supine near term

- **Blood tests.** In normal pregnancy, WCC, platelets, ESR, D-dimers, and fibrinogen are usually raised, and serum creatinine levels reduced. CRP is not significantly affected. D-dimer is increased from about 6 weeks gestation to 3 months post partum

- **CXR** may show increased pulmonary vasculature due to normal increase in cardiac output. Required for diagnosis of pneumonia and pneumothorax. With abdominal shielding, the radiation doses to mother and baby are very small and CXR should be performed if clinically necessary. Lateral CXR carries a greater radiation exposure and should be avoided

- **Ventilation-perfusion scans** are considered relatively safe in pregnancy, and are the investigation of choice if pulmonary embolism is suspected (although some experts suggest performing leg vein ultrasound first; if an asymptomatic DVT is confirmed in the setting of clinical features suggestive of pulmonary embolism, then treatment may be started without the need for radiation exposure from further imaging). If V/Q is non-diagnostic, consider pulmonary angiography; the radiation exposure from the combination of CXR, V/Q, and angiography is not thought to be associated with fetal injury. CT pulmonary angiography carries a greater radiation dose and, in the setting of the hormonal changes within the breast during pregnancy, leads to an increased risk of breast cancer in the mother.

Pre-operative assessment of the respiratory patient

The respiratory physician may be asked to assess a patient prior to elective or emergency surgery. These patients are usually those with pre-existing respiratory disease, such as COPD.

- The usual functional status of the patient should be determined
- Their respiratory function should be optimized if possible, with medication changes where appropriate.

These patients may require ventilatory support post-operatively. Ultimately the decisions regarding fitness for surgery rest with the surgeon and the anaesthetist.

Assessing the pre-operative patient

- Usual functional state and exercise tolerance (those with an exercise tolerance of <5 m will not come off a ventilator)
- Oxygen saturations on air and after exertion, such as walking or climbing up and down a step for 2 minutes
- Arterial blood gas on air, if saturations <94%. **Risk of surgery increases as the CO_2 increases**
- Spirometry, with bronchodilator reversibility testing. **Risk of surgery increased if FEV_1 < 0.8 l**
- CXR—if 65+ and no CXR in last year, or if acute respiratory symptoms
- History of snoring or OSA
- ECG
- Echocardiogram, if cardiac function compromised.

Options for management of the pre-operative patient

- Regular inhaled or nebulized bronchodilators, if air flow obstruction
- Regular inhaled steroid, if evidence of steroid reversibility
- Pre-operative course of oral steroids, if evidence of steroid reversibility
- Pre-operative course of antibiotics, if evidence of infection
- Consider pulmonary rehabilitation
- Consider chest physiotherapy with deep breathing exercises
- Referral for CPAP if OSA present
- Optimize nutrition
- Lose weight
- Advise to stop smoking; reduces post-operative complication rate.

Risk factors for peri-operative complications

- Thoracic or upper abdominal surgery
- Anaesthetic length >3.5 hours
- Smoker
- Chronic lung disease
- Raised $PaCO_2$
- Current respiratory symptoms
- Poor performance status
- Concurrent cardiac disease
- Obesity
- Older age.

Post-operative breathlessness

The respiratory physician is often asked to see patients post-operatively who have become dyspnoeic following an operative procedure. The risk of pulmonary complications is greatest with thoracic or upper abdominal surgery, when a degree of pulmonary dysfunction and consequent breathlessness due to atelectasis is inevitable.

Always rule out upper airway obstruction.

The four most likely common causes are:

- Infection/atelectasis
- Pulmonary emboli
- Left ventricular failure (fluid overload)
- Exacerbation of underlying lung disease, such as COPD or UIP.

Points to consider when assessing these patients

- Is the patient acutely unwell, needing immediate resuscitation and ventilatory support?
- Co-morbid disease and past medical history, especially pulmonary, cardiac, or thromboembolic disease
- Type of surgery
- Time since surgery:
  - *Early complications (hours)* related to residual anaesthetic effect not adequately reversed, atelectasis, respiratory failure, hypovolaemic shock, infection, PE, fat embolism, air embolism, left ventricular failure and fluid overload, myocardial ischaemia
  - *Later complications (hours–days)* related to PE, ARDS, infection, myocardial ischaemia.

Initial tests to consider performing in these patients

- Oxygen saturations and arterial blood gas breathing room air and on oxygen
- ECG
- CXR—compare to pre-operative CXR, if available
- Full blood count and clotting screen
- U&E and bicarbonate
- See if they had pre-operative oximetry and spirometry performed. There should be a record of the oxygen saturation in the anaesthetic room.

A D-dimer level is unhelpful as it will be raised by many different intra- and post-operative mechanisms.

CRP and WCC are also largely unhelpful as these are frequently raised post-operatively.

Possible cause of dyspnoea	Management options
Basal atelectasis (commoner in smokers and following abdominal or trans-thoracic procedures. Mucus in bronchial tree causes small airway obstruction, subsequent alveolar air reabsorption, and collapse of lung segments); collapsed lobe—mucus plugging	Adequate analgesia to encourage expectoration, nebulized saline, chest physiotherapy, deep breathing. If lung does not reinflate, consider bronchoscopy to suction out secretions.
Pneumonia—follows atelectasis and collapse. Possible aspiration also.	If fever and chest signs, give antibiotics for hospital-acquired pneumonia (see page 192), adequate analgesia to encourage expectoration, chest physiotherapy.
Thromboembolic disease	Oxygen as required. Measure A–a gradient on blood gas. Start treatment dose of unfractionated heparin (if not contraindicated by the operation), arrange VQ scan or CTPA, check D-dimers (although unhelpful unless negative). If in extremis consider urgent CT or echocardiogram and thrombolysis (see page 418)
Respiratory failure	Opiate overdose or anaesthetic agents causing neuromuscular block not reversed. Undiagnosed respiratory muscle weakness.
Metabolic acidosis	Check U&E, look for underlying problem, such as renal failure or sepsis.
Myocardial ischaemia	Oxygen, check cardiac enzymes and 12-hour troponin. Sublingual or IV glyceryl trinitrate if required for pain. Start prophylactic heparin (if not contraindicated by the operation).
Myocardial infarction	Thrombolysis likely to be contraindicated by recent surgery, so consider referral for primary angioplasty.
Cardiac failure/Fluid overload	Oxygen, IV frusemide, central line, and ionotropes if required. Echocardiogram to assess left ventricle.
ARDS	Supportive, likely to need mechanical ventilatory assistance. See page 522.
Phrenic nerve damage causing diaphragmatic paralysis. May occur with thoracic operations such as CABG.	Diagnose on lung function tests, CXR, and clinically decreased diaphragm movement. Advise to tilt whole bed (head up) when sleeping. Phrenics may recover but can take 2+ years.
Fat embolism following long bone fracture, especially with reaming and manipulation.	Oxygen, IV fluids, supportive care
Laryngeal spasm	Reassurance, oxygen if required.
Anaemia	Cross-match and transfuse. Identify if ongoing bleeding source.
Myasthenia gravis crisis precipitated by anaesthetic agents	May need intubation and ventilation. Stop all anti-cholinesterases. Consider plasma exchange and IV immunoglobulin. Urgent neurology input.

Part 2

Clinical conditions

Asthma

Definition There is no universally agreed definition; it is usually a clinical diagnosis—a chronic airway inflammatory disorder with inflammation due to complex interactions between inflammatory cells, mediators, and airway cells. This is characterized by airway hyperreactivity to a variety of non-specific stimuli, leading to a variable degree of airway obstruction, some of which may become irreversible over many years.

In susceptible individuals this leads to recurrent episodes of wheeze, chest tightness, breathlessness, and cough (particularly at night).

- The disease is associated with widespread and variable airflow obstruction, which may reverse spontaneously or with treatment
- Airway inflammatory changes lead to increased bronchial responsiveness to a variety of non-specific stimuli.

Epidemiology There is a wide variation in disease prevalence, with highest levels seen in English-speaking countries (where there is also a high prevalence of sensitization to common aeroallergens). The reason for the increasing worldwide prevalence over the last few decades is unclear. It is the commonest chronic respiratory disease in the UK, with a prevalence of 10–15%.

Pathophysiology Best described as chronic eosinophilic bronchitis/bronchiolitis. Airway inflammation is seen, with cellular infiltration (T helper-2 (Th2) cells, lymphocytes, eosinophils, and mast cells). There is large and small airway involvement, and cytokine production (platelet activating factor and leukotrienes).

Airway obstruction occurs due to a combination of:
- Smooth muscle contraction
- Airway lumen secretions
- Airway wall thickening.

May become irreversible over time due to:
- Basement membrane thickening, collagen deposition, and epithelial desquamation
- Airway remodelling occurs in chronic disease, with smooth muscle hypertrophy and hyperplasia.

Aetiology This is due to a combination of genetic and environmental factors, with many different genes identified.

Immunological mechanisms A subgroup of asthmatics are atopic, and therefore react to antigen challenge by producing specific IgE from B lymphocytes. This leads to the formation of IgE–antigen complexes that bind to mast cells, basophils, and macrophages, leading to the release of pre-formed mediators such as histamine, and eosinophil chemotactic factor. These factors cause bronchoconstriction and airway oedema.

Prostaglandins, leukotrienes, kinins, and platelet activating factor (PAF), are all important secondary messengers involved in the inflammatory response.

Genetic factors The hereditary basis of asthma and atopy is well established, and a number of chromosomes and linkages are implicated, in particular chromosomes 5, 13, and 14. However the multiple mechanisms and second messengers involved in asthma, make the contribution of the effects of specific genes difficult to determine.

Hygiene hypothesis This suggests that early life exposure to allergens switches off the allergic response (by reducing Th2-mediated responses), leading to reduced allergen sensitivity later in life, therefore reducing allergen-driven diseases such as asthma. Large epidemiological studies support this hypothesis.

Environmental factors The increasing prevalence of asthma appears to be associated with a rising standard of living worldwide, and not just in westernized societies. This has implicated a number of environmental factors. A number of explanations are speculated (but not proven), including dietary changes, a reduction in childhood infections, increased immunization, or a combination of all three.

Clinical features

- Cough
- Shortness of breath
- Wheeze
- Chest tightness.

Classically these are:
Variable, intermittent, worse at night, and associated with specific triggers e.g. tree and grass pollen, cat and dog dander, and non-specific triggers, e.g. cold air exposure, perfumes, and bleaches, due to airway hypersensitivity.

Examination

- May be entirely normal
- Classically expiratory wheeze is heard
- Chest deformity/hyperinflation (longstanding or poorly controlled disease).
- Severe life-threatening asthma may have no wheeze and a silent chest.

Diagnosis

This is usually a clinical diagnosis. Also important to:

- Identify provoking factors, e.g. cold air, bleach, perfume, and environmental aeroallergens (grasses, pollen, hay), and any occupational exposures
- Assess disease severity. Longitudinal studies show greater decline in lung function in asthmatics than non-asthmatics—greater still in asthmatics who smoke.

Don't forget to look for/ask about:

- Nasal obstruction/postnasal drip
- Atopic dermatitis/eczema/hay fever
- Allergies including food allergy
- Reflux/GORD disease (treating reflux may improve asthma control)
- Triggers
- Social situation/stresses
- Aspirin sensitivity (associated with later onset asthma and nasal polyps)
- Family history.

The diagnosis is based on the presence of:

Symptoms (cough, wheeze, breathlessness)
Day to day peak flow variability (>15% variability, or reversibility to inhaled β_2 agonist)
Airway hyperresponsiveness

Consider the diagnosis of asthma in:

Recurrent cough, episodic breathless, and wheeze
Chest tightness
Isolated or nocturnal cough
Exercised-induced cough or breathlessness
Hyperventilation syndrome (page 535)

Aspirin-induced asthma (AIA)

Defined as chronic rhinoconjunctivitis, nasal polyps, and asthma
Asthma is precipitated by ingestion of aspirin or other NSAIDs
Occurs in up to 20% of asthmatics, and is commoner in women
The mechanism is thought to be via aspirin inhibition of the cyclo-oxygenase pathway, with excess leukotriene production via the lipooxygenase pathway
BAL and urine in AIA patients show excess leukotrienes post-aspirin exposure
Loss of anti-inflammatory prostaglandin E2 may also be important

Oral allergy syndrome

A subset of patients sensitized to aeroallergens such as tree and grass pollens develop localized lip angioedema after ingestion of specific fruits that share cross-reactive epitopes with pollen allergens. The reaction occurs immediately after ingesting the fruit. Cooked fruit is usually tolerated, presumably because the culpable proteins are denatured with cooking. Birch pollens cross-react with apples, hazelnuts, and potato. Ragwort shares epitopes with melon and bananas

Investigations

The number of investigations required depends on the certainty of the diagnosis from the history and simple spirometry and peak flow recordings. Most patients referred for a respiratory opinion will already have completed home peak flow recordings, and have had a CXR. Repeating PEFs may still be of benefit.

Essential investigations (on which the diagnosis is based)

- *Peak flow recording/simple spirometry* to look for variability and response to treatment. Airway obstruction leads to decreased peak expiratory flow rate (PEFR) and forced expiratory volume in one second (FEV_1), but these may be normal between episodes of bronchospasm. If they are persistently normal, the diagnosis must be in doubt. The diagnosis is certain if:
  - 20% diurnal PEF variation on >3 days per week, in a week of peak flow diary measures
  - FEV_1 > 15% decrease after 6 minutes exercise
  - FEV_1 > 15% (and 200 ml) increase after 2 week trial of oral steroid (30 mg prednisolone od)
- *Bronchodilator reversibility testing* FEV_1 > 15% (or 200 ml) increase after short-acting β_2 agonist therapy (e.g. salbutamol 400 μg by MDI with spacer or 2.5 mg by nebulizer).

Non essential/optional investigations

- *Blood tests*
  FBC (eosinophilia—question the diagnosis if high total eosinophil count; consider Churg–Strauss syndrome)
  IgE (associated atopy, i.e. positive skin prick tests to common allergens, often with associated allergic rhinitis and eczema)
- *Aspergillus precipitins* (Aspergillus sensitivity, ABPA) see Chapter 23
  Specific IgE if other environmental triggers suspected
- *CXR* if atypical symptoms. May show hyperinflation or evidence of localized abnormality simulating wheeze, e.g. adenoma (rare)
- *Skin tests* to define atopic constitution, or identify potential triggers
- *Metacholine/histamine challenge* measures bronchial hyperresponsiveness (BHR) as a PC_{20}, the dose of agent provoking a 20% fall in FEV_1. Asthma is indicated by a PC_{20} of below 8 mg/ml. Normal subjects have a $PC_{20} > 16$ mg/ml. The absence of BHR argues against the diagnosis of asthma
- *Bronchial provocation tests* aim to demonstrate bronchospasm to an inhaled agent, usually occupational. The response to an aerosolized sample of a suspected agent may be useful if the diagnosis of occupational asthma is suspected, but PEF recordings at home, work, and on holiday may be more useful. Should only be carried out in a tertiary referral centre, under expert supervision
- *Sputum analysis* Sputum eosinophilia may help confirm the diagnosis
- *Laryngoscopy/ENT examination* Useful if concerns about nasal symptoms or obstruction, e.g. from polyps, or to exclude upper airway obstruction or a vocal cord abnormality

- *Bronchoscopy* Rarely needed. Its main use is to exclude an obstructing airway tumour (e.g. carcinoid)
- *Lung biopsy* is very occasionally needed in those in whom no adequate explanation for persistent and minimally reversible air flow obstruction is seen, to exclude another cause, e.g. bronchiolitis obliterans.

Main differential diagnoses in asthma

Consider especially if unusual features in the history, or poor correlation between objective measures and symptoms, or poor treatment response:

- Upper airway obstruction (breathlessness, noisy, stridulous breathing, low peak flows out of proportion to FEV_1)
- Foreign body aspiration
- Tumour, e.g. carcinoid (but can respond to steroids)
- CCF (young patient with a murmur)
- Vocal cord dysfunction
- Hyperventilation syndrome
- Chronic thromboembolic disease or primary pulmonary hypertension
- Interstitial lung disease
- Churg–Strauss syndrome (and other eosinophilic lung diseases)
- Bronchiolitis (page 463)
- Gastro-oesophageal reflux disease.

Acute severe asthma

Most asthma deaths occur outside hospital and are:
- In patients with chronic severe disease
- In those receiving inadequate medical treatment
- In those who have been symptomatically deteriorating, and may have already sought medical help
- Associated with adverse behavioural and psychosocial factors.

Fatality in asthma is due to cardiac arrest secondary to hypoxia and acidosis—reversal of hypoxia is paramount

Give high flow oxygen

Risk factors for fatal or near fatal asthma
- Previous near fatal asthma, e.g. previous ventilation or respiratory acidosis
- Three or more classes of asthma medication
- Repeated A&E attendances
- Large β_2 agonist use
- Adverse psychosocial features
- Brittle asthma.

Brittle asthma
Type 1—wide PEF variability (>40% diurnal variation for >50% of the time over >150 days), despite appropriate therapy
Type 2—sudden severe attacks on background of apparently good control

Severity of acute asthma
Moderate
- Increasing symptoms
- PEFR 50–75% predicted best
- No features of acute severe asthma
- One hour following treatment in A&E, patients with PEF > 75% predicted or best, may be discharged home with appropriate changes to their asthma medication, in the absence of concerns, e.g.
  - Significant ongoing symptoms
  - Compliance concerns
  - Living alone
  - Psychological problems or learning difficulties
  - Previous near fatal or brittle asthma
  - Nocturnal presentation
  - Pregnant
  - Exacerbation despite adequate oral steroid pre-presentation.

Severe asthma

Defined as any of:
- PEFR 33–50% predicted or best
- RR > 25
- HR > 110
- Inability to complete sentence in one breath.

Life-threatening asthma

Any one of:
- PEFR < 33%
- SaO_2 < 92 % (NB needs ABG)
- PaO_2 < 8 kPa
- Normal CO_2 (4.6–6 kPa)
- Silent chest
- Cyanosis
- Poor respiratory effort
- Bradycardia/arrhythmia/hypotension
- Exhaustion
- Confusion
- Coma.

Near fatal asthma

- Raised $PaCO_2$ and/or
- Needing mechanical ventilation with raised inflation pressures.

In-hospital treatment of acute asthma

Airway—ensure no upper airway obstruction
Breathing—give high flow oxygen
Circulation—gain IV access

Monitoring

- Record PEF on arrival in A&E, and 15–30 minutes after starting treatment
- Record O_2 saturation and maintain $\geq 92\%$
- ABG for pH and $PaCO_2$ if saturation <93% or other severe features
- Record and document heart rate and respiratory rate
- Measure glucose and potassium
- Oxygen—high concentration (40–60%) and high flow mask, e.g. Hudson
- CXR if concerns about infection/pneumothorax.

NB CO_2 retention due to too much oxygen is not a problem in acute asthma. *A high CO_2 indicates a life-threatening attack and should precipitate urgent ITU review for ventilatory support*, not controlled oxygen therapy. CO_2 is often low (due to hyperventilation). A normal CO_2 may indicate a tiring patient.

Treatment

β_2 agonist—inhaled or nebulized, e.g. nebulized salbutamol 2.5–5 mg, driven by oxygen.
Give repeated doses, or continuous, e.g. 5–10 mg per hour.
Use IV only if inhaled therapy cannot be used reliably (rarely the case).
NB risk of hypokalaemia with β_2 agonist and steroids.

Anticholinergic—nebulized ipratropium bromide added to β_2 agonist therapy may improve bronchodilatation in acute severe asthma, if poor initial β_2 agonist response.

Steroids—the earlier given in an attack, the better the outcome.
Oral is as effective as intravenous.
Dose 40–50 mg oral prednisolone, continuing for at least 5 days or until recovery. There is no agreed definition of recovery, but sensible to continue oral steroids until peak flow is maintained for 5–7 days. Dose can be stopped abruptly (assuming the patient continues on inhaled steroid). This does not apply to patients on repeated doses, or long-term steroids, where a longer course may be appropriate.

IV magnesium sulphate—if poor response to above therapies, 1.2–2 g IV infusion over 20 minutes.

IV aminophylline—some patients may respond, give if poor response to initial therapy, in acute severe or life-threatening disease.
Dose 5 mg/kg loading dose over 20 min, followed by continuous infusion of 0.5–0.7 mg/kg (500 mg in 500 ml normal saline or 0.5% dextrose at (0.5 × body weight in kg) ml/hour). If on maintenance therapy, do not give loading dose but start continuous infusion.
NB Needs therapeutic drug monitoring. Side-effects: nausea, arrhythmias, palpitations.

Antibiotics—only if infective element to the exacerbation.

IV fluids—patients are often dehydrated.

IM adrenaline—may be useful if near arrest, whilst waiting for ITU support.

ITU referral
Liaise with ITU early!
Better to discuss early a patient who does not subsequently need ITU input, than to find you and your patient in difficulty, with no ITU bed.

When to discuss with ITU:

Worsening PEF despite treatment
Worsening hypoxia
Hypercapnia
Falling pH
Exhaustion/poor respiratory effort
Drowsiness/confusion
Respiratory arrest

Discharge
Consider discharge when:
- On reducing β_2 agonist dose
- Off nebulized drugs and on inhalers ≥24 hours
- PEF ≥ 75% predicted or best
- Minimal PEF diurnal variation.

Prior to discharge consider
- Reason for the exacerbation, could it have been avoided?
- Checking patient's self-management plan/asthma action plan
- Checking inhaler technique (page 619)
- Booking an appointment with GP or practice nurse for within 24 hours
- Booking chest clinic appointment.

Monitoring morbidity—the 3 RCP questions

In the last week or month:
- Have you had difficulty sleeping because of your asthma symptoms (including cough)?
- Have you had your usual asthma symptoms during the day (cough, wheeze, chest tightness, or breathlessness)?
- Has your asthma interfered with your usual activities (e.g. work, housework)?

Chronic asthma: management

Aim to minimize symptoms and prevent exacerbations, prevent the potential consequences of longstanding airway inflammation leading to airway remodelling and chronic unresponsive airway obstruction, and improve quality of life.

The emphasis should be on education, self-management, and personal asthma action plans. Aim for:

- Minimal day and night symptoms
- No exacerbations
- Normal lung function
- No limit to physical activity
- Minimum steroid dose.

Treatment is based on disease severity using a step up/step down approach, starting treatment at the level appropriate to disease severity, based on the history, spirometry, and medication usage.

The main aims during out-patient review are:

Ensure the diagnosis is correct
Aim for no symptoms/normal lung function on minimal treatment
Ensure an action plan is in place for exacerbations
Identify patients at risk of an adverse outcome

Pharmacological management

British Thoracic Society Guidelines for the Management of Asthma
Step 1—mild intermittent asthma
- Short-acting β_2 agonist
- Check compliance, inhaler technique (including Volumatic or other spacer), and eliminate potential triggers
- 10 puffs per day (2 or more canisters/month) is a marker of poorly controlled disease.

Step 2—regular preventer therapy
- Start at 400 µg/day Beclomethasone (BDP) in a twice daily dose
- Titrate steroid dose to symptoms, aiming for lowest effective dose
- Local steroid side-effects only (oral candida, dysphonia) from BDP ≤ 800 µg per day
- Possible dose-related bone density effects at this dose.

Step 3—add on therapy
- If taking 200–800 µg/day inhaled steroid, consider long-acting β_2 agonist. A combination preparation may be appropriate.

Step 4—Poor control on moderate dose inhaled steroid and add on therapy—addition of fourth drug
- Leukotriene receptor antagonist—about 1/3rd of patients respond. May be useful if atopic or for exercise induced asthma. Trial for one month, and stop if no response
- Theophylline (side-effects, e.g. nausea, and needs therapeutic drug monitoring)
- Slow-release oral β_2 agonist.

Step 5—Continuous or frequent use of oral steroids

- NB risk of side-effects if on oral steroids for >3 months, or 3 to 4 courses per year
- Warn patient of potential side-effects (hypertension, diabetes, cataracts, gastric erosions). Consider osteoporosis prophylaxis with calcium or a bisphosphonate and document baseline bone densitometry (see page 627)
- Aim for lowest possible dose steroid.

Additional treatment options

Steroid-sparing drugs, e.g. methotrexate, gold and cyclosporin—may be useful if other treatments unsuccessful. These need haematological surveillance for side-effects, and there are very few data to support their use. Continuous subcutaneous terbutaline infusion via a portable syringe driver may be useful.

Additional points

Regular review—to ensure patients are on appropriate treatment for their disease severity, and are maintained on the lowest possible inhaled steroid dose. Step down treatment if stable for 3 months or more. Step down inhaled steroid by reducing dose by 25–50% at three-monthly intervals.

Asthma action plan—all patients with severe asthma should have an agreed written asthma action plan (self-management plan), their own peak flow meter, and regular checks of compliance and inhaler technique. This should include a plan for deteriorating symptoms and falling peak flows. Patients on low dose inhaled steroids (200 μg) should have their dose increased by fivefold at the start of an exacerbation. This should not be extrapolated to higher inhaled steroid doses. The previous recommendation of doubling the dose of inhaled steroid at the start of an exacerbation is unproven.

Non-pharmacological management

Allergen avoidance may reduce severity of disease in sensitized individuals. House dust mite control measures need to be comprehensive—there is no current evidence to support it, though trials are ongoing. Pet removal may be useful, if the history is suggestive, and sensitivity has been demonstrated by skin prick testing or raised specific IgE levels.

Smoking cessation may reduce asthma severity.

Complementary therapies No current evidence exists.

Dietary manipulation No consistent evidence, and none supported by interventional trials. Low magnesium intake is associated with increased asthma prevalence. Fish oils may be beneficial.

Weight reduction in obese asthmatics leads to improved control.

Immunotherapy Desensitization using allergen-specific immunotherapy may be beneficial in a small subgroup of patients.

Buteyko breathing technique is a series of breathing exercises that mimic yoga breathing techniques. A number of studies have shown a reduction in the use of inhaled bronchodilator and steroid use in asthmatics carrying out these exercises, with no change in lung function or bronchial hyperresponsiveness.

Future developments

Anti IgE/allergen immunotherapy Omalizamub (not yet licensed in the UK) is a humanized anti-IgE antibody that has been found to be effective in patients with moderate to severe asthma. It may reduce exacerbations and steroid dose and improve lung function. It is given subcutaneously every two to four weeks and may be useful in patients with severe atopic disease, as it is also effective for rhinitis and dermatitis.

New steroids Research for 'dissociated steroids' is ongoing. These are steroids in which the useful, anti-inflammatory effects (mediated by transcription factor inhibition) are dissociated from the side-effects (mediated via glucocorticoid DNA binding). Safer steroids, e.g. Ciclesonide, a new once daily inhaled steroid, appear to have an improved side-effect profile. Ciclesonide is a pro-drug, activated by airway esterases, with fewer side-effects due to high degrees of protein binding.

Eosinophil inhibitors A variety of approaches to inhibit eosinophil recruitment are under investigation, including adhesion molecule inhibition and eosinophil chemotactic receptor inhibition.

Phosphodiesterase-4 inhibitors New generation PDE4 inhibitors, e.g. roflumilast, are being investigated in clinical trials. These drugs have a broad anti-inflammatory action, with neutrophil inhibitory effects. Early clinical trial data looks promising.

Cytokine modulators Tumour necrosis factor (TNF)–alpha plays an important role in the pathogenesis of asthma. Anti-TNF antibodies have been beneficial in the treatment of inflammatory bowel disease and rheumatoid arthritis. It may be useful in the treatment of severe asthma, as may blockage of other important leukotrienes, e.g. IL-13.

Inflammation marker or surrogate-based treatment is treatment based on monitoring surrogate markers of inflammation such as exhaled nitric oxide or sputum eosinophil counts. It may lead to reduced steroid requirements, and improved long-term outcomes.

Further information

British Guideline on the management of asthma. *Thorax* 2003; **58**: S1

www.brit-thoracic.org.uk/sign/index.htm—a good site from which to download copies of the asthma guidelines in various formats and to obtain training information

www.occupationalasthma.com

Difficult/refractory asthma

Patients with refractory asthma are a small subgroup of asthma patients (<5%). They have difficult to treat disease, reflected by high maintenance medication requirements or persistent symptoms and air flow obstruction, with multiple exacerbations, despite high medication use.

They have high numbers of admissions, and cause significant anxiety to their families, and medical staff.

There is a wide range of disease severity, including those with highly labile disease and those with severe, more chronic air flow obstruction.

The disease is usually defined on the basis of
- Medication requirements
- Asthma symptoms
- Frequency of exacerbations
- Severity of airflow limitation.

Patients exhibit the features of asthma, and it is thought that the airflow obstruction, airway hyperresponsiveness, and PEF diurnal variability are more severe in refractory disease, though the physiological reasons for this remain unclear.

These patients typically fail to completely reverse their airflow obstruction following a two week course of oral prednisolone and demonstrate a poor bronchodilator response to inhaled β_2 agonists.

The pathological mechanism is likely to be ongoing airway inflammation, with increasing airway fibrosis, but this is not proven. Other possibilities include steroid resistance (see opposite), β_2 receptor downregulation, or a different disease process altogether.

Diagnosis of refractory asthma
- Confirm the diagnosis is correct—this may mean going back through the notes and retaking a thorough history
- Confirm reversible airflow limitation (as for non-refractory asthma; see page 94)
- Consider other diagnoses for cough, breathlessness, and wheeze and investigate for potential exacerbating diseases:
  - COPD
  - Bronchiectasis/cystic fibrosis
  - Sinus disease—consider ENT review
  - Churg–Strauss syndrome/eosinophilic syndromes—consider ANCA
  - Allergic bronchopulmonary aspergillosis—consider *Aspergillus* precipitans/skin tests/IgE
  - Vocal cord dysfunction
  - Hyperventilation syndrome
  - Gastro-oesphageal reflux—consider OGD/24 hour pH
  - Upper airway obstruction—consider CT or bronchoscopy
  - Obstructive sleep apnoea—consider sleep study
  - Cardiac dysfunction—consider echo and/or cardiological opinion
  - Psychiatric/emotional issues/secondary gain—consider psychiatry or psychology review.

Before labelling a patient as 'refractory', compliance must be confirmed. This may be by checking pharmacy prescription records, using inhaler devices monitoring medication usage, or by measurement of plasma prednisolone levels.

Treatment is that of non-refractory asthma, with inhaled long-acting β_2 agonists and high-dose inhaled corticosteroids.

In patients unable to tolerate a prednisolone dose <20 mg per day, corticosteroid pharmacokinetic studies may be useful. However, <25% of patients with severe asthma show clinically significantly increased prednisolone clearance (usually a specific reason can be identified, such as concomitant use of enzyme inducing medication).

Inflammatory markers, e.g. sputum or plasma eosinophil counts or exhaled nitric oxide levels, may be useful to assess medication response, though no trials have demonstrated their use clinically in this group of patients.

Anti-inflammatory and immunomodulating drugs may be of benefit (specialized centre only). These include methotrexate, cyclosporin, oral gold, intravenous gammaglobulin, and macrolide antibiotics. None of these have been studied in a randomized controlled trial in this group of patients, and none have demonstrated improvement in airway hyperresponsiveness.

'Steroid-resistant' asthma This subgroup of patients represents a very small proportion of refractory asthma patients. Middle-aged, obese women, often with other additional diagnoses, are overrepresented in this group. They require supportive treatment, without high doses of glucocorticoids. Diagnoses other than asthma are likely and investigation should be directed towards these.

Further information

Systematic assessment of difficult-to-treat asthma. Robinson DS *et al*. *ERJ* 2003; **22**: 478–83

Pseudo-steroid resistant asthma. Thomas PS *et al*. *Thorax* 1999; **54**: 352–6

Asthma in pregnancy

- Pregnancy can affect asthma
- Asthma can affect the outcome of pregnancy
- Prognosis—1/3 worsen, 1/3 improve, 1/3 no change
- Asthma course is likely to be similar in successive pregnancies
- Severe asthma is more likely to deteriorate than mild asthma.

Pre-pregnancy counselling

- Asthmatics must continue normal asthma medication
- Smoking cessation advice
- Monitor the pregnant asthmatic closely.

Acute asthma in pregnancy

Risk to fetus of uncontrolled asthma outweighs any small risk of drugs
Asthma medications are generally safe in pregnancy
Steroids should be continued.

- Drug therapy as for non-asthmatics
- Maintain oxygen saturation >95%
- Continuous fetal monitoring for acute severe asthma
- Liaise with obstetrician if acute severe asthma.

Leukotriene receptor antagonists

Limited safety data available in pregnancy. Recommended not to start in pregnancy. Continue in women who have previously demonstrated significant improvement in disease control prior to pregnancy.

Management during labour

- Acute asthma is rare in labour (probably due to high sympathetic drive)
- Regional anaesthetic blockade preferable to general anaesthesia
- Prostaglandin E_2 may be safely used for induction of labour
- Prostaglandin F_2 alpha (for post-partum bleeding) may cause bronchospasm
- Give parenteral hydrocortisone 100 mg 6–8 hourly during labour if on oral prednisolone at >7.5 mg daily for >2 weeks prior to delivery.

Breast-feeding

- An asthmatic mother reduces the chance of atopy in her child by breast feeding
- Prednisolone is secreted in breast mik, but the infant is exposed to only tiny and clinically irrelevant doses.

Occupational asthma

This is asthma due to specific workplace sensitizers and may account for 10% of adult onset asthma.
The diagnosis is often difficult to make.
Early diagnosis is important, as earlier removal from the workplace in affected individuals leads to a better outcome.
It is different to asthma exacerbated by irritants in the workplace.

- Agents induce asthma through IgE and non-IgE mechanisms
- The latency between first exposure and symptom onset can be long, and depends on the sensitizing agent—an accurate history therefore includes current and past exposures
- Once sensitized, re-exposure to very low concentrations can provoke symptoms
- May be associated with rhinitis and urticaria
- Improves away from work, but can take several days to settle.

Risk factors

- Atopy
- HLA type (e.g. HLA-DQB1*0503 associated with isocyanate allergy)
- Smoking (especially for high molecular weight agents.

Diagnosis

- Confirm the diagnosis of asthma
- Confirm the relationship between asthma and work exposures
- Find the specific cause.

Document lung function deterioration in the workplace, usually by serial peak flow recording at work, at home, and on holiday.
  Bronchial provocation/challenge testing using suspected agent—only in specialized centres.
  Skin prick testing/specific IgE for certain sensitizers.

Document

- The range of chemicals used
- Working practices
- Use of personal protective equipment.

Serial PEF recording in occupational asthma

- Record every 2 hours from waking to sleep
- For four weeks, whilst no changes to treatment
- Document home/work periods and any holidays
- Analysis is best made by experts, usually using a criterion-based analysis system, e.g. OASYS (a computer program that plots and interprets serial peak flow recordings; see *www.occupationalasthma.com*)
- Patients may be sensitized to more than one agent.

Causes of occupational asthma

Sensitizing agent	Occupational exposure
Low molecular weight agents (act as haptens)	
Isocyanates	Paint sprayers, adhesives, polyurethane foams
Acid anhydrides	Epoxy paint, varnish, resins
Metals	Welders, plating, metal refiners
Glutaraldehyde and other disinfectants	Health care workers
Drugs	Pharmaceutical industry
High molecular weight agents	
Amine dyes	Cosmetics, hair dyes, rubber works
Wood dusts, bark	Textile workers, joiners, carpenters
Animal-derived antigens	Vets, laboratory workers (20% affected)
Biological enzymes	Detergent industry, pharmaceuticals
Plant products	Bakers, hairdressers
Fluxes, colophony	Solderers, electronics industry

Management of occupational asthma

- Identify the cause
- Remove the worker from exposure
- Continue employment if at all possible
- Early diagnosis and removal from exposure are important factors for a good outcome
- Improvement in FEV_1 may be maintained for one year following last exposure, and for up to 2 years for non-specific responsiveness
- The decision to remove the patient from the workplace should not be taken lightly, and should be made by a consultant with experience of occupational lung disease
- Employee may be eligible for Disablement Benefit (no proof of negligence is required).

Latex allergy is seen in up to 18% of health care workers, and is the leading cause of occupational asthma in this group due to the widespread use of latex gloves. It is potentially serious, with avocado, bananas, kiwi, and chestnuts cross-reacting to give a similar clinical picture. Treatment is absolute avoidance; those affected should wear a medic-alert bracelet and always use non-latex gloves.

Vocal cord dysfunction

A proportion of patients labelled as having severe asthma, will have vocal cord dysfunction or so-called 'upper airway hyperresponsiveness'.

Patients will typically present with asthma symptoms, with associated triggers, e.g. odours, cold air. They typically have no reduction in peak flow or response to asthma medications (though this is possible).

A careful history will reveal shortness of breath that is of short duration, worse on inspiration, and extremely sudden in onset, with symptom-free periods.

Pathogenesis

- Recent URTI, may take months to settle
- Postnasal drip/chronic sinusitis
- Gastro-oesophageal reflux disease with microaspiration
- Chronic laryngitis
- Hyperventilation in association with anxiety/panic
- It is postulated that the vocal cord closure may represent a reflex airway protective mechanism.

Diagnosis is based on excluding other causes of cough and breathlessness. The gold standard is visualization of abnormal vocal cord movement at laryngoscopy. Flow volume loop will show inspiratory flow limitation, with 'stuttering' of the flow.

Treatment (for which there are no randomized controlled trials)
- Panting (autopeep)
- Coughing and cough suppression techniques
- Inspiratory resistance devices
- HELIOX/nebulized saline/lidocaine spray
- Sedatives
- Exercise
- Speech therapy.

Further information

Clinical features of vocal cord dysfunction. Newman KB *et al. AJRCCM* 1995; **152**: 1382–6

Allergic rhinitis (hay fever)

This is the syndrome of nasal discharge or blockage with nasal and/or eye itching, and sneezing. It is often associated with postnasal drip, cough, fatigue, and with significant morbidity. Allergic rhinitis is defined as perennial if the symptoms occur year round, seasonal if occurring at a particular time of year. The prevalence is increasing, and affects up to 15% of the UK population.

Aetiology The lining of the nose is in continuum with the lower respiratory tract, and inflammation of the upper and lower airways often coexists. Common aeroallergens provoking seasonal allergic rhinitis are tree pollen in the spring, and grass pollen in the summer months. Perennial rhinitis usually reflects allergy to indoor allergens such as house dust mite (the provoking allergen is a digestive enzyme that is shed in the faeces), cat salivary protein, cockroaches, or animal dander.

Pathophysiology Symptoms occur following the inhalation of allergen to which the subject is sensitized, and against which they have IgE antibodies. These antibodies bind to mast cell IgE receptors, with the release of mediators, including tryptase and histamine, causing symptoms immediately after exposure.

Diagnosis is usually made from the history, which should identify the triggers to the disease. The main differential diagnosis is with sinusitis due to bacterial infection, and upper airway involvement due to vasculitis. Asthma is common in association with rhinitis, and treatment of rhinosinusitis in association with asthma leads to improved asthma control. Up to 50% of asthma patients will have allergic rhinitis.

Treatment

- Allergen avoidance. This may be easier said than done. It can take up to 20 weeks to remove cat allergen from a house. Keeping car and house windows shut and wearing sunglasses may help avoid pollen. Pollen counts are highest in the afternoon and early evening
- Non-sedating antihistamines, e.g. terfenadine, improve sneezing and itching, but have no effect on nasal blockage
- Topical intranasal steroid, e.g. budesonide, triamcinolone
- Topical anticholinergics, e.g. ipratropium may be useful for rhinorrhea, if uncontrolled with topical nasal steroids
- Topical sodium cromoglycate may be beneficial, particularly for allergic conjunctivitis
- Decongestants, e.g. oxymetazoline, may help, but rebound nasal blockage and tachyphylaxis are a potential problem if used regularly.

Chronic obstructive pulmonary disease (COPD)

COPD is a common and is mostly due to smoking. Patients with COPD represent a large proportion of in-patient (approximately 12% of all general medical admissions) and out-patient work for the chest physician.

Definition
- Fixed airflow obstruction
- Minimal or no reversibility with bronchodilators
- Minimal variability in day-to-day symptoms
- Slowly progressive and irreversible deterioration in lung function, leading to progressively worsening symptoms.

Aetiology 95% of cases are smoking-related, typically >20 pack years. COPD occurs in 10–20% of smokers, indicating that there is probable genetic susceptibility. COPD is increasing in frequency worldwide, particularly in some developing countries, due to high levels of smoking. It can also be caused by environmental and occupational factors such as dusts, chemicals, and air pollution.

Pathology
- *Mucous gland hyperplasia* particularly in the large airways, with mucous hypersecretion and therefore a chronic productive cough. Other mucosal damage from smoke:
  - *Squamous metaplasia* replacement of the normal ciliated columnar epithelium by a squamous epithelium
  - *Loss of cilial function* This leads to impairment of the normal functioning of the mucociliary escalator, another reason for the chronic productive cough.
- *Chronic inflammation and fibrosis* of small airways, characterized by CD8 lymphocyte, macrophage, and neutrophil infiltration, with release of pro-inflammatory cytokines. Recurrent infections may perpetuate airway inflammation
- *Emphysema* due to alveolar wall destruction causing irreversible enlargement of air spaces distal to the terminal bronchiole (the acinus), with subsequent loss of elastic recoil and hyperinflated lungs
  - Panacinar emphysema can occur with dilated air spaces evenly distributed across acinii
  - Centriacinar or proximal emphysema can occur with dilated air spaces found in association with the respiratory bronchioles
  - Periacinar or paraseptal emphysema can occur with dilated air spaces at the edge of the acinar unit and abutting a fixed structure, such as the pleura or a vessel.
- *Thickened pulmonary arteriolar wall and remodelling* occur with hypoxia. Leads to increased pulmonary vascular resistance, pulmonary hypertension, and impaired gas exchange.

The cause of the increase in airways resistance is multifactorial. Small airway inflammation reduces the airway lumen. Emphysema destroys the radial attachments to the small airways, which normally hold them open and resist dynamic compression.

Clinical features
- Dyspnoea
- Decreased exercise tolerance
- Productive cough
- Wheeze.

Significant airflow obstruction may be present before the patient is aware of it.

Signs depend on the severity of the underlying disease.
- Raised respiratory rate
- Hyperexpanded/barrel chest
- Prolonged expiratory time >5 seconds, with pursed lip breathing
- Use of accessory muscles of respiration
- Quiet breath sounds (especially in the lung apices) ± wheeze
- Quiet heart sounds (due to overlying hyperinflated lung)
- Possible basal crepitations
- Signs of cor pulmonale and CO_2 retention (ankle oedema, raised JVP, warm peripheries, plethoric conjunctivae, bounding pulse, polycythaemia. Flapping tremor if CO_2 acutely raised).

α_1-antitrypsin deficiency (α_1-AT) is an autosomal recessively inherited condition that is associated with the early development of emphysema. α_1-AT is a glycoprotein protease inhibitor produced by the liver. It is secreted via the bloodstream into the lungs and opposes neutrophil elastase, which destroys alveolar wall connective tissue. Elastase is produced in increased levels by pulmonary neutrophils and macrophages in response to smoking and lung infections. If α_1-AT is deficient, the elastase cannot be opposed, and subsequently basal emphysema develops. Disease is worse in smokers and can cause COPD at a young age. There is also associated liver dysfunction and cirrhosis, as abnormal protein secretion accumulates in the liver.

So far about 75 different alleles have been identified for this gene on the long arm of chromosome 4. The commonest alleles are the M allele (normal), the partially defective S allele, and the almost fully defective Z allele (lysine is substituted for glutamic acid at position 342, leading to abnormal folding, preventing posttranslational processing with retention within cells), commonest in Scandinavia.
- MM, the normal phenotype
- MS, MZ have 50–70% of normal α_1-protease inhibitor (Pi) levels
- SZ, SS have 35–50% of normal levels
- Homozygous ZZ has only 10–20% of normal levels and is the genotype most strongly associated with developing emphysema.

Screening for the defect should be carried out especially in patients <40 with COPD. Siblings should be screened and the particular importance of not smoking and avoiding passive smoking emphasized. Non-smokers are usually asymptomatic. Treatment with enzyme augmentation to slow decline in lung function is currently under evaluation.

Further information
UK alpha1 antitrypsin deficiency support group *www.alpha1.org.uk/Alpha1*

Investigations

Pulmonary function tests
- Obstructive spirometry and flow-volume loops
- Reduced FEV_1 to <80% predicted (FEV_1 is the measurement of choice to assess progression of COPD)
- $FEV_1/FVC < 0.7$
- Minimal bronchodilator reversibility (<15%, usually <10%)
- Raised total lung volume, FRC, and residual volume because of emphysema, air trapping, and loss of elastic recoil
- Decreased TLCO and kCO because presence of emphysema decreases surface area available for gas diffusion.

CXR is not required for diagnosis and repeated CXR is unnecessary unless other diagnoses are being considered (most importantly lung cancer or bronchiectasis).
- Hyperinflated lung fields with attenuation of peripheral vasculature—'black lung sign'. More than 7 posterior ribs seen
- Flattened diaphragms (best CXR correlate of post-mortem degree of emphysema)
- More horizontal ribs
- May see bullae, especially in the lung apices, which if large can be mistaken for a pneumothorax due to the loss of lung markings (CT can differentiate).

Diagnosis is based on the history of smoking and progressive dyspnoea, with evidence of irreversible airflow obstruction on spirometry.

COPD severity according to NICE guidelines, 2004

(which differ slightly from the GOLD guidelines)

Mild:	FEV_1 50–80% predicted May or may not be symptomatic with cough or sputum
Moderate:	FEV_1 30–49% predicted. Increased FRC, reduced TLCO Likely to be symptomatic (cough, sputum, dyspnoea), often managed by patient's GP
Severe:	FEV_1 <30% predicted. Marked hyperinflation, TLCO usually low. Usually hypoxic, with signs of cor pulmonale. Symptomatic, often needing hospital admissions

---

Differential diagnosis of COPD
- Asthma
- Bronchiectasis
- Bronchiolitis
- Left ventricular failure.

MRC dyspnoea scale

1 Not troubled by breathlessness except on strenuous exercise
2 Short of breath when hurrying or walking up a slight hill
3 Walks slower than contemporaries on level ground because of breathlessness, or has to stop for breath when walking at own pace
4 Stops for breath after walking about 100 m or after a few minutes on level ground
5 Too breathless to leave the house, or breathless when dressing or undressing.

Non-pharmacological management of stable COPD

Aims of COPD management should include:
- ensuring the diagnosis is correct
- stopping smoking
- optimizing treatment by minimizing symptoms where possible
- helping the patient maintain their quality of life.

Management should be delivered by a multi-disciplinary team.

No treatment has yet been shown to modify disease progression in the long term, except for stopping smoking.

Smoking cessation is the only intervention that is proven to decrease the smoking-related decline in lung function. All patients with COPD who smoke should be encouraged to stop at every opportunity. The graph below shows the accelerated decline in FEV_1 in susceptible smokers and the delay in this acceleration from stopping smoking; susceptible smokers, however, never regain the original curve. Nicotine replacement therapy should be used to aid smoking cessation (see page 644).

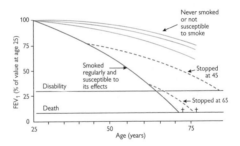

Modification of the Fletcher Peto diagram of FEV_1 decline in susceptible smokers

Education can improve ability to manage illness and stop smoking.

Pulmonary rehabilitation is a multidisciplinary programme, with RCT evidence that it improves exercise tolerance, quality of life, and reduces hospital admissions. The mainstay of rehabilitation is graded exercise, but includes breathing techniques and education. Programmes vary, but are usually run on an out-patient basis over several weeks, with multidisciplinary involvement (see page 637). Should be made available to all appropriate patients with COPD.

Diet Weight loss is recommended if the patient is obese, to minimize respiratory effort. If the patient is very breathless, calorific intake may be low and a catabolic state may exist. Nutritional supplementation may be necessary. Maintaining body weight and muscle mass correlates well with survival.

Psychosocial support Practical support at home, day centres; car disability badge; assess for signs of anxiety and depression.

Pharmacological management of stable COPD

Pharmacological management aims to relieve symptoms and reduce exacerbations, but will not modify disease. Increase treatment in a stepwise fashion. Exacerbations require additional therapeutic support.

Bronchodilators Simple pulmonary function testing may not show significant bronchodilator reversibility of FEV_1, but bronchodilators provide therapeutic benefit in the long term, by reducing dyspnoea.

- Initially prescribe short-acting β_2 agonists as required for symptom relief
- If the patient remains symptomatic, prescribe short-acting β_2 agonist with short acting anti-cholinergic
- If they are still symptomatic, try therapeutic trial of regular long-acting bronchodilator, either with β_2 agonist or anti-cholinergic. Stop if no benefit as it is expensive. Also prescribe this if they have 2 or more exacerbations per year
- Oral methylxanthines, such as theophyllines, can be used as a maintenance therapy and may improve symptoms. Add after inhaled bronchodilators and trial of inhaled steroids; continue only if symptom relief is noted. Their method of action is unclear, but they may have an anti-inflammatory effect. Take care regarding therapeutic/toxic levels, especially in elderly patients
- **Inhaler therapy** provides adequate bronchodilator doses for most patients, especially when used with a spacer device. It is important to check the patient's inhaler technique
- **Nebulizer therapy** is indicated if the patient is unable to use inhalers, or if they are disabled or distressed with breathlessness despite maximal inhaler therapy. Only those with a clear response, with reduction in symptoms or improvement in activities of daily living, should continue with long-term domiciliary nebulized treatment (usually with salbutamol and ipratropium), as there is a significant placebo effect.

Inhaled steroids should be prescribed to all patients with an FEV_1 less than or equal to 50% predicted, who have had 2 or more exacerbations per year requiring treatment with antibiotics or oral steroids. Clinical trials of inhaled steroids have shown a reduction in exacerbation frequency in severe COPD, but no slowing in the decline in lung function. In patients with breathlessness and exercise limitation, inhaled steroids can be given for a 4 week trial, to see if they improve clinical symptoms. Stop if no benefit as expensive. Warn patients regarding steroid side-effects and document.

Oral steroids are not recommended as a maintenance therapy in COPD. It may, however, be difficult to withdraw them in patients with severe COPD following an exacerbation. If so, keep the dose as low as possible and prescribe osteoporosis prophylaxis if indicated. Warn regarding steroid side-effects and document.

Oxygen can be administered via a cylinder for short burst oxygen therapy as required for symptomatic relief, such as after climbing stairs (little trial evidence to support this use), or as long-term oxygen therapy (LTOT) via an oxygen concentrator. The latter is for patients in respiratory failure, with a PaO_2 <7.3 kPa or PaO_2 of 7.3–8 kPa with any of: secondary polycythaemia, peripheral oedema, or pulmonary hypertension present to use for a minimum of 15 hours per day (including sleep). Additional ambulatory cylinders can be provided. Low flow oxygen, such as 2–4 l/min via nasal prongs is usually adequate. Small changes in CO_2 retention with oxygen administration can be tolerated if asymptomatic and no respiratory acidosis. Associated OSA is a risk factor for CO_2 retention. (For further information on prescribing oxygen, see page 634, Chapter 56).

Vaccination Influenza vaccine annually and pneumococcal vaccine.

Antibiotics No trials of antibiotic prophylaxis have been done. Many respiratory physicians prescribe low-dose antibiotics, particularly over the winter. Trials are urgently required. It is likely that this strategy would be more effective than inhaled steroids.

Mucolytics may benefit a few patients with chronic productive cough. Prescribe for a trial period and only continue if there is evidence of improvement.

Palliative care/respiratory sedation Use of low-dose sedatives, such as oramorph 10 mg as required or diazepam 2 mg twice daily, can be used as a palliative care measure. The aim is to relieve the sensation of dyspnoea and associated anxiety, when the patient has severe COPD and is on maximal treatment. Dose may need to be titrated against any rise in CO_2 (surprisingly uncommon).

How to perform a steroid trial to help distinguish asthma from COPD

Measure FEV_1 and slow VC before and after:
- either a high-dose inhaled steroid for 6–8 weeks,
- or a 2 week course of oral prednisolone, 30 mg/day.

>15% increase in FEV_1 implies steroid reversibility and patient is likely to have asthma

>15% increase in slow VC suggests significantly reduced air trapping, and may indicate significant asthma. May occur with a significantly smaller change in FEV_1

Document results of trial clearly in notes.

Further information
Prophylactic antibiotic therapy for chronic bronchitis. Black P et al. Cochrane Database Syst Rev. 2003; (**1**): CD004105

Management of exacerbations

Exacerbations may cause mild symptoms in those with relatively preserved lung function, but may cause considerable morbidity in those with limited respiratory reserves. It has been increasingly recognized that significant numbers of patients do not regain their pre-morbid lung function or quality of life following an exacerbation. An exacerbation is essentially a clinical diagnosis.

Causes may be infective organisms, either viral or bacterial, or non-infective causes, such as pollution or temperature changes. Common bacterial pathogens are *Haemophilus influenzae, Streptococcus pneumoniae*, and *Moraxella catarrhalis* and the commonest viral pathogens are rhinovirus, influenza, coronavirus, and adenovirus.

Symptoms include increased sputum volume and/or purulence, increasing dyspnoea or wheeze, chest tightness, fluid retention.

Management

Assess the severity of the exacerbation: increase in dyspnoea, tachypnoea, use of accessory muscles, new cyanosis, pedal oedema, or confusion. Can the patient self-care and self-medicate? In the presence of severe symptoms, with possible co-morbid disease and decreased functional activities, the patient is likely to need hospital management.

Investigate with CXR, ABGs, ECG, FBC, and U&Es. *Admission arterial pH is the best predictor of survival.* A pH <7.25 is associated with a rapidly rising mortality. A *raised* pH may imply an alternative diagnosis, not associated with worsening airways obstruction, such as pulmonary oedema. Check theophylline level if patient is taking them regularly; send sputum for culture if it is purulent.

Antibiotics if sputum purulent, pyrexial, ↑CRP, new changes on CXR.

Systemic steroids for all patients with exacerbations of COPD who are admitted to hospital or are significantly more breathless than usual. Give prednisolone 30 mg/day for 1–2 weeks, unless there are specific contra-indications. This shortens the recovery time. Long-term steroid treatment should be avoided due to side-effects.

Inhaled or nebulized bronchodilators Breathless unwell patients may benefit from nebulizer therapy in the acute period.

Controlled oxygen therapy 24–35% via facemask, with oximetry, arterial blood gases, or capillary gas monitoring. **Prescribe oxygen to maintain saturations between 80 and 90%,** balancing hypoxia, hypercapnia, and pH. Too little oxygen (SaO_2 < 80% causes anaerobic metabolism and metabolic acidosis, too much oxygen (SaO_2 > 90%) can cause hypercapnia and a respiratory acidosis. A deteriorating pH to below 7.25 has a much poorer prognosis. Make sure your instructions to the ward staff are clear as to the need to keep the SaO_2 within this window, by changing the % O_2 delivered as necessary. Falling conscious level is the best clinical marker of significant CO_2 retention and acidosis.

Intravenous aminophylline Evidence is lacking regarding the effectiveness of IV aminophylline, but it may be beneficial, particularly if the patient is wheezy and has not improved with nebulizers alone. Give a loading dose, unless the patient is on regular oral aminophylline, followed by a maintenance infusion. Need to monitor aminophylline levels daily. Main side-effects are tachycardia and nausea.

Non-invasive ventilation (NIV) Effective in supporting patients during an exacerbation, when maximal medical treatment has not been effective. Appropriate for conscious patients with ongoing respiratory acidosis (pH 7.3 or less), hypoxia, and hypercapnia. May avoid intubation. Ceiling of treatment should be determined before its use. (See page 600.)

Doxapram Intravenous respiratory stimulant drug. Can be used to drive respiratory rate (if below 20 per minute) and depth in COPD exacerbation and hence improve hypoxia, hypercapnia, and respiratory acidosis. Too much doxapram can overdrive breathing to the point of respiratory muscle fatigue, collapse, and death. Should therefore be used with caution and the aim would be to reduce $PaCO_2$ (and raise pH) by only a small amount. Best thought of as reversing the hypoventilation/hypercapnia secondary to oxygen therapy. Doxapram can cause metabolic acidosis, agitation, and cardiac arrhythmias and should only be used at the lowest possible dose (0.5 to 3 mg/min) in the short term (usually 24–36 hours). Its use has largely been replaced by NIV, but may be used if NIV is not available or not tolerated.

Intubation/intensive care If the patient is not responding to medical therapy, a decision regarding invasive mechanical ventilation needs to be made. This may be considered to be appropriate if the patient usually has a good functional status, with minimal other co-morbidity. This would suggest supportive care may help patient survive the exacerbation. These decisions should ideally be discussed with the patient, their family, their consultant, and the ITU consultant and documented in the medical notes. Resuscitation decisions should also be made.

Acute respiratory assessment service (ARAS)/'Hospital at home' Respiratory nurse-led service supporting early discharge of COPD patients after hospital assessment and providing ongoing respiratory care at home. Suitable patients are those without acidotic respiratory failure or other ongoing medical problems. Decreases in-patient stay and hence is an economic alternative.

Further information

Hospital at home for patients with acute exacerbations of COPD: systematic review of the evidence. Ram FSF et al. BMJ 2004; **329**: 315–18

Summary of approaches to medical treatment

An approach to a patient with exacerbation of COPD in the hospital setting

- Assess the severity of the exacerbation by measuring respiratory rate, oxygen saturations, degree of air entry, tachycardia, BP, peripheral perfusion
- Exclude a tension pneumothorax clinically
- If hypoxic, give controlled 24–35% oxygen via Venturi facemask to achieve SaO_2 80–90%, salbutamol nebulizer, establish venous access.
- Check a blood gas
- Order a CXR
- Perform ECG
- Check bloods for WCC, CRP, potassium, etc.
- Optimize volume status
- Take a *brief history* if possible. Important to know what patient's normal functional status is like, such as exercise tolerance and the need for help with activities of daily living. Old hospital notes are helpful regarding severity of disease and whether previous decisions have been made regarding ventilation or resuscitation
- Nebulized bronchodilators—salbutamol 2.5–5 mg and ipratropium 500 µg on arrival and 4–6 hourly
- Continued oxygen therapy-aiming to maintain saturations between 80 and 90%. Repeat blood gases after 60 minutes to ensure improvement if hypoxic or acidotic. Repeat if clinical deterioration
- Consider antibiotics
- Oral steroids
- Consider intravenous aminophylline if not improving with nebulizers
- Consider non-invasive ventilation—pH 7.3 or less, hypoxia, hypercapnia, conscious and not improving after 4 hours of medical management
- Consider doxapram if NIV not available, or not tolerated
- Consider intensive care—ideally consultant-led decision with the patient, their family, and ITU regarding invasive mechanical ventilation. Document in the medical notes. Consider resuscitation status
- DVT prophylaxis.

An approach to COPD in the out-patient clinic

- Establish diagnosis and severity—pulmonary function tests, CXR
- Ensure there are no other causes for symptoms, e.g. anaemia, pulmonary emboli, heart failure, UIP, thyroid dysfunction, pneumothorax, large bulla, depression
- Stop smoking
- Review current treatment—optimize bronchodilatation and inhaled steroids
- Assess whether there is any need for a nebulizer
- Check oxygen saturation and perform blood gas if <92%. Consider LTOT
- Consider pulmonary rehabilitation
- Check vaccinations up to date
- Involve respiratory nurse specialist for input in the community if appropriate
- Follow up in clinic if ongoing medical issues, including if patient may be a lung transplant candidate (see page 382). Otherwise discharge back to GP
- Inform GP of all the above decisions.

Surgical treatment

Lung transplant In young patients (below 60–65), with severe disease, often due to α_1-antitrypsin deficiency, single lung transplant may be an option. Local transplant teams will advise regarding local criteria.

Bullectomy Suitable for selected patients with isolated bullae. Improves chest hyperinflation.

Lung volume reduction surgery (LVRS) Resection of areas of bullous emphysema to reduce chest hyperinflation, improve diaphragmatic function, elastic recoil, physiology of the lungs, and hence functional status of the patient. Patients who may be considered are those with FEV_1 20–30% predicted, with symptomatic dyspnoea despite maximal medical therapy, and with heterogeneous areas of emphysema on CT, giving target areas to resect. Pre-operative assessment: PFTs, 6 minute walk test, quality of life, and dyspnoea indicators. Surgery is performed in specialist centres via median sternotomy or by thoracoscopy. Usually the upper lobe is stapled below the level of the emphysema and then removed. Improvements are seen in FEV_1 and RV, dyspnoea, and quality of life scores. These effects are maximal between 2 and 6 months post-surgery. Symptomatic improvement is sustained for about 2–4 years. Post-operative complications: persistent air leak >7 days in 30–40%, pneumonia in up to 22%, respiratory failure in up to 13%. Post-operative mortality 2.4–17% reported.

The National Emphysema Treatment Trial (Michigan, USA) has shown that there is increased mortality from LVRS for patients with FEV_1 or TLCO <20% predicted, or with homogeneous emphysema. They are also less likely to benefit from surgery. Surgery is not therefore recommended for this group. Trials are ongoing to fully assess which patients with COPD are most likely to benefit and to determine whether open thoracotomy or video-assisted minimally invasive surgery (VATS) is the most effective approach.

Bronchoscopic lung volume reduction is under evaluation, with valve implants placed within the segmental bronchi that supply the hyper-inflated lobes. It is a minimally invasive variation on lung volume reduction surgery, with the aim of improving lung function and quality of life.

Further information

National clinical guideline on management of COPD in adults in primary and secondary care. *Thorax* 2004; **59** (suppl. 1): 232

ERS Consensus Statement—Optimal assessment and management of COPD. *ERJ* 1995; **8**: 1398–1420

Management of COPD. MacNee W and Calverley PMA. *Thorax* 2003; **58**: 261–5

Bronchoscopic volume reduction with valve implants in patients with severe emphysema. Toma TP *et al. Lancet* 2003; **361**: 931–3

LVRS for severe emphysema: appraisal of its current status. Trow TK *Curr Opin Pulm Med* 2004; **10**(2): 128–32

Surgical therapies for COPD. Benditt JO. *Respir Care* 2004; **49**(1): 53–63

Prospective randomised trial comparing bilateral LVRS to pulmonary rehabilitation in severe COPD. Criner GJ *et al. Am J Resp Crit Care Med* 1999; **160**: 2018–27

Effect of LVRS in patients with severe emphysema. Geddes D *et al. NEJM* 2000; **343**: 239–45

www.copd-international.com patient information website

www.copd-support.com for families of patients with COPD

Cor pulmonale

Definition Cor pulmonale is the traditional term for changes in the cardiovascular system resulting from the chronic hypoxia (and usually hypercapnia) of chronic lung disease, mainly pulmonary hypertension and fluid retention. It does not include the similar changes seen in some left-sided disorders such as mitral incompetence.

Causes and pathophysiology Cor pulmonale can occur in most situations where there is chronic hypoxia.

• Most often in the setting of hypoxic and hypercapnic COPD
• Hypoventilation syndromes (scoliosis, neuromuscular diseases)
• Much less common when there is no associated rise in $PaCO_2$.

Cor pulmonale is often also referred to as right heart failure which is misleading as the cardiac output in cor pulmonale is usually *normal or high* and there is often *increased* peripheral perfusion. This is in contrast to true right heart failure when the right ventricle (RV) fails to develop an adequate cardiac output, e.g. following a right-sided myocardial infarction, or pulmonary emboli that occlude a large proportion of the pulmonary vascular bed. This produces a raised JVP, *low* cardiac output and *poor* peripheral perfusion.

Cor pulmonale results from the following sequence of events

• Lung disease causes hypoxia with cyanosis and often polycythaemia
• Hypoxia is sensed both within the kidney, and via the carotid body, generating increases in sympathetic activity and renal vasoconstriction
• Increased sympathetic activity (and other mechanisms) lead to renal retention of salt and water
• This extra salt and water is mainly held in the capacitance vessels (the large veins) with often a raised JVP
• If vascular permeability rises (particularly when the $PaCO_2$ rises, producing peripheral vasodilatation and an increase in capillary pressure), extra fluid accumulates in dependant tissues, mainly the ankles
• A raised JVP and ankle oedema in this setting are NOT due to impaired right ventricular function, but fluid overload and increased vascular permeability.

Patients often present with their first episode of ankle swelling during an exacerbation of their COPD, when for the first time the $PaCO_2$ rises and the PaO_2 falls far enough to provoke the above events. Body weight may not rise suddenly with the onset of ankle oedema; however the extra salt and water retained leading up to the exacerbation moves into the subcutaneous tissues, probably from the CO_2-induced vasodilatation.

The hypoxia also raises the pulmonary artery pressure (PAP), but to relatively minor levels that the RV can manage, particularly if it builds up slowly. Loss of pulmonary vascular bed from emphysema will also raise PAP. The ECG is likely to show right ventricular hypertrophy. However, the RV can cope with much higher pressures than usually occur in cor pulmonale, such as in primary pulmonary hypertension (PPH). During an exacerbation, the extra hypoxia will produce further rises in PAP with which the RV usually copes, helped by the raised JVP providing a larger pre-load to increase RV filling. Thus excessive diuresis in these patients can lead to true fall in right-sided output due to inadequate filling of the RV.

Clinical features
- The underlying disease causing the hypoxia, e.g. COPD/bronchiectasis
- Easily visible veins and a raised JVP
- Cyanosis and a suffused conjunctiva (polycythaemia and vessel dilatation from the raised CO_2)
- Peripheral vasodilatation with full pulse
- Ankle swelling and pitting oedema
- Right ventricular hypertrophy (sternal heave uncommon, masked by hyperinflated lung between heart and chest wall; more often seen with the higher pressures of PPH)
- Tricuspid incompetence (not usually severe).

Investigations
- CXR—enlarged pulmonary arteries/underlying lung disease
- FBC—may have associated polycythaemia
- Oximetry—cor pulmonale unlikely if awake SaO_2 over 92 or 93%
- Blood gases—cor pulmonale progressively more likely as PaO_2 drops below 8 kPa, and $PaCO_2$ rises above 6 kPa
- ECG—may indicate right axis deviation, p pulmonale (right atrial hypertrophy), and right bundle branch block
- Echo—dilated or hypertrophied RV, tricuspid regurgitation, raised PAP, and to exclude other diagnoses such as a patent ASD
- Overnight oximetry—to reveal unexpected degrees of hypoxia, e.g. from OSA.

Management Minimal ankle oedema needs no treatment. 'Trimming' the ankles to normal is unnecessary and may reduce RV output by reducing filling. If the oedema is more substantial then the following may help.
- Treat underlying condition to raise PaO_2 and lower $PaCO_2$
- Raise PaO_2 through added oxygen, provide long-term oxygen at home
- In hypoventilation syndromes, home overnight NIV likely to be the correct management
- Promote a *limited* diuresis with judicious use of diuretics.

In general cor pulmonale is overtreated. It is more a relatively harmless byproduct of hypoxia, than a problem in its own right. Treating the blood gas disturbance, and making it easier for the patient to get his shoes on, are the main therapeutic aims. The long-term oxygen trials showed that *improving the PaO_2* was useful, not lowering the pulmonary artery pressure.

Further information
Hormonal, renal, and autonomic nerve factors involved in the excretion of sodium and water during dynamic salt and water loading in hypoxaemic chronic obstructive pulmonary disease. Stewart AG et al. Thorax 1995; **50**: 838–45

Lung cancer

Epidemiology and types

Epidemiology
- Commonest cause of cancer death in men and women in the UK
- Nearly 38 000 new cases diagnosed per annum in UK
- 2:1 Male:female, but numbers decreasing in men, increasing in women, because of increasing smoking
- 90% smoking-related
- Stopping smoking decreases the risk, but the risk remains higher than in non-smokers
- Risk of lung cancer may be increased by asbestos exposure, arsenic and heavy metal exposure, and coexistent usual interstitial pneumonitis (UIP).

Types of lung cancer In practical terms, lung cancer is divided into two groups, which influence management and treatment decisions:

Non-small cell lung cancer (NSCLC)
- Accounts for 75–80% of all lung cancers
- *Squamous cell carcinoma* is the commonest histological type. Usually presents as a mass on CXR, but may cavitate and look radiologically like a lung abscess. Rarely there may be multiple cavitating lesions. Patients with hypercalcaemia are most likely to have squamous cell carcinoma
- *Adenocarcinoma* may not necessarily be smoking-related. Can occur in scar tissue or sites of fibrosis. Can be a lung primary, or a secondary from adenocarcinomas at other sites, especially if causing pleural infiltration and subsequent pleural effusion
- *Alveolar cell carcinoma* is rare. It can rarely cause copious sputum production (bronchorrhoea). Fluffy air space shadowing on CXR.

Small cell lung cancer (SCLC)
- Accounts for 20–25% of all lung cancers
- Usually disseminated by the time of diagnosis (haematogenous spread)
- Frequently *metastasizes* to liver, bones, bone marrow, brain, adrenals, or elsewhere
- Syndrome of inappropriate secretion of antidiuretic hormone (SIADH) is common in small cell lung cancer
- Surgery usually not appropriate
- Chemo- and radiosensitive
- Untreated extensive small cell lung cancer is rapidly progressive and has a median survival of 6 weeks.

WHO classification of lung tumours, 1999

Squamous cell carcinoma
Small cell carcinoma
Adenocarcinoma
Large cell carcinoma
Adenosquamous carcinoma
Pleomorphic/sarcomatoid
Carcinoid tumour

Clinical features

Smokers with chest symptoms, especially those aged over 50, need investigation.

Symptoms and signs

These may be due to local tumour effects, metastatic tumour effects, or paraneoplastic manifestations. Many patients have no specific signs. In some, they may be found to have lung cancer as an incidental finding on CXR performed for another reason.

Local tumour effects

- Persistent cough, or change in usual cough
- Haemoptysis
- Chest pain (suggests chest wall or pleural involvement)
- Unresolving pneumonia or lobar collapse
- Unexplained dyspnoea (due to bronchial narrowing or obstruction)
- Wheeze or stridor
- Shoulder pain (due to diaphragm involvement)
- Pleural effusion (due to direct tumour extension or pleural metastases)
- Hoarse voice (tumour invasion left recurrent laryngeal nerve)
- Dysphagia
- Raised hemi-diaphragm (phrenic nerve paralysis)
- SVCO (see page 154)
- Horner's syndrome (meiosis, ptosis, enopthalmos, anhidrosis) due to apical or Pancoast's tumour
- Pancoast's tumours can directly invade sympathetic chain and brachial plexus and rib. Cause weakness of small muscles of the hand—C5/6, T1 motor loss and shoulder pain.

Metastatic tumour effects

- Cervical/supraclavicular lymphadenopathy (common, present in 30%, and may be an easy site for diagnostic biopsy)
- Palpable liver edge
- Bone pain/pathological fracture due to bone metastases
- Neurological sequelae secondary to cerebral metastases (median survival of NSCLC with brain metastases is 2 months)
- Hypercalcaemic effects (due to bony metastases or direct tumour production of parathyroid hormone related peptide)
- Dysphagia (compression from large mediastinal nodes).

Paraneoplastic syndromes

- Cachexia and wasting
- Clubbing (any cell type, more common in squamous and adenocarcinoma)
- Syndrome of inappropriate ADH (SIADH; mainly SCLC)
- Ectopic ACTH (Cushing's syndrome, but due to rapid development; biochemical changes predominate, mainly SCLC)
- Hypertrophic pulmonary osteo-arthropathy (HPOA, often in association with clubbing, any cell type; more common in squamous and adenocarcinoma)

- Eaton–Lambert myasthenic syndrome—with SCLC. Affects proximal limbs and trunk, with autonomic involvement and hyporeflexia and only a slight response to edrophonium. Repeated muscle contraction may lead to increasing strength and reflexes. Symptoms may predate lung cancer by up to 4 years
- Cerebellar syndrome (usually SCLC)
- Limbic encephalitis (usually SCLC).

Lymphangitis carcinomatosa

Infiltration of pulmonary lymphatics by tumour. May be due to lung cancer or breast, prostate, stomach, or pancreatic malignancies. Causes shortness of breath, cough, and is often associated with systemic signs of advanced malignancy. May be visible on CXR as fine linear shadowing throughout both lung fields. Septal lines present. May look like pulmonary oedema. Easily diagnosed on CT. Oral steroid treatment and diuretics can give symptomatic relief, but it is usually a short-lived response. Often part of a rapid decline.

Investigations

Patients should be referred under the '2-week cancer wait' scheme and should be seen within 14 days of referral. The aim of the investigations is to reach a histological diagnosis and tumour stage, in order to determine the most appropriate treatment.

In out-patients

- **History and examination**, including smoking and occupational histories
- **Spirometry** pre-biopsy or surgery
- **CXR** (PA and lateral)—location of lesion, pleural involvement, pleural effusion, rib destruction, intrathoracic metastases, mediastinal lymphadenopathy. CXR can be normal
- **Blood tests**, including sodium, calcium, and liver function tests. Check clotting if biopsy planned
- **Sputum cytology** only indicated in patients who are unfit for bronchoscopy or biopsy
- **Diagnostic pleural tap**, if effusion present
- **Fine needle aspiration** of enlarged supraclavicular or cervical lymph nodes.

Radiology

- **CT chest, liver, adrenals (contrast-enhanced) to assess tumour site and size** Lung cancers frequently metastasize to the mediastinal lymph nodes, liver, and adrenals. CT can locate lesions amenable to biopsy (either the primary tumour or a metastasis). Assesses size of local and regional lymph nodes. Poor at assessing whether enlarged nodes are reactive (inflammatory), or represent metastatic spread (79% sensitive, 78% specific). Can assess tumour invasion to mediastinum and chest wall
- **Ultrasound scan** of neck or liver may provide information about enlarged lymph nodes or metastases suitable for biopsy
- **MRI** Used to answer specific questions relating to tumour invasion/borders. Good for assessing brachial plexus involvement. No role in nodule assessment
- **Bone scan** Indicated if any suggestion of metastatic disease, such as bony pain, pathological fracture, hypercalcaemia, raised alkaline phosphatase. Highly suggestive of bony metastases if multiple areas of increased uptake. Solitary lesion may require further evaluation
- **CT head** Only indicated if any neurological evidence of metastatic disease, such as persistent vomiting, fit, focal neurological signs, headache, unexplained confusion, or personality change
- **Positron emission tomography (PET scanning)** Imaging technique, where metabolically active tissues such as tumours, take up more of a radiolabelled 18-fluorodeoxyglucose (FDG) molecule. They then show as a 'hot-spot'. Improves the rate of detection of local and distant metastases in patients with NSCLC. Useful for assessing regional and mediastinal lymph nodes (88% sensitive, 93% specific). Becoming more widely used and should be interpreted with the CT. PET positive nodes that would exclude a patient from surgery should be confirmed as malignant with a biopsy, unless the pre-test probability of malignancy is high. False negatives occur in tumours with a low

metabolic activity, small nodules, and hyperglycaemic patients. False positives in patients with benign pulmonary nodules with a high metabolic rate, such as infective granulomata.

Multidisciplinary team (MDT)

Should include a chest physician, radiologist, thoracic surgeon, oncologist, pathologist, lung cancer nurse, and palliative care specialist, who meet regularly in order to discuss patients and plan the most appropriate course of management.

The Department of Health in the UK has produced guidelines for performance in lung cancer care. These encourage access to the MDT in decision making for the treatment and investigation of all patients with lung cancer.

Diagnostic procedures

Aspects of further investigation may be inappropriate if the patient has advanced disease, is frail with co-morbid conditions, or does not want to pursue diagnosis. This should be documented in their notes, to aid audit and cancer service evaluation.

Bronchoscopy Method of obtaining histological and cytological specimens. Suitable for central tumours. Tumours can be washed, brushed, and biopsied. Transbronchial needle aspiration of lymph nodes can be performed to aid staging. Bronchoscopic samples are more likely to be histologically positive if there is:
• An ill-defined lesion on the CXR
• An endobronchial component to the tumour
• Tumour less than 4 cm from the origin of the nearest lobar bronchus
• A segmental or larger airway leading to the mass.

Greater diagnostic yield if performed after CT scan, as radiologically abnormal areas can be targeted. Tumour position bronchoscopically may contribute to operative decisions: tumour confined to a lobar bronchus may be resectable with lobectomy, tumour <1 cm from the main carina requires pneumonectomy, left vocal cord paralysis indicates inoperability due to tumour infiltration of the left recurrent laryngeal nerve, and a splayed carina occurs secondary to enlarged mediastinal nodes.

CT/USS-guided biopsy of tumour or of an enlarged lymph node, especially in the neck, or of a metastasis (see box opposite). 85–90% sensitivity in lesions >2 cm.

Mediastinoscopy Biopsy of enlarged mediastinal lymph nodes to determine whether they are inflammatory or have malignant invasion. Suprasternal notch incision under general anaesthetic, blunt dissection, palpation, and endoscopic visualization and biopsy of nodes: paratracheal, prevascular, tracheobronchial, and anterior subcarinal. 93% sensitivity, 96% specificity. Technically more difficult if SVCO. Bleeding in <0.3%, left recurrent laryngeal nerve injury in 1%, pneumothorax, mediastinal emphysema, infection, oesophageal perforation (all rare). Repeat mediastinoscopies have lower positive yield and higher complication rate.

Mediastinotomy Biopsy of aorto-pulmonary, sub-aortic, phrenic, or hilar nodes. Metastatic involvement of these nodes does not necessarily preclude curative surgical resection with a pneumonectomy. Also can assess direct tumour invasion of central pulmonary artery or thoracic aorta, which would preclude curative surgery. Right or left parasternal incision, blunt dissection, palpation, and endoscopic visualization and biopsy of nodes.

Thoracoscopy May be required to determine whether a pleural effusion contains malignant cells or is inflammatory, for example due to pneumonia caused by an obstructing lesion. Malignant effusions are evidence of T4 disease and are hence a contraindication to surgery.

Operative It is sometimes difficult to obtain definitive cytology or histology pre-operatively. If there is a high suspicion of malignancy, surgery can be performed regardless. Patients undergoing surgery are given a pathological stage, which is sometimes different to the clinical stage. This is because resection margins, lymph nodes, and the pleura can be sampled histologically.

Radiologically guided lung biopsy

Indications
- New or enlarging mass, not amenable to bronchoscopy
- Multiple chest nodules in patient not known to have malignancy
- Persistent undiagnosed single or multiple focal infiltrates
- Hilar mass.

Pre-biopsy preparation
- Discuss with MDT
- Recent spirometry, with $FEV_1 > 35\%$ predicted
- Check APTT and PT < 1.4 and platelets >100, 000/ml. If not, discuss with haematologist to determine whether it is safe to proceed.
- Recent imaging available
- High risk patients should have overnight admission following the biopsy
- Written information for patient, with informed signed consent.

Biopsy preparation
- Perform without sedation if possible
- Use USS if possible
- Local anaesthetic to skin and subcutaneous tissue
- Perform at least two passes, may use FNA or cutting needle. FNA high diagnostic yield for malignant lesions (95%), but less for benign (10–50%). Cutting needles as good for malignancy and better for benign diagnoses. Operator decision.

Post-biopsy
- Observation by staff for 1 hour in case of complications
- Erect CXR 1 hour after biopsy and reviewed by doctor
- Manage any pneumothorax according to BTS guidelines (page 290) Small pneumothoraces often resolve spontaneously, but may need in-patient admission if there are concerns.

Complications
- 20% chance of pneumothorax, 3% require chest drain
- Haemoptysis 5%, death 0.15%.

Guidelines for radiologically guided lung biopsy. Manhire A *et al. Thorax* 2003: **58** (11): 920–34

Staging

Clinical and radiological tools categorize tumour size, location, regional and distant spread. They can also therefore give prognostic information.

- **Small cell lung cancer** is staged as:
  - *Limited* confined to ipsilateral hemi-thorax and supraclavicular lymph nodes
  - *Extensive* everything else
- **Non-small cell lung cancer** is commonly classified using TNM staging system (see box below). Frequency of patient stage at diagnosis:
  - I and II–20%
  - III–35%
  - IV–45%

TNM Staging of Lung Cancer (American Joint Committee on Cancer and the Union Internationale Contre le Cancer)

Extent of primary tumour (T)

Tx	Primary tumour cannot be assessed, or tumour proven by presence of malignant cells in sputum or bronchial washings but not visualized by imaging or bronchoscopy
T0	No evidence of primary tumour
Tis	Carcinoma *in situ*
T1	Tumour <3 cm surrounded by lung or visceral pleura, without bronchoscopic evidence of invasion more proximal than the lobar bronchus
T2	Tumour >3 cm, or in main bronchus, >2 cm distal to carina or invading visceral pleura or associated with atelectasis or obstructive pneumonitis that extends to the hilar region, but does not involve whole lung
T3	Tumour of any size which invades chest wall, diaphragm, parietal pericardium, mediastinal pleura, or tumour in main bronchus < 2 cm distal to carina, or associated atelectasis or obstructive pneumonitis of the entire lung
T4	Tumour of any size invading: mediastinum, heart, great vessels, trachea, oesophagus, carina, vertebral body, or separate nodules in the ipsilateral lobe as primary tumour, or malignant pleural or pericardial effusion

Regional lymph nodes (N)

Nx	Cannot be assessed
N0	No regional lymph node metastasis
N1	Ipsilateral peribronchial and/or ipsilateral hilar nodes and intrapulmonary nodes involved by direct extension of tumour
N2	Ipsilateral mediastinal and/or subcarinal nodes
N3	Contralateral mediastinal, hilar nodes, or any scalene or supraclavicular nodes

Distant metastasis (M)
Mx Cannot be assessed
M0 No distant metastasis
M1 Distant metastasis present, including separate nodules in different
lobes

Lung cancer clinical staging and survival

Stage	TNM subset	After treatment survival (%)	
		1 year	5 years
0	Tis	?	?
IA	T1 N0 M0	91	61
IB	T2 N0 M0	72	38
IIA	T1 N1 M0	79	34
IIB	T2 N1 M0	61	24
	T3 N0 M0	55	22
IIIA	T1 N2 M0	50	13
	T2 N2 M0	50	13
	T3 N1–2 M0	56	9
IIIB	T4 N0–2 M0	37	7
	T1–4 N3 M0	32	3
IV	Any T, Any N, M1	20	1

Further information

Revisions in the International System for staging lung cancer. Mountain CF. *Chest* 1997; **111**: 1710–17

Regional Lymph Node Classification for Lung Cancer Staging. Mountain CF and Dresler CM. *Chest* 1997; **111**: 1718–23

Non-small cell lung cancer (NSCLC): surgery

Much of the investigation of lung cancer is to determine whether a patient has potentially curable disease by surgery. Other treatment options consist of chemotherapy, radiotherapy, and best supportive care, i.e. symptom-based conservative management. The MDT decides the most appropriate choice of treatment to then be discussed with the patient.

Surgery

The aims of surgery for lung cancer are to completely excise the tumour and local lymphatics, with minimal removal of functioning lung parenchyma.

- Stages I and II non-small cell lung cancers are usually amenable to surgery if the patient is fit enough (see below). This has a high chance of cure in stage I (70% in IA), and a reasonable chance in stage II. 10–20% of NSCLC patients undergo resection
- In stage IIIA tumours, surgery alone is unlikely to be curative, but adjuvant chemotherapy and radiotherapy can improve survival rates. These patients should be in clinical trials
- Stages IIIB and IV are inoperable
- Stages 0/tumour *in situ* often will have no defined primary lesion amenable to resection. The natural progression of these tumours is still unknown, as they may progress or regress with time.

Resectability of a tumour implies likelihood of complete removal by surgery and this is different from patient operability, which is determined by the patient's fitness for surgery.

Fitness for surgery

- *Age:* not a contraindication, but increasing age associated with an increased peri-operative morbidity. Higher mortality risk if over 80 and if pneumonectomy rather than lobectomy (14% mortality versus 7% respectively). Right pneumonectomy has higher mortality than left pneumonectomy (more lung removed). 2-year post-operative survival similar to that of other age groups
- *Lung function:* $FEV_1 > 1.5$ l post-bronchodilators for lobectomy, >2 l post-bronchodilators for pneumonectomy or more than 60% of predicted. Borderline cases may require further lung function assessment (arterial saturations, full PFTs including TLCO, isotope perfusion scan, exercise testing), in order to calculate whether predicted post-operative $FEV_1 > 40\%$ in association with TLCO > 40%
- *Cardiovascular:* postpone surgery if patient has had MI within 6 weeks. Cardiology opinion if patient has had MI within 6 months. Echo if they have heart murmur. Pre-operative ECG for all
- *CNS:* If any history of TIAs, strokes, or carotid bruits: need carotid Doppler studies and vascular surgeon opinion if necessary
- *Nutritional:* requirements should be optimized, with advice from a dietician if necessary.

Types of surgery Lobectomy or bi-lobectomy for localized tumour, or pneumonectomy for tumour involving more than one or two lobes. If hilar nodes are infiltrated by tumour a more radical lobectomy or a pneumonectomy is required. The local lymph nodes are removed in each procedure for pathological staging. *Wedge excision* removes only the tumour with minimal surrounding lung parenchyma, and may be performed for a localized peripheral lesion with clear regional lymph nodes, especially if the post-operative respiratory function is predicted to be borderline: there is a higher local recurrence rate however (up to 23%). *Sleeve resections* involve a lobectomy and the removal of a section of bronchus affected by tumour, forming an anastomosis between the airway proximal and distal to it. This may avoid a pneumonectomy. Resection margins should be macroscopically free from tumour. If there is limited local tumour invasion to the chest wall, this can be resected with a 5 cm margin. Reconstruction with prosthetic material may be necessary if 2 or more ribs are resected, aiming to preserve the chest wall function.

Post-operative complications Broncho-pleural fistula, respiratory failure, infection, phrenic nerve damage causing diaphragmatic paralysis, recurrent laryngeal nerve damage causing hoarse voice, prolonged chest wall pain. Mortality: 1–3.5% for wedge excision, 2–4% for lobectomy, 6–8% for pneumonectomy. Risk increases with increasing age, associated ischaemic heart disease, impaired respiratory function, and poor performance status.

Following surgery
Patients are often followed-up by the chest clinic on a 6 monthly basis for CXR review. This is to ensure they are radiologically clear of tumour recurrence, and there is not a second primary tumour. They should also be advised to seek earlier review if they have symptoms of persistent haemoptysis or new cough, weight loss, new chest pain.

Further information
Guidelines on the selection of patients with lung cancer for surgery. BTS/SCTS. *Thorax* 2001; **56**: 89–108

NSCLC: chemotherapy

- Consider in patients with stage III to IV disease, WHO performance status 0 to 2, even if they are asymptomatic from their cancer (greater toxicity in those with poorer performance status)
- 40% respond temporarily
- Small improvement in symptom control and quality of life compared to best supportive care
- Limited survival gains, 6–7 weeks compared to best supportive care
- Combination chemotherapy (the use of more than one drug) is superior to single agent chemotherapy, improving survival rates when compared to single agent at 6 and 12 months (51 vs. 49% and 25 vs. 22%, respectively)
- Commonly used first-line regimens include gemcitabine or vinorelbine plus a platinum drug (carboplatin or cisplatin), usually given for 4 cycles. Side-effects: nausea, myelosupression, ototoxicity, peripheral neuropathy, nephropathy if dehydrated. No alopecia
- Patients are monitored during chemotherapy with repeat CT, usually after 2 cycles, to establish whether they have partial response, stable disease, or progressive disease, despite chemotherapy. This CT influences decisions regarding further chemotherapy
- Second-line treatments can be given in patients who relapse and are of good performance status. Taxanes (paclitaxel, docetaxel) are the most commonly used agents. These cause alopecia
- Adjuvant chemotherapy following surgery has been found to have significant survival advantages compared to surgery alone in recent International Adjuvant Lung Cancer Trial (IALT). No consensus yet on how this should come in to clinical practice
- Pre-operative chemotherapy currently under clinical trial
- Neo-adjuvant chemotherapy used with surgery in stage IIIa disease, in some centres, usually as part of a clinical trial.

ECOG performance status

0 = Fully active, able to carry on all pre-disease performance without restriction

1 = Restricted in physically strenuous activity but ambulatory and able to carry out work of a light or sedentary nature, e.g. light house work, office work

2 = Ambulatory and capable of all self-care but unable to carry out any work activities. Up and about more than 50% of waking hours

3 = Capable of only limited self-care, confined to bed or chair more than 50% of waking hours

4 = Completely disabled. Cannot carry on any self-care. Totally confined to bed or chair.

Toxicity and response criteria of the Eastern Cooperative Oncology Group. Oken MM et al. Am J Clin Oncol 1982; **5**: 649–55

Response evaluation criteria in solid tumours (RECIST)—method of measuring response of a tumour to treatment (particularly in chemotherapy trials)

Target lesion = all measurable lesions up to a maximum of 5 lesions per organ and 10 lesions in total, representative of all involved organs. Record and measure sum of their longest diameter.

Non-target lesions = all other sites of disease, which are recorded at baseline. Measurements of these lesions are not required, but presence or absence of each is noted during follow-up.

Evaluation of target lesions

- **Complete response (CR)**—disappearance of all target lesions
- **Partial response (PR)**—at least a 30% decrease in the sum of the longest diameter of target lesions
- **Progressive disease (PD)**—at least a 20% increase in the sum of the longest diameter of target lesions
- **Stable disease (SD)**—neither sufficient shrinkage to qualify for PR, nor sufficient increase to qualify for PD.

Evaluation of non-target lesions

- **Complete response (CR)**—disappearance of all non-target lesions and normalization of tumour marker level
- **Incomplete response/stable disease (SD)**—persistence of one or more non-target lesion(s) or/and maintenance of tumour marker level above the normal limits
- **Progressive disease (PD)**—appearance of one or more new lesions and/or unequivocal progression of existing non-target lesions.

Further information

Chemotherapy and NSCLC. *Drug and Therapeutics Bulletin* 2002, volume **40**; no 2

Chemotherapy in NSCLC: a meta-analysis using updated data on individual patients from 52 randomised clinical trials. NSCLC Collaborative Group. *BMJ* 1995; **311**: 899–909

NSCLC: radiotherapy

May be given for:
- Curative intent (high dose)
- Palliative control (high dose)
- Symptom relief (low dose).

CHART (continuous hyperfractionated accelerated radiotherapy) is high-dose radiotherapy given with curative intent.
- Recommended for patients with localized chest disease > 5 cm, stage I to II with performance status 0 to 1, who are resectable, but unfit for surgery or do not want surgery
- Small radiation doses three times a day for 12 days (54 Gy in 36 fractions over 12 days)
- Patients are often in-patients for the duration of their therapy to facilitate their frequent radiotherapy sessions
- Less morbidity than conventional radical radiotherapy
- A large randomized control trial has shown an improvement in 2-year survival from 20% with conventional radical radiotherapy to 29% with CHART. The largest benefits were in patients with squamous cell carcinoma
- Severe dysphagia more likely with CHART in the first 3 months than with conventional radiotherapy
- Not performed in all UK centres.

High-dose palliative radiotherapy is given to patients with symptomatic disease, good performance status, no evidence of metastases, and who will be able to tolerate a high-dose regime. An example of such a regime would be 36–39 Gy in 12–13 fractions over 6 weeks.

Low-dose radiotherapy is given for symptom relief in patients who would be unable to tolerate high-dose palliative radiotherapy or those with evidence of metastases. Symptoms may include pain, haemoptysis, breathlessness, or cough.

Urgent radiotherapy is used in combination with oral steroids for relief of superior vena cava obstruction by tumour, though stenting performed via CT angiography is the treatment of choice. Radiotherapy has no benefit following complete primary tumour surgical resection.

Chemoradiotherapy is used to improve tumour radiosensitization for localized disease. There may be some additional advantages with treatment of potential distant micrometastases. Some early survival benefits have been shown, and further studies are underway.

Further information
CHART vs. conventional radiotherapy. Saunders M *et al. Lancet* 1997; **350**: 161–5

Small cell lung cancer: treatment

Surgery Limited small cell lung cancer may benefit from surgical resection if there is no evidence of metastases. This is rare. It requires further assessment with brain and bone scanning. The patient should also be considered for post-operative chemotherapy for treatment of micro-metastases, especially if histology was only determined at operation.

Chemotherapy

Combination chemotherapy is used for limited and extensive SCLC.

- Etoposide with either cisplatin or carboplatin is the standard regime
- Given 3 weekly, commonly for 6 cycles
- Different regimes are selected according to performance status
- Patients with performance status 3 may benefit from less intensive out-patient chemotherapy on a 3 weekly basis
- Patients are carefully assessed and, if there is no sign of a response to treatment based on CXR or CT scan, they are switched to second-line agents
- 80–90% response if limited disease; 60–80% if extensive disease
- Chemotherapy may increase survival to 14 months in limited disease.

Radiotherapy

- Patients with limited stage disease who are reasonably well and obtain a partial response or better from chemotherapy should go on to have consolidation radiotherapy to the chest disease
- Prophylactic cranial radiotherapy is advised at completion of chemotherapy. This improves survival by 5.4%
- In patients with extensive disease, including cerebral metastases, or poorer performance status, chemotherapy is given first. If there is a good response, palliative radiotherapy may be given on an individual patient basis.

Lung cancer: emerging areas

Autofluorescent bronchoscopy (see page 672)

Biological therapies such as oral thalidomide acting as an angiogenesis inhibitor are being tried. These may offer medium-term survival benefits in both SCLC and NSCLC.

Molecular biology Aiming to find specific molecular targets at which to aim new therapies in NSCLC, e.g. epidermal growth factor receptor (EGFR) inhibitors such as gefitinib (a quinozaline) and cetuzimab (monoclonal antibody).

Further information

BTS Recommendations to respiratory physicians for organising the care of patients with lung cancer. *Thorax* 1998: **53** (suppl. 1): S1–8

www.bacup.org.uk

www.cancerguide.org

www.cancerresearchuk.org

www.lungcanceronline.org

www.nice.org.uk/CG024NICEguideline

www.roycastle.org, patient network, telephone 0800 358 7200

Superior vena caval obstruction (SVCO): aetiology and clinical assessment

Obstruction of the flow of blood in the superior vena cava results in the symptoms and signs of SVCO. It is caused by two different mechanisms (which may coexist): *external compression* or *invasion* of the superior vena cava by tumour extending from the right lung (four times more common than the left lung), lymph nodes, or other mediastinal structure; or due to *thrombosis* within the vein.

Aetiology The commonest cause is malignancy. Lung cancer and lymphoma together cause 94% of SVCO.

Malignant causes

Lung cancer Up to 4% of lung cancer patients will develop SVCO at some point during their disease. Up to 10% of small cell lung cancers present with SVCO.

Lymphoma Up to 4% of lymphoma patients will develop SVCO, most commonly in non-Hodgkin's lymphoma. This usually occurs due to extrinsic compression of the SVC by enlarged lymph nodes.

Other malignant causes Thymoma, mediastinal germ cell tumours, tumours with mediastinal metastases (commonest is breast cancer).

Benign causes include granulomatous disease, intrathoracic goitre, and central venous lines, port-a-caths, and pacemaker wires (causing thrombosis). In the past SVCO was commonly due to untreated infection, e.g. syphilitic thoracic aortic aneurysm or fibrosing mediastinitis (due to actinomycosis, tuberculosis, blastomycosis, or aspergillus). These are all now rare.

Clinical features
- Facial and upper body oedema with facial plethora, often with increased neck circumference, and a cyanotic appearance
- Venous distension of the face and upper body. SVCO due to malignancy usually develops over days to weeks, so an adequate collateral circulation does not have time to develop. Pemberton's sign, facial plethora, distress, and sometimes stridor after lifting the arms above the head for a few minutes may clarify the diagnosis
- Breathlessness
- Headache—worse on bending forwards or lying down
- Cough/haemoptysis or other signs of an underlying lung malignancy
- Hoarse voice
- Dysphagia
- Syncope/dizziness (reduced venous return)
- Confusion.

Diagnosis is usually made clinically from the signs of facial and upper body swelling, with distension of superficial veins across the chest wall, neck, and upper arms.

Investigations The investigation and treatment of SVCO was previously considered a medical emergency. SVCO is now not considered to be immediately life-threatening, making treatment less urgent, and allowing a definitive diagnosis to be made prior to treatment. The exception to this rule is the patient who presents with stridor or laryngeal oedema, which is a medical emergency.

- **CXR** Up to 85% have an abnormal CXR (as lung malignancy is the commonest underlying disorder). Mediastinal widening is common
- **CT chest with contrast** can stage the underlying malignancy and image the venous circulation and collateral blood supply
- **Tissue diagnosis** Usual practice is to obtain a tissue diagnosis of the underlying disease before starting treatment, as the underlying diagnosis can alter treatment markedly. Symptomatic obstruction will have been developing for some weeks prior to presentation and, in the clinically stable patient, a delay of 24 to 48 hours whilst the correct underlying diagnosis is obtained is warranted. Radiotherapy prior to biopsy can lead to problems making a subsequent histological diagnosis, and, similarly, high-dose steroids can make the diagnosis of lymphoma difficult
- **Cytological diagnosis** may be obtained from:
  - Pleural fluid
  - Biopsy of an extrathoracic lymph node (e.g. supraclavicular nodes)
  - Bronchoscopy, or mediastinoscopy if no endobronchial disease, may be needed, depending on CT features. There may be increased risk of bleeding post-biopsy because of venous congestion, and anaesthesia is theoretically more risky because of possible associated tracheal obstruction or pericardial effusion (potentially leading to haemodynamic compromise due to cardiac tamponade), though these can be anticipated from the CT scan
  - Sputum.

SVCO: management

This is usually in two phases:
- Initial general treatment: oxygen, analgesia, sitting the patient up (to reduce venous pressure), and steroids (in some)
- Followed by treatment of the underlying disease causing the SVCO, which depends on the tissue diagnosis. The major differential in terms of treatment is small cell carcinoma (initial chemotherapy), non-small cell carcinoma (initial radiotherapy), and lymphoma (chemotherapy). The presence of SVCO usually means that surgical resection of a NSCLC is not possible.

Steroids There are limited trial data to support the use of steroids in SVCO, prior to definitive treatment, but most would start them fairly promptly. They may be useful in reducing oedema, and improving symptoms. Ideally a tissue diagnosis should be obtained before commencing steroids, but this may not always be possible. The problem arises where the underlying diagnosis is lymphoma, where steroids may alter the histology, making a definitive diagnosis more difficult. In an older smoker, with an obvious CXR mass (in whom the diagnosis is likely to be lung cancer), steroids can probably be started without risk to the underlying histology.

Radiotherapy 90% patients are oedema-free by 3–4 weeks. In those with a poor response to radiotherapy, only 25% survive 1 year.

Intraluminal stents are used for malignant SVCO, and will often be a first-line treatment whilst radiotherapy is planned. These are successful in 90% of cases, with relief of symptoms in most patients within 48 hours. They do not preclude subsequent radiotherapy or chemotherapy. It is not clear whether post-procedure anticoagulation is required. Some centres advocate the use of low-dose warfarin anticoagulation (i.e. 1 mg a day), aiming for an international normalized ratio (INR) of < 1.6. Thrombosis in the superior vena cava is not a contraindication to the procedure, as clot can be dispersed mechanically or with thrombolysis at the time or the procedure.

  Stent complications Stent migration is the major complication, but most patients do not live long enough for this to be a major problem.

Anticoagulation Some recommend prophylactic anticoagulation in the presence of SVCO. There is a small increased risk of intracerebral bleeding, but the benefits of SVCO treatment may be limited by subsequent SVC thrombus if anticoagulation is not started. This is controversial.

SVCO due to thrombosis is usually in association with central venous lines or pacemaker wires. If the clot is less than 5 days old (as judged by symptoms) thrombolysis is warranted. Subsequent oral anticoagulation may reduce recurrence.

Prognosis depends on the underlying disease, and is unrelated to the duration of SVCO at presentation. The majority of SVCO is due to mediastinal spread of carcinoma of the lung, so the overall prognosis is generally poor, but depends on the patient's performance status, stage and extent of disease, and the cell type.

Further information

Steroids, radiotherapy, chemotherapy and stents for SVCO in carcinoma of the bronchus: a systematic review. Rowell NP and Gleeson FV. *Clin. Oncol.* (R Coll. Radiol.) 2002; **14**: 338–51

Hypercalcaemia

Definition and aetiology A serum calcium level over 2.75 mmol/l is considered abnormal; borderline values need repeating. In malignancy a raised calcium is due to increased osteoclast activity, either from bony metastases or the ectopic production of a PTH-like hormone. A serum level over 3.25 mmol/l is rare outside malignancy, although can occur in sarcoidosis.

Clinical features Values over 3 mmol/l are usually symptomatic. Common symptoms are confusion, weakness, nausea, reduced fluid intake, and constipation. There may be a short QT interval on ECG, and renal failure.

Investigations Exclude other causes of hypercalcaemia and identify the tumour, although in most patients with malignant hypercalcaemia the diagnosis of malignancy will already be known. The PTH will be suppressed in malignant hypercalcaemia, but raised in hyperparathyroidism. The phosphate will tend to be low in hyperparathyroidism and hypercalcaemia due to ectopic PTH, and low/normal in sarcoidosis, metastatic bone disease, and with excess vitamin D. Check for renal failure.

Management
- Isotonic saline infusion (250 ml/h initially, to reverse dehydration, but avoid fluid overload, reducing to 150 ml/h) with furosemide to increase calcium excretion
- Steroids help, but less so than in sarcoid-associated hypercalcaemia, partly through reduced intestinal absorption

In addition to this initial management:
- Reduce bone reabsorption with biphosphonates (take a few days to work maximally).
  - *Intravenous preparations.* Disodium pamidronate, 10 ml vial of 3 mg/ml, or 10 ml vial of 6 mg/ml infused over two hours. Works for several weeks. Sodium clodronate, 300 mg (one x 5 ml vial of 60 mg/ml) daily for 7 days or 1.5 grams single dose (five x 5 ml vials of 60 mg/ml). Zoledronic acid, 4 mg vial reconstituted in water and given over two hours, repeated monthly if required
  - *Oral preparations.* Clodronate, one 800 mg tablet twice a day. The biphosphonates can also reduce the pain of secondary bony deposits and may reduce pathological fracture rate.

Syndrome of inappropriate ADH (SIADH) secretion

Definition and aetiology Excessive retention of water relative to electrolytes due to inappropriate production of ADH. Hence there is hyponatraemia (<135 meq/l), hypo-osmolality, a urine osmolality >100 mosmol/kg, a urine sodium concentration usually above 40 meq/l, normal acid–base (and potassium), and usually a low plasma urea concentration. Diuretic-induced hyponatraemia will be accompanied by evidence of dehydration, e.g. raised urea. Causes of SIADH include:

- Drugs, e.g. carbamezepine, fluoxetine, high-dose cyclophosphamide
- Post major surgery
- Pneumonia
- HIV infection
- CNS disorders, e.g. stroke, infection, psychosis
- Small cell lung cancer, either ectopic ADH production or rarely stimulation of normal ADH production.

Clinical features Lethargy and confusion often when sodium levels fall below 130 meq/l and nearly always when below 120 meq/l.

Investigations A low sodium in the presence of a low urea and an appropriate clinical setting may be adequate to make a diagnosis. If sodium depletion/water overload are a possible alternative cause of hyponatraemia, they should be accompanied by a urine osmolarity <100 mosmol/kg (or a specific gravity <1.003, or a urine sodium <40 meq/l). Therefore values increasingly above this are suggestive of SIADH (unless the patient is on loop diuretics when of course the urinary sodium concentration will be higher).

Management
- Fluid restriction (0.5 to 1.0 l/day) will help, but is often unpleasant for the patient
- Demeclocycline (450 mg bd, tetracycline derivative) blocks ADH action at the distal renal tubules and can be used long-term
- Salt tablets/extra-dietary salt
- May resolve over a few weeks following chemotherapy
- Hypertonic saline is rarely indicated and can provoke brainstem damage (demyelination) through rapid changes in osmolality.

Future developments
New drugs specifically blocking the ADH receptor in the distal tubule are under investigation.

Spinal cord compression

Prompt treatment is needed for spinal cord compression to prevent irreversible paraplegia and loss of bowel and bladder function.

Definition and aetiology Spinal cord compression occurs commonly in patients with metastatic cancer (in about 5% of all cancer patients, particularly breast, lung, and prostate cancer). It may be the first presentation of cancer, but often occurs with a known primary tumour. Cord compression is commonly caused by direct spread from a vertebral metastasis into the extradural space, or less commonly from pressure on the cord from a primary tumour in the posterior mediastinum or the retroperitoneum, or by pressure from a mass of retroperitoneal nodes. It is unusual to have a metastasis within the cord itself, although meningeal spread can occur. Spinal cord compression causes interruption of the arterial supply to the cord and subsequent infarction.

Clinical features Patients frequently experience back pain initially, due to associated vertebral collapse. This precedes any neurological signs. Pain is not, however, universal. Neurological signs may be non-specific: weak legs, constipation, urinary incontinence. Leg weakness develops over hours to days, with associated sensory loss. Loss of bladder and bowel sensation is a late sign and usually heralds irreversible paraplegia within hours or a few days. Examination reveals bilateral upper motor neurone signs in the legs, with increased tone, weakness, brisk reflexes, and extensor plantars. There may be sensory loss in the legs, particularly with a loss of proprioception and a sensory level on the trunk. Sensory loss in the saddle area, with decreased rectal tone suggests a cauda equina lesion. The bladder may be palpable.

Investigations

Have a low threshold for investigating a patient with known cancer with back pain

- **MRI** of the spine is the investigation of choice to demonstrate the level of the cord compression
- **CT** is less reliable, but can also be helpful, if MRI is not available
- **Plain spine XR** may show vertebral metastases, but this is usually unhelpful, as there is no imaging of the spinal cord. Time should not be wasted in getting a plain XR
- **Bone scan** shows vertebral metastases, but again does not image the spinal cord. Earlier scans showing bony metastases may alert the physician to the possibility of future cord compression
- If patient is not known to have underlying malignant disease, a search for a primary tumour should be performed, but must not delay treatment of the spinal cord compression. Take full history (weight loss, anorexia, specific symptoms) and perform full examination, CXR, blood tests, PSA, and myeloma screen.

Management depends on tumour type and overall prognosis. Discuss with oncologist and/or neurosurgeon to determine which definitive treatment(s) are the most appropriate for the patient.

- High-dose steroids (dexamethasone IV 4 mg/6 hours). These should be started whilst waiting for MRI scan, if the clinical picture suggests cord compression
- Radiotherapy to the metastasis or tumour causing cord compression, particularly if there are multiple sites of cord compression or if surgery is not advised
- Surgical decompression of the cord, reconstruction, and stabilizing the spinal column
- Catheter if in urinary retention
- Care for pressure areas
- DVT prevention
- Consider chemotherapy if appropriate, for underlying cancer causing the spinal cord compression, once the initial treatment has taken place
- Rehabilitation, ideally in unit with spinal cord expertise.

A recent Dutch study showed 66% of patients with metastatic cord compression (from all cancers) admitted to rehabilitation centres were discharged and average survival post-discharge was 808 days. 52% were alive at one year.

Prognosis Patients who are mobile at presentation have the best prognosis and are likely to have preserved neurological function following treatment. If there is some preserved motor function, 25% will be able to walk post-treatment. If paraplegia is present pre-treatment, less than 10% will be able to walk afterwards. Loss of bladder function for more than 24–48 hours cannot be reversed.

Further information

Epidural metastatic spinal cord compression: functional outcome and survival after in-patient rehabilitation. Eriks IE et al. Spinal Cord 2004; **42**(4): 235–9

Pulmonary carcinoid tumours

These are uncommon primary lung tumours, 1–2% of all lung tumours. Equal male/female incidence, typical age at presentation is 40–50 years. They are a form of neuroendocrine tumour and can have similar histological appearances to small cell lung cancer.

Pathophysiology Although typically slow growing benign tumours, more aggressive subtypes exist, with metastatic potential. Commonly they are located endobronchially, but can also be located peripherally in the lung parenchyma.

Clinical features

- Endobronchial carcinoids can cause isolated wheeze, dyspnoea, infection, haemoptysis, or persistent lobar collapse
- Parenchymal carcinoids are often asymptomatic, being detected on routine CXR
- Carcinoid syndrome, with flushing, tachycardia, sweats, diarrhoea, wheeze, and hypotension, occurs in 1% of pulmonary carcinoid tumours
- Carcinoid tumours can also be associated with Cushing's syndrome, due to ectopic tumour ACTH production.

Investigations

- *CXR* may reveal a well-defined tumour, which should be further characterized on CT. *Tumourlets* is the description given to multiple endobronchial or parenchymal carcinoid tumours
- *Bronchoscopy* is performed for accessible endobronchial carcinoid tumours. They typically appear to be intraluminal, cherry red, and covered with intact epithelium. Bronchial brushings may be adequate for a histological diagnosis. Bronchial biopsy can be associated with brisk or torrential bleeding, so care should be taken. Some avoid biopsy altogether and proceed to surgical resection based on a clinical diagnosis. CT-guided biopsy may be preferred for peripheral tumours
- *Histological diagnosis* can be difficult as the appearances can be similar to those of small cell lung cancer. Special stains and immunohistochemistry are used to help differentiate between the two. Clinically, however, these tend to be quite different conditions and clinical details can aid pathological diagnosis. Carcinoid tumours are characterized as being *typical* or *atypical*. They each have a characteristic pattern:
  - *Typical carcinoids* have no necrosis, occasional nuclear pleomorphism, and absent or late mitoses. Distant metastases are rare and metastasis to lymph nodes occurs in 5–15% of cases. The 5-year survival is 100% and 10-year survival is 87%
  - *Atypical carcinoids* may show focal necrosis and often have nuclear pleomorphism. There is increased mitotic activity. They have distant metastases in 20% and metastasize to the lymph nodes in up to 48% of cases. The 5-year survival is 69% and 10-year survival is 52%.

Management

- Patients with isolated pulmonary carcinoid tumours should be considered for surgical resection. Resection is ideally limited, removing minimal amounts of normal lung parenchyma. Tumour resection is associated with resolution of any features of the carcinoid syndrome
- If the tumour is atypical or close to the resection margin, patients should be followed up with repeat CXR on an annual basis. Radiotherapy is not performed
- Tumour size does not relate to the presence of lymph node metastases and therefore local lymph nodes should be sampled peri-operatively
- In the 1% with carcinoid syndrome, serotonin antagonists, such as octreotide, can be used for treatment. Isolated liver metastases can be treated with arterial embolization. Metastatic aggressive carcinoid tumours can be treated with chemotherapy, such as etoposide, cisplatin, 5-fluorouracil, and streptozotocin.

Further information

Update in pulmonary carcinoid tumours: a review article. Hage R et al. Ann Surg Oncol. 2003; **10**: 697–704

Pulmonary nodules

Definition These are focal, round, or oval areas of increased opacity in the lung, measuring less than 3 cm in diameter. They are detected on CXR or CT. Greater use of CT and thinner slice spiral CT scanning has led to increased detection rates. CT allows the precise localization of a nodule and reliable determination of its features. It has a high sensitivity of detecting nodules of <5 mm in diameter. Volumetric analysis using CT-aided software means that a 3D nodule can be simulated, to aid nodule characterization and assess whether its volume has increased over time.

Causes of pulmonary nodules

Benign
Infectious granulomata
Non-infectious granulomata
Bronchial adenoma
Benign hamartoma (developmental
abnormality, containing cartilage, epithelium,
and fat. Can contain smooth muscle. Slowly
growing. Can be seen at any age, especially 40+;
often calcify.)

Malignant
Lung cancer
Solitary metastasis

- The majority of pulmonary nodules are benign, although exact numbers depend on the characteristics of the population screened
- 20–30% of patients with lung cancer may present with a solitary pulmonary nodule
- Of the nodules detected on CT in smokers with a normal CXR, between 1 and 2.5% will be malignant
- The Early Lung Cancer Action Project screening programme of CT scans in 60+ year olds, with at least a 10-pack year history of smoking in the USA, found non-calcified nodules in 23%, which were seen on CXR in 7%. 11% of these nodules were malignant on biopsy
- Early detection of these malignant nodules might alter the management of the patient, with surgical resection of a stage 1 cancer.

Management options for patients with pulmonary nodules

Observation Baseline CT scan, then repeat after an arbitrary time interval, such as 3 and 12 months, or 3, 6, and 12 months. If the nodule has increased in size or is showing features of malignancy, consider biopsy or proceed straight to surgical resection. PET scan may be helpful in combination with CT if the nodule is increasing in size, but cannot be biopsied.

Biopsy Difficult on small nodules <7 mm.

Resection If nodule has features of malignancy and biopsy not possible.

Chemotherapy or radiotherapy If nodule proven to be malignant, but surgical treatment is not indicated due to performance status.

Combined modality treatment

Factors that suggest a pulmonary nodule is malignant

- Size >1 cm
- Smokers, older age
- Increasing volumetrically determined growth rates over time
- Increased enhancement with contrast, suggesting increased vascularity (>15 Hounsfield units)
- Irregular or spiculated margin, with distortion of adjacent vessels
- Associated ground-glass shadowing
- Cavitation with thick irregular walls
- Pseudocavitation within nodule—bronchoalveolar cell carcinoma.

Factors that suggest a pulmonary nodule is benign

- Stable or decreasing size for 2 years
- Nodule resolves during follow-up
- Non-smoker
- Lack of enhancement with contrast
- Smooth, well-defined margins (although 21% of smooth nodules may be malignant)
- Benign pattern of calcification: central, diffuse solid, laminated, or 'popcorn like'—related to prior infections or calcification in a hamartoma
- Intranodular fat—likely hamartoma
- Cavitation with thin smooth walls
- Younger age
- Resident in histoplasmosis endemic areas, such as North America.

Pulmonary nodule with extrathoracic malignancy

In a patient with pre-existing malignancy, a pulmonary nodule could be a metastasis, new lung cancer, or benign disease. The histology of the extra-pulmonary neoplasm and the patient's smoking history influence this. These cases need discussion within the cancer MDT to determine whether nodule biopsy or treatment of the underlying primary cancer would be the most appropriate management.

One study determined the likelihood of a pulmonary nodule being a new primary or metastasis based on the site of the original cancer:

- **New lung primary more likely** if the primary tumour is: head and neck, bladder, breast, bile ducts, oesophagus, ovary, prostate, stomach
- **Metastasis more likely** if the primary tumour is: melanoma, sarcoma, testes
- **Either new primary or metastasis possible** if the primary tumour is: salivary gland, adrenal, colon, parotid, kidney, thyroid, thymus, uterus.

Further information

Solitary pulmonary nodules. Erasmus J et al. Radiographics 2000; **20**: 43–66

Solitary pulmonary nodule with extra pulmonary neoplasms. Quint L et al. Radiology 2000; **217**: 257–61

Early lung cancer action project: overall design and findings from baseline screening. Henschke et al. Lancet 1999; **354**: 99–105

Lung cancer screening

This is an area that is currently being developed. Screening programmes are based on the theory that early detection of lung cancer and any subsequent intervention will improve the patient's outcome. There is no evidence yet of reduction in lung cancer mortality from screening studies. To be detectable on CXR, a lung cancer needs to be 1 cm diameter, and 3–4 mm diameter to be detectable on CT.

Screening studies

- Four previous CXR screening studies in the 1970s were negative, of which the **Mayo Lung Project** has been the most studied. This compared 4 monthly CXR and sputum cytology for 6 years in 45+ year old smokers of 20+ per day, with infrequent or no screening in a control group. 206 cancers were found in the study group and 160 in the control group, but all-cause mortality was not affected by screening, even at 20 years
- More recent studies have used low-dose spiral CT scanning. The **Early Lung Cancer Action Project (ELCAP)** in New York recruited 1000 symptom-free volunteers aged 60+ with a 10 pack-year history of smoking, who would be fit for a thoracotomy. There was no control group. Baseline CXR and CT were performed. Non-calcified nodules were present in 23% of patients at baseline on CT. Repeat CT was performed for nodules <5 mm; nodules >6 mm were biopsied and nodules >11 mm received standard care. 2.7% of all the patients entered had malignant nodules; with stage 1 disease in 2.3%. All but one patient had their cancer surgically resected
- Further research is needed to demonstrate a clear detection survival benefit, before national screening programmes should be instituted.

Further information

Lung cancer screening. Ellis JRC et al. British Journal of Radiology 2001; **74**: 478–85

Lung cancer screening: an update. Marcus PM. Journal of Clinical Oncology 2001; **19**: 83s–86s

Screening for lung cancer. Kawahara M. Curr Opin Oncol 2004; **16**:141–5

Mediastinal abnormalities

The mediastinum is the area within the centre of the chest containing the heart, great vessels, nerves, lymph nodes, trachea, oesophagus, and thymus. Common symptoms of mediastinal disease include cough, chest pain, and dyspnoea, as well as symptoms relating to any structure being compressed, such as dysphagia, stridor, or SVCO. Mediastinal disorders can also be asymptomatic. They may be found incidentally following a CXR.

Anatomy

Anterior mediastinum The area behind the body of the sternum and in front of the fibrous pericardium. Contains the thymus, which also extends superiorly.

Posterior mediastinum The area in front of the vertebral bodies and behind the fibrous pericardium. Contains the spinal nerve roots, the descending aorta and oesophagus, the azygos and hemiazygos veins, the thoracic duct, and vagus and splanchnic nerves.

Superior mediastinum The area located between the thoracic inlet superiorly, the manubrium of the sternum anteriorly, by the superior 4 thoracic vertebrae posteriorly and inferiorly where a horizontal plane would cross through the sternal angle. It contains the aortic arch and its large branches and the upper half of SVC. It also contains the trachea, the oesophagus, the thoracic duct, the phrenic, vagus, cardiac, and left recurrent laryngeal nerves.

Middle mediastinum The area containing the heart and pericardium, the ascending aorta, the lower half of the SVC, part of the azygos vein, the pulmonary arteries and veins, the tracheal bifurcation, phrenic nerves, and the IVC.

These areas are easily seen on a lateral CXR

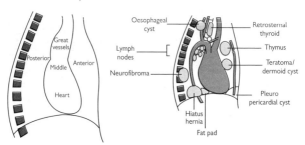

Likely nature of mediastinal mass according to anatomical site

Anterior mediastinal mass
- Thymoma (superior)
- Thyroid (superior)
- Germ-cell tumour
- Lymphoma
- Ascending aortic aneurysm
- Pleuropericardial cyst
- Pericardial fat pad
- Morgagni anterior diaphragmatic hernia (page 594).

Superior mediastinal mass
- Bronchogenic cyst.

Posterior mediastinal mass
- Neural tumour
- Foregut duplication or cyst
- Lipoma
- Descending aortic aneurysm
- Bochdalek posterior diaphragmatic hernia (page 594).

Approach to the patient with a mediastinal mass

- Full history
- Examination, including skin and lymphadenopathy (neck, axillae, groins)
- Examine testes
- Look for fatigability: ptosis, opthalmoplegia, unable to maintain upward gaze
- Look for signs of SVCO or stridor
- Blood tests, including AFP, beta HCG, anti-acetyl choline receptor antibody
- Arrange CT scan of chest
- Try and locate old CXRs.

Mediastinal abnormalities 1

Neural tumours mostly occur in the posterior mediastinum. 75% are benign in adults.

- *Schwannomas and neurofibromas* are benign peripheral nerve sheath tumours. They may be multiple. Usually asymptomatic, although can cause segmental pain. Slowly enlarge and rarely can cause cord compression, with dumb-bell shaped tumours straddling the intervertebral foramen. Can be surgically excised
- *Malignant peripheral nerve sheath tumours, or neurosarcomas,* include new malignant growths and benign neurofibromas that have undergone malignant change. They may cause systemic features of malignancy and can invade locally and metastasize
- *Autonomic nervous system tumours,* including neuroblastomas and ganglioneuromas, range from benign to malignant. Surgical removal is the treatment of choice, with radiotherapy and chemotherapy if the tumour is malignant.

Thymoma Tumour of epithelial origin arising in the thymus. May contain functioning thymic tissue. M = F. Rare below age 20. Myasthenia gravis is present in 30–40% of patients with a thymoma; this is often unimproved after thymectomy and may even develop after the thymoma is removed. 20% of patients presenting with myasthenia gravis are found to have a thymoma, particularly if patients are over 50 and male. This group is likely to have positive acetylcholine receptor (AChR) autoantibodies, which bind to acetylcholine receptors at the postsynaptic motor endplate, decreasing available acetylcholine binding sites, causing nerve fatigability.

Patients with thymomas are usually symptomatic with pain, dyspnoea, dysphagia, or myasthenia gravis symptoms. Thymomas contained within the thymic capsule tend to be benign, although they do have malignant potential; those that have extended outside the capsule are malignant, and may involve local structures or metastasize. Diagnose with CT and treat with surgical excision of the thymus, avoiding prior FNA or biopsy as this may cause tumour seeding outside the capsule. Consider post-operative radiotherapy for invasive tumours, especially those not completely excised. Thymectomy is indicated in patients with myasthenia gravis even without thymoma, as it may lead to symptomatic improvement. This gives best results in those with detectable AChR antibody levels and younger patients early in the disease course, particularly those with severe disease.

Thymic cyst may be congenital, or acquired secondary to inflammation. Asymptomatic unless large and causing symptoms of compression. Benign, but usually treated with surgical excision, as diagnostic certainty may be difficult.

Thymic carcinoid Not associated with myasthenia gravis and behaves aggressively, with local recurrence and metastasis. May be associated with Cushing's syndrome. Treatment with surgery or chemotherapy or octreotide.

Also: thymic carcinoma, thymic lipoma, and thymic hyperplasia.

Germ cell tumour Arise from immature germ cells during development. Tend to be in an anterior and mid-line location.

- *Mature cystic teratomas* represent 80% of germ cell tumours. These are benign and occur in young adults. M = F. Often asymptomatic, but can erode surrounding structures and cause symptoms. CXR shows well-defined mass, which may contain flecks of calcification. Treatment is by surgical excision

- *Seminoma* occurs in men age 20–40 years. Mediastinal seminomas are malignant and almost always arise within the thymus and are histologically indistinguishable from those occurring in the testes. Can be primary mediastinal tumour or metastasis from testicular tumour; therefore always examine testes. Patients frequently present with chest pain. CXR shows non-calcified lobulated anterior mediastinal mass, confirmed with CT. Serum AFP is normal and this aids diagnosis. Diagnose with surgical biopsy. Surgical excision is not recommended as is usually incomplete. Treatment is with cisplatin-based chemotherapy initially, which can cause infertility and therefore patients may wish to consider sperm banking before treatment. Tumours are radiosensitive, so radiotherapy used if they are bulky. Long-term survival expected in 80%. Better prognosis than non-seminomatous germ cell tumours

- *Non-seminomatous germ cell tumours* (including choriocarcinoma, teratocarcinoma, and yolk sac tumours) are all malignant and occur in men in their 30s. They are symptomatic due to local invasion and they metastasize. CXR shows mediastinal mass and diagnosis is with surgical biopsy. βHCG and AFP are raised. Treatment is with cisplatin-based chemotherapy. βHCG and AFP are markers of disease and fall with tumour response.

Thyroid Retrosternal goitre occurs, especially in older women. Usually asymptomatic unless large and compressing the trachea, causing dyspnoea and stridor. May be seen on plain CXR. CT and radioactive iodine isotope scans are helpful in diagnosis. Flow-volume loops are abnormal if there is tracheal compression. Surgery is recommended if there is airway compromise, but can lead to tracheomalacia afterwards.

Also: parathyroid adenoma

Mediastinal abnormalities 2

Lymphoma The mediastinum is frequently involved in patients with Hodgkin's lymphoma. CT scan is necessary to assess the extent of this and to assess response to treatment. To establish the histological diagnosis of lymphoma, an adequate tissue sample is required; this should be from a biopsy, rather than a fine needle aspirate. This may be best achieved surgically, via mediastinoscopy. Examine patient for peripheral lymph nodes, as these may be easier to biopsy. Treatment is with chemotherapy initially.

Enlarged lymph nodes

- *Metastases* from breast, lung, and oesophageal cancer
- *Castleman's disease* Giant lymph node hyperplasia. Rare. Two forms:
  - *Angio-follicular hyperplasia* causing mediastinal or hilar lymph node mass. Often asymptomatic or may cause cough or wheeze due to localized compression. Non-progressive. May have fever and raised ESR. Nodal biopsy shows follicles of pericapillary lymphocytes and proliferation of the plump and eosinophilic capillary endothelial cells. Removal of nodes may improve symptoms. Can also occur on pleura
  - *Multicentric Castleman's disease* is a more aggressive disease that occurs in association with HIV infection. Lymphoproliferative disorder with prominent systemic symptoms, as well as generalized lymph node enlargement, hepatosplenomegaly, paraproteinaemia, and skin rash. Biopsy shows prominent plasma cell infiltration. Related to IL-6 overproduction and human herpes virus-8 infection. Treatment is with steroids ± chemotherapy (doxorubicin, vincristine, and cyclophosphamide), but prognosis is poor. Can progress to non-Hodgkin's lymphoma. Rapidly fatal without treatment.

Cysts

- *Foregut duplications or cysts* can be related to the oesophagus or the airways, especially near the carina. Lined by respiratory epithelium. Often diagnosed in childhood, as they cause dyspnoea, stridor, or cough due to limited space to expand. Seen on CXR and CT and treated with surgical excision
- *Pleuropericardial cysts* mostly occur at the cardiophrenic angles and can measure up to 25 cm diameter. M = F. Usually asymptomatic, but may cause chest pain. CXR shows smooth round shadow abutting the heart. Excision can be carried out at thoracoscopy, but conservative management is favoured. Also known as springwater cysts.

Inflammation

- *Mediastinitis* occurs after oesophageal perforation or rupture, due to malignancy, instrumentation, or vomiting (Boerhaave's syndrome). Patients are ill, with pain and fever. CXR may show widened mediastinum or air in the mediastinum. Pneumothorax or pleural effusion may also be seen. Treatment includes repairing the defect, parenteral feeding, and antibiotics. High morbidity and mortality

- *Mediastinal fibrosis* Rare, idiopathic condition that occurs in middle age. Symptoms depend on which aspects of the mediastinum are involved, but may include dyspnoea, wheeze, haemoptysis, hoarse voice, dysphagia, pulmonary hypertension, SVCO. CXR shows a widened mediastinum. Diagnosis made on biopsy, particularly to exclude malignancy. Treatment is supportive; steroids and surgical debulking ineffective. Prognosis variable, depending on sites involved. May be associated with retroperitoneal fibrosis, radiotherapy, methysergide, auto-immune disease, or infection with TB, histoplasmosis, aspergillus, or nocardia.

Mediastinal emphysema or pneumomediastinum. Can be caused by sneezing, straining, Valsalva manoeuvres, vomiting, substance abuse, parturition, positive pressure ventilation, instrumentation, or trans-bronchial biopsy. Usually symptomless, but occasional pain. Hamman's sign positive (click with each heart beat on auscultation over lung). Treat with high flow oxygen. Resolves spontaneously.

Vascular Aortic aneurysms are usually asymptomatic, but symptoms relate to compression of adjacent structures. May diagnose on CXR as a widened mediastinum. This is best imaged via CT or MRI. Surgery should be considered to prevent death from rupture.

Bacterial respiratory infection

Community-acquired pneumonia

Community-acquired pneumonia (CAP) is a common disease, associated with significant morbidity and mortality.

Definition A syndrome of infection that is usually bacterial with symptoms and signs of consolidation of part(s) of the lung parenchyma. This is different to bronchitis (see page 533).

Epidemiology

- CAP is the commonest infectious cause of death and the 6th leading cause of death in the UK and USA (with quoted age-adjusted death rates of between 1 and 24/100,000)
- Up to 40% of UK adults with CAP require hospital admission. Hospital mortality varies between 5 and 12%
- A BTS multicentre UK study showed that 5–10% of patients with CAP require ICU admission
- Mortality up to 50% in those admitted to ICU
- CAP managed in the community has a mortality of 1%.

Pathophysiology The lung and tracheobronchial tree are usually sterile below the level of the larynx, so an infecting agent must reach this site via a breach in host defences. This may be by microaspiration (which occurs in around 45% of healthy individuals overnight), haematogenous spread, direct spread from an adjacent structure, inhalation, or activation of previously dormant infection.

Aetiology Broadly similar pathogens are seen in patients managed in the community and in hospital. A single pathogen is identified in 85% of cases. The proportion of cases with more than one pathogen is unknown.

Risk factors for CAP

- *Aspiration* Typically caused by anaerobes and Gram-negative organisms
- *Alcoholism and diabetes* Typically associated with bacteraemic pneumococcal pneumonia. Anaerobes and mixed infections are more common in alcoholics
- *Oral steroids/immunosuppression* Legionella infection may be more common
- *COPD* Haemophilus influenzae and Moraxella catarrhalis are more common, and COPD is more common in those with bacterial pneumonia
- *Nursing home residents* have an increased frequency of CAP, with aspiration, Gram-negative organisms, and anaerobes more common than in age-matched elderly people. Haemophilus influenzae is the most common causative organism. Mycoplasma pneumonia and legionella are less common.

Organisms causing community-acquired pneumonia

- *Streptococcus* or *pneumococcus pneumoniae*—the most frequently identified organism, commonest in winter. Epidemics in the UK are associated with overcrowding, e.g. in prisons
- *Legionella pneumophilia*—most common in the autumn. 52% are travel-related. Epidemics occur related to water containing systems in buildings, typically in the Mediterranean
- *Staphylococcus aureus*—commonest in winter months. Coincident influenza infection in 39% of those requiring hospital admission, and 50% of those admitted to ICU
- *Influenza*—annual epidemics in the winter months, complicated by pneumonia in 3% of community cases. 10% of those admitted to hospital have coincident *Staphylococcus aureus* infection
- *Mycoplasma pneumoniae*—epidemics occur every 4 or 5 years in the UK
- *Chlamydia pneumoniae* (Q fever)—epidemics in the community; whether it has a direct pathogenic role, or is an associated infectious agent is not clear
- *Chlamydia psittaci*—infection acquired from birds and animals, with 20% of cases having a history of bird contact. Human-to-human spread may occur. Uncommon
- *Chlamydia burnetti*—epidemics in relation to animal sources (usually sheep), but occupational exposure only present in 8%. Uncommon.

CAP: clinical features

- Fever
- Cough
- Sputum
- Shortness of breath
- Pleuritic chest pain
- Non-specific features in the elderly. May present 'off legs' or with confusion, in the absence of fever.

Examination

- Raised respiratory rate (may be the only sign in the elderly)
- Tachycardia
- Localizing signs on chest examination. Reduced chest expansion on the affected side, with signs consistent with consolidation (reduced air entry, with bronchial breathing, reduced percussion note, increased vocal resonance) and crackles. A normal chest examination makes the diagnosis unlikely.

Diagnosis of CAP is made on the basis of:

- Symptoms and signs of an acute lower respiratory tract infection
- New focal chest signs
- New radiographic shadowing, for which there is no other explanation
- At least one systemic feature (e.g. sweating, fevers, aches, and pains)
- No other explanation for the illness.

Most helpful in diagnosis:

- Fever, pleuritic pain, dyspnoea, and tachypnoea
- Signs on chest examination.

Specific clinical features of pathogens The aetiological agent cannot be accurately predicted from the clinical features alone, although some features are more statistically likely with one pathogen than another. The exception to this is the presence of chest pain or fever (>39°C) in those admitted to ICU, which predicts a higher likelihood of streptococcal pneumonia.

- *Streptococcus pneumoniae* Increasing age, co-morbidity (especially cardiovascular), acute onset, high fever, and pleuritic chest pain
- *Bacteraemic Streptococcus pneumoniae* Alcohol, diabetes, COPD, dry or no cough, female
- *Legionella* Younger patients, smokers, absence of co-morbidity, more severe infection, neurological symptoms, evidence of multisystem disease (e.g. abnormal liver enzymes and raised creatine kinase)
- *Mycoplasma pneumoniae* Younger patients, prior antibiotics, less multisystem involvement, but extrapulmonary involvement, including haemolysis and skin and joint problems
- *Staphylococcus aureus* Recent influenza-like illness
- *Chlamydia psittaci* Longer duration of symptoms prior to admission, headache

- *Chlamydia burnetti* Dry cough, high fever, male
- *Klebsiella pneumoniae* Low platelet count and leucopenia, male.

Rare causes
- *Acinetobacter* Older patients, history of alcoholism, high mortality
- *Streptococcus milleri* Dental or abdominal source of infection
- *Streptococcus viridans* Aspiration is a risk factor.

CAP: severity assessment

- CAP has a wide range of severity. An assessment of severity enables the most appropriate care to be delivered in the most appropriate clinical setting
- Early identification of patients at high risk of death allows early decisions about hospital admission and possible need for assisted ventilation to be made
- Assessment of disease severity depends on the experience of the clinician, and a number of predictive assessment models have been trialled. These predictive models of severity should be regarded as adjuncts to clinical assessment, and regular reassessment of the disease is needed.

Poor prognostic factors Those with two or more adverse prognostic factors are at high risk of death, and should be managed as for severe CAP.

- **Age** (≥65)
- **Coexisting disease** — including cardiac disease, diabetes, COPD, stroke
- **Respiratory rate** ≥ 30/minute—this is one of the most reliable predictors of disease severity
- **Confusion**—abbreviated mental test score ≤ 8
- **Blood pressure**—systolic ≤ 90 mmHg and/or diastolic ≤ 60 mmHg
- **Hypoxaemia**—respiratory failure with PaO_2 < 8 kPa and the need for ventilation predicts mortality
- **Urea** ≥ 7 mmol/l
- **Albumin** < 35 g/l
- **White cell count**—a WCC > 20 or < 4 x 10^9/l are both predictive
- **Radiology**—bilateral or multilobe involvement. In patients admitted to ICU, progression of CXR changes is a poor prognostic marker
- **Microbiology**—positive blood culture, whatever the pathogen isolated.

Severity assessment can be summarized as **CURB** or **CURB-65.**

CURB score core factors

- **C**onfusion—new mental confusion defined (AMTS ≤ 8)
- **U**rea—≥7 mmol/l
- **R**espiratory rate raised ≥30/min
- **B**lood pressure—systolic BP ≤ 90 and/or diastolic BP ≤ 60
- **65** age ≥ 65.

The presence of the 4 'core' CURB factors correlates with mortality:
- 4 factors present gives a mortality of 83%, 3 factors 33%, 2 factors 23%, 8% with one, and 2.4% in the presence of no core factors
- Low risk of death: age <50, no coexisting disease, CURB score zero.

**Abbreviated mental test score
(1 point per question, max = 10)**

Age
Date of birth
Time (to nearest hour)
Year
Hospital name
Recognition of 2 people (e.g. nurse, doctor)
Recall address
Date of First World War
Name of monarch
Count backwards 20 to 1

CAP: investigations

General investigations are aimed at confirming the diagnosis, assessing disease severity, guiding appropriate treatment, assessing the presence of underlying disease, enabling identification of complications, and monitoring progress.

- **Oxygenation assessment** Those with an oxygen saturation of <92% on admission, or with features of severe pneumonia should have arterial blood gases measured. The inspired oxygen concentration must be documented
- **CXR**
  - Consolidation, most commonly in the lower lobes. Also interstitial infiltrates and cavitation
  - Multilobe involvement, more common in bacteraemic pneumococcal infection
  - Pleural effusion, more common in bacteraemic pneumococcal infection
  - Lymphadenopathy, uncommon, but most likely with mycoplasma infection
  - Multilobe involvement, cavitation, or spontaneous pneumothorax suggest *Staphylococcus aureus* infection
  - Upper lobe preponderance—*Klebsiella.*
- **CT chest** Unlikely to add additional information. May be useful if the diagnosis is in doubt or the patient is severely ill and failing to respond to treatment, in order to exclude abscess formation, empyema, underlying malignancy, or other interstitial disease process
- **Blood tests**
  - FBC—a white cell count (WCC) > 15×10^9 suggests bacterial (particularly pneumococcal) infection. Counts of >20 or <4 indicate severe infection
  - Deranged renal and liver function tests can be indicative of severe infection, or point to the presence of underlying disease. LFTs may be abnormal, particularly with right lower lobe pneumonia. A raised urea is a marker of more severe pneumonia
  - Metabolic acidosis is associated with severe illness
  - C-reactive protein may be useful in management, with high levels being a more sensitive marker of infection than the white cell count or temperature. Serial measures may be useful in assessing response to treatment.

Microbiological investigations The microbiological cause for CAP is not found in 25–60% of patients, and therefore often does not contribute to patient management. Microbiological investigations can help to aid selection of optimal antibiotics, hence limiting antibiotic resistance, and the possible problems of *Clostridium difficile* associated diarrhoea. They also inform public health or infection control teams, aiding in the monitoring of pathogen trends causing CAP over time.

- **Blood cultures** Recommended for all patients with CAP, ideally before antibiotics are started
- **Sputum culture and sensitivity** Useful for those patients who have failed to improve with empirical antibiotic treatment, and in those with

non-severe pneumonia admitted to hospital, who are expectorating purulent samples and have not received prior antibiotics. Also useful in severe pneumonia. Not routinely recommended for those treated in the community.

Sputum examination is recommended for possible tuberculosis in those with weight loss, a persistent cough, night sweats, and risk factors for TB, e.g. ethnic origin, social deprivation

- *Pleural fluid* (if present) for M, C, & S and pH to exclude empyema (see page 308)
- *Viral and atypical pathogens* In severe CAP
- *Serological testing* Paired samples (from within 7 days of the onset of the illness, repeated 7–10 days later) should be tested together, in those with severe CAP, and in those unresponsive to β-lactam antibiotics.

Specific serological tests

- **Legionnaires' disease** A number of immunological tests exist to aid in the prompt and accurate diagnosis of *Legionella pneumophilia*:
  - Urinary antigen detection is sensitive and specific, and rapid results can be obtained early
  - Direct immunofluorescence tests (DIF)—*Legionella pneumophilia* can be detected on bronchial aspirates
  - Culture is 100% specific (sputum, endotracheal aspirate, BAL, pleural fluid, lung)
  - Serology—antibody levels and PCR are also available.
- *Mycoplasma pneumonia*
  - The complement fixation test (CFT) is the commonest serological assay and is regarded as the gold standard. Culture of *Mycoplasma pneumoniae* is not generally available.
- *Chlamydia*
  - Chlamydial antigen can be detected by DIF in respiratory samples or by CFT.
- *Others*
  - Influenza A and B, adenovirus, respiratory syncytial virus.

CAP: management

General management

- *Oxygen* Hypoxia is due to V/Q mismatching, as blood flows through unventilated lung. Aim for oxygen saturation > 92%. If there is severe concomitant COPD, controlled oxygen therapy and close monitoring of blood gases are mandatory. A rising CO_2 in a patient without prior respiratory disease may indicate they are tiring, and need respiratory support—discuss with ITU early
- *Fluids* Assessment of volume status, by JVP (with or without central venous access) and blood pressure is paramount. Encourage oral fluids. Intravenous fluids may be needed if volume depleted and severely unwell. Monitor urine output
- *Analgesia* Paracetamol or NSAIDs initially if required. Paracetamol also has an antipyretic role
- *Nutrition* Nutritional status is important to the outcome and nutritional supplements may be of benefit in prolonged illness. Poor nutritional status may increase the risk of acquiring pneumonia
- *Physiotherapy* is of no proven benefit in acute pneumonia.

Additional treatments

Bronchoscopy May be helpful, especially after intubation on ITU, to suction retained secretions, particularly if these are causing lobar collapse, obtain further samples for culture, and to exclude an endobronchial abnormality.

Steroids There is no evidence that these are of any benefit in bacterial pneumonia.

Monitoring Temperature, respiratory rate, heart rate, blood pressure, mental status, oxygen saturation, and inspired oxygen concentration should be monitored twice daily, and more often in the severely ill.

ICU admission Those fulfilling criteria for severe CAP on admission, or who fail to respond rapidly to treatment should be considered for transfer for close monitoring, either to a high dependency unit or to ICU. Persisting hypoxia ($PaO_2 \leq 8$ kPa), acidosis, hypercapnia, hypotension, or depressed conscious level, despite maximal therapy, are indications for assisted ventilation. CPAP may be of benefit whilst awaiting for the arrival of the anaesthetist (although this may just be a more effective way of delivering 100% oxygen).

When to discuss patient with CAP with ITU

- Always sooner rather than later
- Respiratory failure ($PaO_2 < 8$ kPa), despite high flow oxygen
- Tiring, with a rising CO_2
- Worsening metabolic acidosis, despite antibiotics and optimum fluid management
- Hypotension despite adequate fluid resuscitation.

CAP: antibiotics

- Most antibiotics are used empirically at diagnosis of CAP, in the absence of microbiological information. The clinical scenario also guides antibiotic choice, such as the addition of anaerobic cover in an alcoholic who has a high chance of aspiration
- Severity assessment guides antibiotic therapy, and the method of antibiotic administration
- Local protocols and antibiotic resistance patterns may also guide choice.

General points

- Early administration of antibiotics is associated with an improved outcome
- Antibiotics given before admission can influence the results of subsequent microbiological investigations, but this should not delay antibiotic administration in the community if the patient is unwell
- It is vital that there is no delay in the administration of the first antibiotic dose in patients admitted to hospital. The admitting doctor should oversee its administration.

  IV antibiotics will be needed in 30–50% of patients admitted to hospital. Consider IV antibiotics if:
  - Severe pneumonia
  - Loss of swallow reflex
  - Impaired absorption
  - Impaired conscious level

  Oral antibiotics should be used in those with community-managed pneumonia, or those with non-severe hospital-managed pneumonia, with no other contraindications.

  Add anaerobic antibiotic cover, e.g. metronidazole if possible aspiration pneumonia in an unconscious patient, or if suspicion of a lung abscess on CXR/CT.
- Switch from IV to oral antibiotics as soon as possible, usually when a patient has shown clear response to treatment, with a normal temperature for 24 hours.

Length of treatment

There is no evidence to guide treatment length, but consensus suggests
- 7 days—non-severe, uncomplicated pneumonia
- 10 days—severe microbiologically undefined pneumonia
- 14–21 days—legionella, staphylococcal, or if Gram-negative pneumonia suspected.

Suggested initial antibiotics for CAP treatment

	Preferred treatment	Alternative (if intolerant of, or allergic to preferred treatment)
Community treatment	amoxicillin 500 mg–1 g tds PO	erythromycin 500 mg qds PO or clarithromycin 500 mg bd PO
Hospital treatment: not severe pneumonia		
Oral	amoxicillin 500 mg–1 g tds PO ± erythromycin 500 mg qds PO or clarithromycin 500 mg bd PO	erythromycin 500 mg qds PO or clarithromycin 500 mg bd PO or levofloxacin 500 mg od PO
If intravenous treatment needed	ampicillin 500 mg qds IV or benzylpenicillin 1.2 g qds IV *plus* erythromycin 500 mg qds IV or clarithromycin 500 mg bd IV	levofloxacin 500 mg od IV
Hospital treatment: severe pneumonia	co-amoxiclav 1.2 g tds IV or cefuroxime 1.5 g tds IV or cefotaxime 1 g tds IV or ceftriaxone 2 g od IV *plus* erythromycin 500 mg qds IV (or clarithromycin 500 mg bd IV)	Levofloxacin 500 mg bd IV *plus* benzylpenicillin 1.2 g qds IV

CAP: treatment failure

A CRP that does not fall by >50% at 4 days suggests either treatment failure, or the development of a complication such as a lung abscess or empyema.

Causes of failure to improve

- Slow clinical response, particularly in the elderly patient
- Incorrect initial diagnosis
  - Pulmonary thromboembolic disease
  - Pulmonary oedema
  - Bronchial carcinoma
  - Bronchiectasis
  - Also consider eosinophilic pneumonia, foreign body aspiration, alveolar haemorrhage, cryptogenic organizing pneumonia, vasculitis or connective tissue disease, drug-induced lung disease
  - Review the history, examination, and radiology
  - Consider repeat imaging, e.g. CT chest.
- Secondary complication
  - Pulmonary, e.g. parapneumonic effusion (occurs in 36–57%, most resolve spontaneously, thoracentesis is recommended), empyema, abscess formation, ARDS
  - Extrapulmonary, e.g. septicaemia, metastatic infection (e.g. meningitis, endocarditis, septic arthritis), sequelae of initial insult, e.g. renal failure, myocardial infarction.
- Inappropriate antibiotics or unexpected pathogen
  - Review dose, compliance, and route of administration. Send further microbiological specimens
  - Review microbiological data, exclude less common pathogens, e.g. legionella, mycoplasma, staphylococcal disease
  - Pathogen may be resistant to common antibiotics; 10% of CAP will have a mixed infection
  - Consider tuberculosis, fungal infection.
- Impaired immunity
  - Systemic, e.g. hypogammaglobulinaemia, HIV infection, myeloma
  - Local, e.g. bronchiectasis, aspiration, underlying bronchial carcinoma
  - Overwhelming infection.

Recommended antibiotic treatment of specific causative organisms

Pathogen	Preferred antibiotic	Alternative antibiotic
Streptococcus pneumoniae	amoxicillin 500 mg–1 g tds PO or benzylpenicillin 1.2 g qds IV	erythromycin 500 mg qds PO or clarithromycin 500 mg bd PO or cefuroxime 0.75–1.5 g tds IV or cefotaxime 1–2 g tds IV or ceftriaxone 2 g od IV
Mycoplasma pneumoniae and Chlamydia pneumoniae	erythromycin 500 mg qds PO / IV or clarithromycin 500 mg bd PO or IV	tetracycline 250–500 mg qds PO or fluoroquinolone PO or IV
Chlamydia psittaci and Chlamydia burnetti	tetracycline 250–500 mg qds PO or 500 mg bd IV	erythromycin 500 mg qds or clarithromycin 500 mg bd, both PO or IV
Legionella species	clarithromycin 500 mg bd PO or IV ± rifampicin 600 mg od or bd, PO or IV	fluoroquinolone PO or IV
Haemophilus influenzae	Non β-lactamase producing amoxicillin 500 mg tds PO or ampicillin 500 mg qds IV β-lactamase producing co-amoxiclav 625 mg tds PO or 1.2 g tds IV	cefuroxime 750 mg–1.5 g tds IV or cefotaxime 1–2 g tds IV or ceftriaxone 2 g od IV or fluoroquinolone PO or IV
Gram-negative enteric bacilli	cefuroxime 1.5 g tds or cefotaxime 1–2 g tds IV or ceftriaxone 1–2 g bd IV	fluoroquinolone IV or imipenem 500 mg qds IV or meropenem 0.5–1.0 g tds IV
Pseudomonas aeruginosa	ciprofloxacin 500–750 mg bd PO ceftazidime 2 g tds IV plus gentamicin or tobramycin (NB therapeutic drug monitoring)	ciprofloxacin 400 mg bd IV or piperacillin 4 g tds plus gentamicin or tobramycin
Staphylococcus aureus	Non MRSA flucloxacillin 1–2 g qds IV ± rifampicin 600 mg od / bd, PO or IV MRSA vancomycin 1 g bd (NB therapeutic drug monitoring)	teicoplanin 400 mg bd IV ± rifampicin 600 mg od or bd PO/IV linezolid 600 mg bd PO/IV

CAP: follow-up

CXR resolution Radiographic improvement lags behind clinical improvement. There is no need to repeat a CXR before hospital discharge in those who have made a satisfactory clinical recovery.
- In one study of CAP, complete radiographic resolution occurred after 6 weeks in 74% of patients, but only in 51% at 2 weeks
- Radiographic resolution is slower in the elderly, those with multilobe involvement at presentation, smokers, and hospital in-patients
- Legionella and pneumococcal pneumonia are slower to resolve (may take 12 weeks or more).

CXR follow-up is recommended around 6 weeks after CAP:
- In all patients with persisting symptoms or clinical signs
- In all patients at higher risk of underlying lung malignancy, i.e. smokers and those over the age of 50.

This is to exclude an underlying condition that may have led to CAP, such as lung cancer. Further investigations such as bronchoscopy should be considered at this time in patients with persisting symptoms and/or a persistently abnormal CXR.
- One study showed lung cancer is diagnosed on follow-up in 17% of smokers aged over 60 treated for CAP in the community
- Other studies have shown an incidence of lung cancer of 11% in current and ex-smokers aged over 50, who are in-patients with CAP and who undergo bronchoscopy prior to discharge.

Vaccination

Influenza vaccination This reduces hospital deaths from pneumonia and influenza by about 65% and respiratory deaths by 45%. It also leads to fewer hospital admissions.
Recommended for 'high risk' individuals
- Chronic lung disease
- Cardiac, renal, and liver disease
- Diabetes
- Immunosuppression due to disease or treatment
- Those aged over 65
- Long stay residential care
- Health care workers
- Contraindicated in people with hen egg hypersensitivity (the virus is cultured in chick embryos).

The vaccination contains both A and B subtype viruses and provides partial protection against influenza illnesses. It is modified annually, based on recent viral strains. The protection rate from influenza by vaccination is over 75% for influenza A and 51–97% for influenza B; it gives protection of around 66%, though antibody levels appear to reduce about 6 years after vaccination.

Pneumococcal vaccination
Recommended for
- Asplenic individuals (including coeliac disease and sickle cell disease)
- Chronic renal, cardiac, and liver disease
- Diabetes
- Immunodeficiency or immunosuppression (due to disease, including HIV infection, or drugs).

It should not be given during acute infection, or in pregnancy.
Re-immunization is contraindicated within 3 years.

Further information

British Thoracic Society Guidelines for the management of community acquired pneumonia in Adults. *Thorax* 2001; **56** S: VI
An updated version of the 2001 guidelines is on the BTS website: *www.brit-thoracic.org.uk/docs/MACAPrevisedApr04.pdf*

Community acquired pneumonia. Thomas MF. *Lancet* 2003; **362**: 1991–2001

Hospital-acquired pneumonia: clinical features

Definition New radiographic infiltrate in the presence of evidence of infection (fever, purulent sputum, leucocytosis) with onset at least 72 hours after hospital admission. It represents around 15% of hospital-acquired infections. Most occur outside the ICU, but those at highest risk are mechanically ventilated patients. Hospital-acquired pneumonia is expensive, and prolongs hospital stay. It requires different antibiotic treatment to community-acquired pneumonia, and is the leading cause of death from hospital-acquired infection. It is also known as nosocomial pneumonia.

Pathophysiology Hospital-acquired pneumonia occurs from haematogenous spread of organisms, aspiration of infected upper airway secretions, or from the inhalation of bacteria from contaminated equipment.

Aspiration is thought to be the most important cause. Around 45% of normal people aspirate during sleep, and this is increased in hospital in-patients (who may be more frail) and in those with chronic disease. These patients' upper airways become colonized with Gram-negative bacteria (in up to 75% within 48 hours of admission) and this proportion is even higher in those who have received broad spectrum antibiotics. In addition, the severely ill may have impaired host defences, making them more susceptible to hospital-acquired pneumonia. Alteration in the gastric pH with illness, and various drugs, mean that the gastrointestinal tract is no longer sterile, thereby providing a potential source of bacterial infection. A cerebrovascular event and reduced conscious level are the major risk factors for aspiration.

Risk factors for nosocomial pneumonia

Age > 70
Chronic lung disease and/or other co-morbidity (especially diabetes)
Reduced conscious level/Cerebrovascular accident
Chest/abdominal surgery
Mechanical ventilation
Nasogastric feeding
Previous antibiotic exposure
Poor dental hygiene
Steroids and cytotoxic drugs

Risk factors for specific organisms

Streptococcus pneumoniae and *Haemophilus influenza*—increased risk in trauma.
Staphylococcus aureus—increased risk in ventilated neurosurgical patients (especially closed head injury), blunt trauma, and coma.
Pseudomonas aeruginosa—increased risk with intubation > 8 days, COPD, prolonged antibiotics.
Acinetobacter species—increased risk with prolonged ventilation and previous broad spectrum antibiotics.
Anaerobic bacteria—increased with recent abdominal surgery, aspiration.

Clinical features It presents typically with:
- Fever
- Productive cough
- Raised inflammatory parameters
- New CXR infiltrate
- Deterioration in gas exchange.

Diagnosis is often a clinical one, and identification of the infecting agent can be difficult, especially if the patient has already received broad spectrum antibiotics.

Investigations
- *CXR* usually shows a non-specific infiltrate
- *Blood, sputum, and pleural fluid* should be cultured
- *Arterial blood gas* to determine severity
- *Renal and liver function tests* to assess other organ dysfunction
- *Serological tests* are of little use in nosocomial pneumonia.

Hospital-acquired pneumonia: management

Severity assessment The CURB or CURB-65 pneumonia severity score (see page 180) for community-acquired pneumonia has not been validated in hospital-acquired pneumonia, but may be useful in guiding the treatment needed.

Microbiology

- About 50% are mixed infections
- 30% are due to aerobic bacteria alone (most commonly Gram-negative bacilli and pseudomonas)
- Anaerobes alone are found in about 25%
- *Pseudomonas aeruginosa* and *Staphylococcus aureus* are common causes
- *Peptostreptococcus, Fusobacteroides,* and *Bacteroides* species are commonly isolated, as well as *Enterobacter* species, *Escherichia coli, Serratia marcescens, Klebsiella,* and *Proteus* species
- *Acinetobacter* is a new emerging pathogen
- MRSA is increasing in prevalence
- Viruses are recognized as causes.

Management

- Patients developing pneumonia within 48 hours of arrival in hospital can be treated with standard community-acquired pneumonia antibiotics (see page 186), as the pneumonia is likely to be due to bacteria acquired in the community
- Patients developing pneumonia more than 48 hours after hospital admission need antibiotics to cover different organisms
- Intravenous, prolonged treatment is usually needed, with cover for Gram-negative anaerobic bacteria. This is best done by using a second-generation cephalosporin, e.g. cefuroxime 750 mg–1.5 g tds, with an aminoglycoside, e.g. gentamicin 7 mg/kg od (unless renal impairment), with levels at 8 to 12 hours, to determine dose interval
- Supportive treatment is also required, with oxygen, fluids, and ventilation if necessary
- In penicillin-allergic patients clindamycin or ciprofloxacin can be used (as long as *Streptococcus pneumoniae* is not thought to be the infecting agent). Levofloxacin has better pneumococcal cover
- Complications of nosocomial pneumonia are the same as for community-acquired pneumonia, including lung abscess and empyema. Drug fever, sepsis with multiorgan failure, and pulmonary embolus with secondary infection are all more common in nosocomial pneumonia
- In this situation, chest ultrasound (to look for empyema) or CT scanning may demonstrate abscess, underlying tumour, or infection at extrathoracic sites.

Prognosis It has a high mortality, ranging between 20 and 50%.

Prevention Meticulous hygiene and hand washing by medical staff, in addition to careful infection control measures have been shown to reduce hospital-acquired pneumonia.

Post-operatively, early mobilization and careful cleaning and maintenance of respiratory equipment, and pre-operative smoking cessation reduce infection rates. Some intensive care units use antibiotics to selectively decontaminate the gastrointestinal tract of Gram-negative bacilli. This has been shown to reduce infection rates, but there is no proven effect on mortality, or length of ITU admission.

Ventilator-acquired pneumonia (VAP)

Definition Pneumonia in a mechanically ventilated patient, which develops 48 hours after intubation. It has a prevalence of up to 65% in some units. It is an independent predictor of mortality, with mortality up to 50% in some series.

The major cause is bacterial contamination of the lower respiratory tract from the aspiration of oropharyngeal secretions, which is not prevented by cuffed endotracheal tube or tracheostomy.

Diagnosis suggested by
- New or progressive CXR infiltrate
- Associated with fever, high WCC, and purulent secretions.

There are many non-infectious causes of fever and CXR infiltrate in ITU patients, so the diagnosis is not always straightforward.

Differential diagnosis of fever and CXR infiltrate in ITU

- Chemical aspiration without infection
- Atelectasis
- ARDS
- Left ventricular failure
- PE with lung infarction
- Pulmonary haemorrhage
- Cryptogenic organizing pneumonia (COP)
- Drug reaction
- Tumour
- Lung contusion.

Investigations
- *CXR* often shows a non-specific infiltrate, with air bronchograms being the best predictor of the disease
- *Airway sampling for microbiology*
  - *Bronchoscopic sampling* Protected specimen brush (PSB) samples (with the tip of the bronchoscope placed opposite the orifice of an involved segmental bronchus, and the PSB advanced through its protective sheath into the airway); or BAL samples (from a sub-segmental bronchus, with the end of the bronchoscope wedged into the airway, ideally >150 ml saline wash) are the best methods to obtain lower airway samples with minimal contamination.

    VAP is diagnosed when an arbitrary threshold of organisms is grown on a BAL or PSB sample. The usual cut-offs are 1000 colony-forming units/ml (cfu/ml) for PSB samples, and >10,000 cfu/ml for BAL samples. The thresholds will vary from unit to unit, and the threshold for starting treatment will also vary. Airway neutrophil counts may also aid in making the diagnosis
  - *Non-bronchoscopic airway sampling*, e.g. blind bronchial sampling of lower respiratory tract secretions, is less sensitive and specific than bronchoscopic sampling. It does not need an expert operator, and is cheaper

- *Serial sampling* is favoured in some units. Regular non-invasive serial airway sampling may aid early diagnosis of VAP. It needs careful interpretation, as the microbiology of the respiratory tract changes over time in critically ill mechanically ventilated patients
- *Tracheal aspiration samples* are easy to obtain, but non-specific in diagnosing VAP, as upper airway colonization is very common.
- Additional sources of fever are common in ventilated patients, including infected lines, sinusitis, urinary tract infection, and pseudomembranous colitis and may warrant further investigation.

Antibiotic treatment Problems with the emergence of resistant bacteria mean that empirical treatment with antibiotics is used less commonly. Local policies are often in place, and advice should always be sought from microbiology.

Risk factors for resistant organisms include:

- Ventilation >7 days
- Prior broad spectrum antibiotic use (e.g. third-generation cephalosporin).

Antibiotics should be chosen on the basis of
- Recent antibiotic treatment
- Local policy and known local flora
- Culture data.

Antibiotics should cover anaerobes and MRSA, Legionella (if long hospital stay), *Pseudomonas aeruginosa*, and *Acinetobacter*.

Failure to respond should lead to a change of antibiotics, and a search for additional infection, or another cause of the radiographic infiltrate. Further cultures should be sent.

Aspiration pneumonia

Definition Pneumonia that follows the aspiration of exogenous material or endogenous secretions into the lower respiratory tract.

Epidemiology Aspiration pneumonia is the commonest cause of death in patients with dysphagia due to neurological disorders, and is the cause of up to 20% of pneumonias in nursing home residents. It occurs in about 10% of patients admitted to hospital with a drug overdose.

Pathophysiology Micro-aspiration is common in healthy individuals, but for an aspiration pneumonia to occur, there must be compromise of the normal defences protecting the lower airways (i.e. glottic closure, cough reflex), with inoculation of the lower respiratory tract of a significant amount of material. Most pneumonias are a result of aspiration of micro-organisms from the oral cavity or nasopharynx.

Situations predisposing to aspiration pneumonia

- *Reduced conscious level* (cough reflex and impaired glottic closure)
  - Alcohol
  - Drug overdose
  - Post-seizure
  - Post-anaesthesia
  - Massive CVA.
- *Dysphagia*
  - Motor neurone disease
  - Following a neurological event; those with impaired swallow reflex post-CVA are seven times more likely to develop a pneumonia than those in whom the gag reflex is unimpaired.
- *Upper gastrointestinal tract disease*
  - Surgery to the stomach or oesophagus
  - Mechanical impairment of glottic or cardiac sphincter closure, e.g. tracheostomy, nasogastric feeding, bronchoscopy.
  - Pharyngeal anaesthesia
- *Increased reflux*
  - Large volume vomiting
  - Large volume nasogastric feed
  - Feeding gastrostomy
  - Recumbent position.
- *Nursing home residents*
  - The risk of aspiration is lower in those without teeth, who receive aggressive oral hygiene
  - There is a higher incidence of silent aspiration in the otherwise healthy elderly
  - High correlation between volume of aspirate and the risk of developing pneumonia.

Aspiration pneumonia: clinical features

Three pulmonary syndromes result from aspiration. The amount and nature of the aspirated material, the site and frequency of the aspiration, and the host's response to it will determine which pulmonary syndome occurs.

1. Chemical pneumonitis

This is aspiration of substances toxic to the lower airways, in the absence of bacterial infection.

This causes a chemical burn of the tracheobronchial tree causing an intense parenchymal inflammatory reaction, with release of inflammatory mediators, that may lead to ARDS. Animal studies show that an inoculum with a pH < 2.5 is needed to initiate an inflammatory reaction, if of a relatively large volume, about 25 ml in adults. Animal models show rapid pathological changes within 3 minutes, with atelectasis, pulmonary haemorrhage, and pulmonary oedema. (This was first described by Mendelson, referring to the aspiration of sterile gastric contents, and its toxic effects. The original case series was in obstetric anaesthesia.)

Clinical features
- Rapid onset of symptoms, with breathlessness (within 1 to 2 hours)
- Low grade fever
- Severe hypoxaemia and diffuse lung infiltrates involving dependent segments
- CXR changes within 2 hours.

Treatment
- If aspiration is observed—suction and/or bronchoscopy to clear aspirated secretions or food. This may not prevent chemical injury from acid, which is similar to a flash burn
- Support of cardiac and respiratory function—with intravenous fluids, oxygen ± ventilation
- Steroids—controversial. No benefit has been shown in human studies, but there is some evidence to support their use in ARDS
- Antibiotics—usually given, even in the absence of evidence of infection, because secondary bacterial infection is common, and may be a contributing, or primary factor in the aspiration. Acid-damaged lung is more susceptible to the effects of secondary bacterial infection; up to 25% will develop secondary bacterial infection. Activity against Gram-negative and anaerobic organisms needed, e.g. cefuroxime plus metronidazole, penicillin plus clindamycin.

2. Bacterial infection
Aspiration of bacteria normally resident in the upper airways or stomach. The normal bacterial flora are anaerobes, in a host susceptible to aspiration, and less virulent than the bacteria causing CAP.

Clinical features depend on the infecting organism:
- Cough, fever, purulent sputum, breathlessness
- The process may evolve over weeks and months rather than hours
- May be more chronic, with weight loss and anaemia
- Absence of fever or rigors

- Foul smelling sputum
- Periodontal disease
- Involvement of dependent pulmonary lobes
- Anaerobic bacteria are more difficult to culture, so may be present, but not identified in microbiological culture
- May present with later manifestations, e.g. empyema, lung abscess.

Major pathogens are *Peptostreptococcus*, *Fusobacterium nucleatum*, *Prevotella* and *Bacteroides* species. Mixed infection is common.

Treatment
- Antibiotics, to include anaerobic cover, e.g. co-amoxiclav or metronidazole plus penicillin
- Swallow assessment / neurological review if no obvious underlying cause found.

3. Mechanical obstruction Aspiration of matter that is not directly toxic to the lung may lead to damage by causing airway obstruction or reflex airway closure. Causative agents include:
- Saline
- Barium
- Most ingested fluids, including water
- Gastric contents with a pH > 2.5
- Mechanical obstruction, such as occurs in drowning, or those who are unable to clear a potential innoculum, e.g. neurological deficit, impaired cough reflex, reduced conscious level
- Inhalation of an object, with the severity of the obstruction depending on the size and site of the aspirated particle. This is commoner in children, but does occur in adults, e.g. teeth, peanuts.

Treatment
- Tracheal suction
- No further treatment is needed if no CXR infiltrates.

Lung abscess: clinical features

Definition A localized area of lung suppuration leading to necrosis of the pulmonary parenchyma, with or without cavity formation.

Lung abscesses may be single or multiple, acute or chronic (>1 month), primary or secondary. They may occur spontaneously, but, more commonly, an underlying disease exists. Lung abscess is now rare in the developed world, but has a high mortality of 20–30%. They are most common in alcoholic men aged >50.

Pathophysiology Most are the result of aspiration pneumonia. Predisposing factors for abscess are those for aspiration pneumonia (page 198).

- Dental disease
- Impaired consciousness—alcohol, post-anaesthesia, dysphagia
- Diabetes
- Bronchial carcinoma (with bronchial obstruction)
- Secondary to pneumonia (cavitation occurs in about 16% of *Staphylococcus aureus* pneumonia)
- Immunocompromise—abscesses due to *Pneumocystis jiroveci* (PCP), *Cryptococcus neoformans*, *Rhodococcus* species, and fungi in HIV positive patients
- Septic embolization (right heart endocarditis due to *Staphylococcus aureus* in intravenous drug abusers).

The bacterial inoculum reaches the lung parenchyma, often in a dependent lung area. Cavitation occurs when parenchymal necrosis leads to communication with the bronchus, with the entry of air and expectoration of necrotic material, leading to the formation of an air fluid level. Bronchial obstruction leads to atelectasis with stasis and subsequent infection, which can predispose to abscess formation.

Presentation

- Often insidious onset
- Productive cough ± haemoptysis
- Breathlessness
- Fevers
- Night sweats
- Non-specific feature of chronic infection—anaemia, weight loss, malaise (especially in the elderly)
- Foul sputum, or purulent pleural fluid.

Lemierre's syndrome (necrobacillosis) Jugular vein suppurative thrombophlebitis. This is a rare pharyngeal infection in young adults, most commonly due to the anaerobe *Fusobacterium necrophorum*. It presents with a classical history of painful pharyngitis, in the presence of bacteraemia. Infection spreads to the neck and carotid sheath, often leading to thrombosis of the internal jugular vein. This may not be obvious clinically (neck vein USS or Doppler may be needed). Septic embolization to the lung with subsequent cavitation, leads to abscess formation. Empyema and abscesses in the bone, joints, liver, and kidneys can complicate.

Lung abscess: diagnosis

The diagnosis is usually made from the history along with the appearance of a cavity with an associated air fluid level on CXR.

Investigations

- *Microbiological culture*, ideally before commencing antibiotics. Useful to exclude tuberculosis
  - Blood cultures
  - Sputum or bronchoscopic specimen (BAL or brushings rarely needed)
  - Transthoracic percutaneous needle aspiration (CT-or ultrasound-guided) may provide samples. Risk of bleeding, pneumothorax and seeding of infection to pleural space, if abscess not adjacent to the pleura.

In practice, blood cultures and sputum microbiology usually suffice. Samples are usually only obtained by more invasive means if appropriate antibiotics are not leading to an adequate clinical response.

- *Imaging*—exclude aspirated foreign body, underlying neoplasm, or bronchial stenosis and obstruction
  - **CXR** may show consolidation, cavitation, air-fluid level (if patient is unwell, the CXR likely to be taken in semi-recumbent position, so an air-fluid level may not be visible). 50% of abscesses are in the posterior segment of the right upper lobe, or the apical basal segments of either lower lobe
  - **CT** is useful if the diagnosis is in doubt and cannot be confirmed from the CXR appearance, or if the clinical response to treatment is inadequate. It can also help to define the exact position of the abscess (which may be useful for physiotherapy, or if surgery is being considered—rarely needed).

CT also is useful to differentiate an abscess from a pleural collection—a *lung abscess* appears as a rounded intrapulmonary mass, with no compression of adjacent lung, with a thickened irregular wall, making an acute angle at its contact with the chest wall. An *empyema* typically has a 'lenticular' shape, and compresses adjacent lung, which creates an obtuse angle as it follows the contour of the chest wall.

CT can determine presence of obstructing endobronchial disease, due to malignancy or foreign body, and may be useful in defining extent of disease in a very sick patient who has had significant haemoptysis. Even with CT, differentiating an abscess from a cavitating malignancy can be very difficult (no radiological features differentiate them).

Microbiology Commonly mixed infection, usually anaerobes.

- The most common organisms are those colonizing the oral cavity and gingival crevices—*Peptostreptococcus*, *Prevotella*, *Bacteroides*, and *Fusobacterium* species
- Aerobes—*Streptococcus milleri*, *Staphylococcus aureus*, *Klebsiella species*, *Streptococcus pyogenes*, *Haemophilus influenzae*, *Nocardia*
- Non-bacterial pathogens are also reported—fungi (*Aspergillus*, *Cryptococcus*, *Histoplasma*, *Blastomyces*) and mycobacteria.

Opportunistic infections in immunocompromised—*Nocardia*, *Mycobacteria*, *Aspergillus*.

Differential diagnosis of a cavitating mass, with or without an air/fluid level

- Cavitating carcinoma—primary or metastatic
- Cavitatory tuberculosis
- Wegener's granulomatosis
- Infected pulmonary cyst or bulla (can produce a fluid level, usually thinner walled)
- Aspergilloma
- Pulmonary infarct
- Rheumatoid nodule
- Sarcoidosis
- Bronchiectasis.

Lung abscess: management

Antibiotics to cover aerobic and anaerobic infection, including β-lactamase inhibitors, e.g. co-amoxiclav and clindamycin. Long courses are needed. Risk of *Clostridium difficile* diarrhoea.
- Infections are usually mixed, therefore antibiotics to cover these
- Metronidazole to cover anaerobes
- No data to guide length of treatment. Common practice would be 1–2 weeks intravenous treatment, with a further 2–6 weeks oral antibiotics, often until out-patient clinic review.

Drainage Spontaneous drainage is common, with the production of purulent sputum. This can be increased with postural drainage and physiotherapy.
- No data to support use of bronchoscopic drainage
- Percutaneous drainage with radiologically placed small percutaneous drains for peripheral abscesses may be useful in those failing to respond to antibiotic and supportive treatment. These are usually placed under ultrasound guidance (though are rarely indicated).

Surgery is rarely required if appropriate antibiotic treatment is given. It is usually reserved for complicated infections, failing to respond to standard treatment, after at least 6 weeks of treatment.
   May be needed if:
- Very large abscess (>6 cm diameter)
- Resistant organisms
- Haemorrhage
- Recurrent disease
- Lobectomy or pneumonectomy is occasionally needed, if severe infection with an abscess leaves a large volume of damaged lung that is hard to sterilize.

Complications Haemorrhage (erosion of blood vessels as the abscess extends into the lung parenchyma). This can be massive and life-threatening (see page 25), and is an indication for urgent surgery.

If slow to respond, consider
- Underlying malignancy
- Unusual microbiology, e.g. mycobacterium, fungi
- Immunosuppression
- Large cavity (>6 cm)—may rarely require drainage
- Non-bacterial cause-e.g. cavitating malignancy, Wegener's granulomatosis
- Other cause of persistent fever, e.g. *Clostridium difficile* diarrhoea, antibiotic-associated fever.

Prognosis 85% cure rate, in the absence of underlying disease. Mortality is reported as high as 75% in immunocompromised patients. The prognosis is much worse in the presence of underlying lung disease, with increasing age and large abscesses (>6 cm) with *Staphylococcus aureus* infection.

Nocardiosis

Definition *Nocardia* are Gram-positive, partially acid-fast, aerobic bacilli that form branching filaments. They are found in soil, decaying organic plant matter, and water, and have been isolated from house dust, garden soil, and swimming pools. Infection typically follows inhalation, although percutaneous inoculation also occurs. The *Nocardia asteroides* species complex accounts for the majority of clinical infections.

Consider *Nocardia* infection when soft-tissue abscesses and/or CNS manifestations occur in the setting of a pulmonary infection. The combination of respiratory, skin, and/or CNS involvement may lead to a misdiagnosis of vasculitis, and the respiratory manifestations may mimic cancer, tuberculosis, or fungal disease.

Epidemiology *Nocardia* occurs worldwide, and the frequency of subclinical exposure is unknown. Clinically apparent infection is rare, and usually occurs in patients with immunocompromise (haematological malignancy, steroid therapy, organ transplant, diabetes, alcoholism, and HIV infection, especially IV drug users) or pre-existing lung disease (particularly pulmonary alveolar proteinosis, tuberculosis). Infection also occurs in apparently healthy people (10–25% of cases). Nosocomial infection and disease outbreaks have been reported.

Clinical features

Pulmonary disease
- The lung is the most common site of involvement
- Patients typically present with productive cough, fever, anorexia, weight loss, and malaise; dyspnoea, pleuritic pain, and haemoptysis may occur but are less common
- Empyema occurs in up to a quarter of cases, and direct intrathoracic spread causing pericarditis, mediastinitis, rib osteomyelitis, or SVCO is also reported.

Extrapulmonary disease
- Dissemination from the lungs occurs in 50% of patients
- Central nervous system is the most common site of dissemination, occurring in 25% of pulmonary nocardiosis cases. Single or multiple abscesses occur, and may be accompanied by meningitis
- Other sites include the skin and subcutaneous tissues, kidneys, bone, joints and muscle, peritoneum, eyes, pericardium, and heart valves.

Investigations
- Identification by smear and culture is the principal method of diagnosis. *Nocardia* grow on routine media usually within 2–7 days, although more prolonged culture (2–3 weeks) may be required
- Direct smear of appropriate specimens (e.g. aspirates of abscesses, biopsies) is highly sensitive and typically shows Gram-positive, beaded branching filaments, which are usually acid-fast on modified ZN stain. Examination of BAL fluid may also be diagnostic

- Sensitivity testing of isolates and identification to species level is done by reference laboratories
- Biopsies typically show a mixed cellular infiltrate; granulomata occur rarely, and may result in misdiagnosis as tuberculosis or histoplasmosis
- CXR and CT may demonstrate parenchymal infiltrates, single or multiple nodules (sometimes with cavitation), or features of pleural infection
- Sputum smear is usually unhelpful. Sputum culture has a greater yield but *Nocardia* growth may be obscured in mixed cultures. The significance of *Nocardia* growth on sputum culture in asymptomatic patients is unclear; it may represent contamination or colonization in the setting of underlying lung disease
- Blood cultures are almost always negative, although *Nocardia* bacteraemia may occur in the setting of profound immunocompromise
- Consider MRI of the brain to exclude asymptomatic CNS involvement in patients with pulmonary nocardiosis.

Management

- Discuss treatment with an infectious diseases specialist
- Drug treatment choices include sulphonamides/co-trimoxazole, minocycline, imipenem, cefotaxime, ceftriaxone, or amikacin. Sulpha drugs, in particular co-trimoxazole, have traditionally been the mainstay of therapy. Imipenem and amikacin combination therapy has been shown to be active *in vitro* and in animal models, and is recommended for pulmonary nocardiosis and for very ill patients. Extended spectrum cephalosporins such as ceftriaxone and cefotaxime have the advantages of good CNS penetration and low toxicity
- Optimal treatment duration is unclear: typically given for 6 months in non-immunocompromised patients, and for 12 months or longer for CNS involvement or immunocompromised patients
- Surgery may be required for abscess drainage.

Prognosis Clinical outcome is dependent on the site and extent of disease and on underlying host factors. Disease remissions and exacerbations are common. Cure rates are approximately 90% in pleuropulmonary disease, and 50% in brain abscess. Mortality of *Nocardia* infection is generally low, although it approaches 50% in cases of bacteraemia.

Further information

Nocardiosis: review of clinical and laboratory experience. Saubolle MA, Sussland D. *J Clin Micro* 2003; **41**: 4497–01

Nocardiosis. Lerner Pl. *Clin Inf Dis* 1996; **22**; 891–905

Actinomycosis

Definition Actinomycosis is caused by a group of anaerobic Gram-positive bacilli, of which *Actinomyces israelii* is the commonest. These organisms are present in the mouth, gastrointestinal tract, and vagina. Clinical infection may follow dental procedures or aspiration of infected secretions. Infection is slowly progressive and may disseminate via the bloodstream or invade tissue locally, sometimes resulting in sinus tract formation.

Consider this diagnosis particularly in patients with pulmonary disease accompanied by soft tissue infection of the head and neck. The diagnosis of actinomycosis is often unsuspected, and the clinical and radiological features may mimic cancer, tuberculosis, or fungal disease.

Epidemiology Actinomycosis is rare. It can occur at any age, and is more common in men. Predisposing factors include corticosteroid use, chemotherapy, organ transplant, and HIV infection.

Clinical features

Thoracic disease Thoracic disease occurs in about 15% of cases. Symptoms of pulmonary involvement are non-specific, and include cough, chest pain, haemoptysis, fever, anorexia, and weight loss. Chest wall involvement may occur, with sinus formation or rib infection, and empyema is common. Mediastinal involvement is documented.

Extrathoracic disease Soft tissue infection of the head and neck, particularly the mandible, is the commonest disease presentation (about 50% of cases). Discharging sinuses may form. Other extrathoracic disease sites include the abdomen (particularly the ileocaecal region), pelvis, liver, bone, and CNS (manifest as single or multiple abscesses).

Investigations
- CXR and CT appearances are variable, including masses (sometimes with cavitation), parenchymal infiltrates, consolidation, mediastinal disease, and/or pleural involvement
- Diagnosis is based on the microscopy and anaerobic culture of infected material. Warn the microbiology laboratory if the diagnosis is suspected, as specific stains and culture conditions are required. Examination of infected material may reveal yellow 'sulphur granules' containing aggregated organisms. Sample sputum, pleural fluid, and pus from sinus tracts; inoculate into anaerobic transport media, and rapidly transport to lab. Endobronchial biopsies have a low sensitivity. Most infections are polymicrobial, with accompanying aerobic or anaerobic bacteria.

Management
- Discuss treatment with an infectious diseases specialist
- Drug treatment choices include penicillin, amoxycillin, clindamycin, or erythromycin. Administration should initially be intravenous. Optimal treatment duration is unclear (typically given for 6–12 months)
- Surgery may be required for abscess drainage
- Monitor response to treatment with serial CT or MRI scans
- Treat any associated periodontal disease.

Prognosis Disease relapse is common if prolonged treatment is not administered.

Further information
Pulmonary actinomycosis. Mabeza GF and Mcfarlane J. *Eur Respir J* 2003; **21**: 545–51

Anthrax

Definition and epidemiology

- *Bacillus anthracis* is an aerobic, Gram-positive spore-forming bacterium that causes human disease, principally following either inhalation or cutaneous contact. Spores can survive in soil for many years. Person-to-person transmission does not occur
- Considerable recent interest has focused on the use of anthrax in bioterrorism: five envelopes containing anthrax spores were sent through the US postal service in 2001, and there were 11 confirmed cases of inhalational anthrax (including 5 deaths) and 7 confirmed cases of cutaneous anthrax. A previous outbreak occurred in Sverdlovsk in the former Soviet Union in 1979, following the release of spores from a biological weapons plant, and resulted in 68 deaths
- Anthrax infection also occurs very rarely in association with occupational exposure to *Bacillus anthracis* in animal wool or hides. The majority of occupational cases result in cutaneous disease, and a diagnosis of inhalational anthrax strongly suggests a bioterrorist attack.

Clinical features

Inhalational anthrax

- Incubation period is variable, although in the USA in 2001 it typically ranged 4–6 days following exposure from opening mail
- Patients typically experience a prodrome of flu-like symptoms such as fever and cough. Gastrointestinal symptoms (vomiting, diarrhoea, abdominal pain), drenching sweats, and altered mental status are often prominent symptoms. Breathlessness, fever, and septic shock develop several days later. Haemorrhagic meningitis is a common complication
- Large haemorrhagic pleural effusions are a characteristic feature.

Cutaneous anthrax

- Initial symptoms include itch and development of a papule at the infection site. A necrotic ulcer with a black centre and often surrounding oedema subsequently develops. Systemic symptoms such as fever and sweats may be present.

Investigations

- *Bacillus anthracis* grows on conventional media, and is readily cultured if sampling precedes antibiotic treatment; a definitive diagnosis requires specialized laboratory tests, however
- Blood tests typically reveal leucocytosis
- Blood cultures are positive in nearly all cases of inhalational anthrax when taken prior to antibiotic treatment. Staining and culture of pleural fluid may be diagnostic
- CXR in inhalational anthrax classically shows a widened mediastinum; pleural effusions and pulmonary infiltrates may be present. CT may also demonstrate mediastinal and hilar lymphadenopathy
- Gram stain and culture of the ulcer is usually diagnostic in cutaneous anthrax, although biopsy is sometimes required.

Management

- Discuss with infectious diseases and public health specialists if the diagnosis is suspected
- Antibiotic treatment should be administered immediately after taking blood cultures. Recent recommendations are for initial treatment with either ciprofloxacin or doxycycline IV, in combination with 1–2 additional antibiotics (choices include clindamycin, vancomycin, meropenem, or penicillin). Subsequent treatment should be with either ciprofloxacin or doxycycline orally for 60–100 days. Oral treatment alone may be sufficient in cases of mild cutaneous disease
- Corticosteroid treatment should be considered in patients with meningitis, or severe neck or mediastinal oedema
- Supportive care, including ventilatory support, treatment of shock with intravenous fluids and/or inotropes, and chest tube drainage of large pleural effusions may be needed.

Prognosis Inhalational anthrax is associated with a high mortality: 5 of the recent 11 cases in the USA died. The mortality of previously documented cases has been even higher, perhaps reflecting a delay or lack of antibiotic treatment.

Prophylaxis Recent USA recommendations advise prophylaxis with oral ciprofloxacin or doxycycline for individuals considered to have been exposed to anthrax spores in contaminated areas. A vaccine is available, although its value in post-exposure prophylaxis is unknown.

Viral respiratory infection

Viral pneumonia: overview

- Viral upper respiratory tract infections are common but typically self-limiting, and are usually managed in the community. Viral pneumonia is much less common but is more serious and usually requires hospitalization. Viral pneumonia in the immunocompetent is rare and typically affects children or the elderly; influenza strains are the commonest cause in adults
- Viruses may also cause serious respiratory infection in the immunocompromised (particularly patients with depressed T-cell function, e.g. following organ transplantation). CMV is the commonest serious viral pathogen that affects immunocompromised patients. Influenza, parainfluenza, RSV, measles, and adenovirus may also cause pneumonia in the immunocompromised, although diagnosis of these viruses is difficult and infection is commonly undetected
- The clinical and radiological features of viral pneumonia are non-specific. Worsening cough and breathlessness following an upper respiratory tract infection suggest the development of pneumonia; wheeze may accompany bronchiolitis. CXR typically shows non-specific diffuse, interstitial infiltrates, and hypoxia may occur. Secondary bacterial infection may complicate viral pneumonia
- A variety of diagnostic techniques are available, including viral culture and immunofluorescence staining (e.g. of BAL fluid), and serology
- Treatment consists of supportive care and in some cases antivirals. Infection with certain viruses may require isolation. Treat secondary bacterial infection with antibiotics
- Specific features of the common and/or important viruses are noted below and in the remainder of the chapter.

Influenza

- Commonest cause of viral pneumonia in immunocompetent adults. It is transmitted via respiratory secretions and is extremely contagious
- Two pathogenic serotypes: A and B. Type A causes more severe disease and occurs in annual epidemics and intermittent pandemics. Type B causes epidemics. Sporadic cases may also occur
- The surface antigens haemagglutinin and neuraminidase determine influenza serotype. Genetic mutations may result in antigenic shifts (major genetic rearrangements between strains, associated with pandemics) and antigenic drifts (more minor genetic variations associated with epidemics). Genetic rearrangement of virus occurs in animal and bird reservoirs, and the virus may then be transferred to humans, e.g. avian strains H5N1 and H9N2 have recently infected individuals in Hong Kong, raising fears of a new pandemic
- May affect previously well individuals, although occurs more commonly in the setting of chronic lung disease, immunocompromise, and in the elderly and institutionalized. Mitral stenosis may particularly increase susceptibility.

Clinical features The clinical picture following infection is very variable: asymptomatic, 'flu' (myalgia, fevers, cough), bronchitis/bronchiolitis, pneumonia (either primary from influenza virus itself, or secondary from bacterial infection), ARDS. Progresses very rapidly.

Diagnosis is often made clinically based on knowledge of a local outbreak. Diagnostic investigations include viral culture, immunofluorescence or ELISA of nasopharyngeal washes, throat swabs, sputum, or lung tissue. Rapid, effective PCR-based tests are becoming available.

Treatment In addition to supportive care, antiviral treatment of pneumonia with amantadine or rimantadine may shorten the duration of illness if started within 48 hours of symptom onset. Early treatment with inhaled zanamivir or oral oseltamivir may also shorten symptom duration. Treat secondary bacterial infection.

Vaccination

- The influenza inactivated vaccine is modified annually based on recent viral strains, and provides partial protection against influenza illness, hospitalization, and death. Vaccination if age > 65, chronic co-morbidity, nursing home residents, or health workers. The benefits of vaccination to asthmatics are uncertain
- Administration of amantadine or rimantadine to high-risk individuals throughout periods of exposure may also prevent infection
- Live attenuated influenza vaccines are currently under investigation.

Respiratory syncytial virus

- Very common cause of bronchiolitis and pneumonia in children. Role in adult respiratory disease is more significant than previously appreciated, and infection often goes unrecognized
- Adult infection occurs particularly in the setting of underlying cardiac or respiratory disease or malignancy; outbreaks affecting adults in hospitals and nursing homes also occur. RSV may be a relatively common viral cause of pneumonia in patients who have recently undergone bone marrow transplantation
- Bronchoscopy with BAL is often diagnostic: detection of RSV antigen in BAL fluid has a sensitivity of nearly 90%. PCR-based diagnostic techniques are being investigated
- Bacterial superinfection may be a frequent complication
- Treatment is principally supportive. Role of aerosolized ribavirin and steroids in the treatment of severe disease in adults is unclear. Reports of successful outcomes in bone marrow transplant recipients following treatment with ribavirin and immunoglobulin.

Further information

Respiratory viral infections in adults. Greenberg SB. *Curr Opin Pulm Med* 2002; **8**: 201–8

Cytomegalovirus pneumonia

Epidemiology
- CMV is the commonest serious viral pathogen in the immunocompromised, and is a particular problem following transplantation, where prophylaxis is now widely used
- Individuals are described as 'seropositive' for CMV if they have evidence of IgG antibodies indicating latent infection following previous exposure; seropositivity increases with age. Infection in transplant recipients results from either transmission from a CMV-positive donor to a CMV antibody-negative recipient (via the organ or a blood transfusion) or reactivation of latent CMV in a seropositive recipient as a result of immunosuppression
- Infection occurs most frequently during the first 4 months following organ or bone marrow transplantation, corresponding to the period of maximal T-cell suppression. Graft-versus-host disease increases the risk of CMV infection.

Clinical and laboratory features
- 'Flu-like' symptoms in immunocompetent patients
- Symptoms of CMV pneumonia in the immunocompromised are non-specific: fever, dry cough, dyspnoea, and malaise
- Extrapulmonary manifestations of CMV infection (e.g. gastro-oesophagitis; hepatitis) may suggest the diagnosis
- Hypoxia may occur. Leucopenia, thrombocytopenia, and abnormal liver function tests are characteristic.

Imaging
- *CXR* typically bilateral diffuse interstitial infiltrate, although lobar consolidation and localized haziness also described; can be normal. A nodular infiltrate may suggest co-infection with *Aspergillus*
- *CT* features include localized or diffuse ground-glass and nodular shadowing that may progress to airspace consolidation.

Diagnosis Antibody tests are used to estimate risk following transplantation, but diagnosis of active disease requires evidence of either viraemia (by antigen or PCR testing of blood) or tissue invasion (by biopsy). A wide range of diagnostic tests are available, and the choice of tests varies between centres—discuss with your local virologist. The nature of the transplant and immunosuppression also influence the interpretation of test results. Methods include:
- Early antigen fluorescence test on BAL fluid (high sensitivity, low specificity)
- Qualitative PCR on blood or BAL fluid (highly sensitive, but unable to differentiate between latent and replicating CMV; negative result practically excludes the diagnosis, positive result is unhelpful)
- CMV antigenaemia on blood (rapid, differentiates between latent and replicating virus)
- Quantitative PCR on blood or BAL fluid (rapid, differentiates between latent and replicating virus)

- Indirect immunofluorescence with monoclonal antibodies to CMV in BAL fluid (rapid, highly sensitive, and specific)
- Histology of lung tissue from transbronchial or surgical biopsies (demonstrate CMV inclusion bodies—the 'owl's eye' appearance—within infected cells; considered gold standard investigation).

In some cases a definitive diagnosis is not possible, and treatment is empirical.

Treatment Ganciclovir 5 mg/kg IV bd for 2–4 weeks (side-effects include neutropenia, anaemia). Consider additional treatment with anti-CMV hyperimmune globulin or prolonged oral valganciclovir in cases of severe or relapsed disease. Foscarnet 60 mg/kg tds for 2–3 weeks is an alternative to ganciclovir for resistant cases, but toxicity (nephrotoxicity, metabolic disturbance) can limit treatment.

Complications

- Opportunistic infection (e.g. PCP, aspergillosis), due to further suppression of T-cell function by the CMV infection itself
- Increased risk of organ rejection, as allografts are more susceptible to CMV infection than native organs.

Outcome The reported mortality from CMV pneumonia varies, although may be as high as 85%. Relapse occurs in up to one-third of patients.

Varicella pneumonia

- Pneumonia occurs in a small proportion of adults with chicken pox or shingles. Risk factors for its development include pregnancy, steroid treatment, and immunocompromise
- There is typically a history of recent exposure to a contact infected with chicken pox or shingles. Chest symptoms tend to occur several days after the onset of rash (erythematous macules progressing to papules and then vesicles). Cough is common, and pleuritic pain and haemoptysis may occur
- CXR typically shows a diffuse small nodular infiltrate; hilar lymphadenopathy and pleural effusions may uncommonly occur. Nodules may subsequently calcify and persist
- Multiorgan involvement may occur
- Diagnosis is usually suspected on the basis of the history of exposure, presence of rash, and CXR features. Cytological examination of smears from skin lesions, serology, or viral culture or PCR on BAL fluid may confirm the diagnosis
- Treatment of varicella pneumonia is with early administration of aciclovir 10–12.5 mg/kg, IV tds for 7 days. Varicella is very infectious until lesions enter the 'crusting' stage; in-patients should be isolated. Consider zoster immune globulin for immunocompromised patients exposed to varicella
- Most cases resolve spontaneously, but a minority progress to respiratory failure and death. Mortality may be as high as 40% in pregnancy.

Measles

- Very rare in adults. Bronchiolitis and pneumonia affect 50% of patients infected with measles, and are a common cause of mortality in children
- Symptoms of fever and upper respiratory tract infection are followed by a diffuse maculopapular rash. Leucopenia is common
- CXR may show reticulonodular infiltrates, hilar lymphadenopathy, and pleural effusions
- Secondary bacterial infection is common
- Treatment is supportive. Treat secondary bacterial infection with antibiotics.

Hantavirus pulmonary syndrome

- Hantavirus pulmonary syndrome was first described following an outbreak in the south-western USA in 1993. Several different hantaviruses (e.g. Sin Nombre virus) have been associated with this syndrome. Previously described hantavirus-associated diseases occurred more commonly in Scandinavia and north-eastern Asia, and tended to cause haemorrhagic fever and renal failure with relative sparing of the lung
- Very rare, and affected individuals are almost exclusively from the USA, particularly from the 'Four Corners Region' where Arizona, Colorado, Utah, and New Mexico meet
- Disease develops following inhalation of aerosolized viruses from rodent faeces, urine, or saliva
- Typically affects previously well young adults
- Common presenting symptoms are fever, chills, cough, myalgia, and gastrointestinal symptoms such as vomiting and abdominal pain. Breathlessness occurs later in the disease course, and is often quickly followed by respiratory failure and the development of ARDS. Shock may occur and is associated with a poor prognosis
- Laboratory testing classically reveals neutrophilia and thrombocytopenia, sometimes with renal impairment and mildly abnormal liver function tests
- CXR typically shows initially bilateral, basal infiltrates that progress to involve all regions of the lung; a minority are normal
- The diagnosis may be confirmed using serology, PCR for the virus, or by detection of viral antigen using immunochemistry
- Treatment is supportive within an intensive care unit. It is unclear if person-to-person transmission occurs, and patients should be in respiratory isolation. Intravenous ribavirin is commonly administered, although it is unclear if this improves outcome
- Mortality 30–50%, with death usually occurring within several days of presentation.

Severe acute respiratory syndrome (SARS): epidemiology and pathophysiology

This rapidly progressive acute respiratory illness was first recognized in November 2002, in the Guangdong Province of China. By late February 2003 it had spread internationally. It was termed SARS by the World Health Organisation (WHO), whose involvement has been (in association with health authorities from the United States, Canada, Singapore, Hong Kong, and other Asian countries) to determine an aetiology, establish infection control measures to prevent further spread, establish a laboratory test for diagnosis, and evaluate treatments.

Epidemiology Cases of SARS were first recognized in the Guangdong province of China in November 2002, with 792 cases reported by February 2003. This first outbreak mainly affected health care workers and their contacts. The disease spread to Hong Kong via a Guangdong province physician, who infected individuals in a Hong Kong hotel lift. The disease rapidly spread to Singapore, Thailand, Vietnam, and Canada via travellers from Guangdong province and Hong Kong. Case numbers fell by mid May 2003, and by July 2003, the worldwide epidemic had ended. Further cases have subsequently been reported. An isolated case of laboratory-acquired SARS was reported in Singapore in September 2003. A further laboratory outbreak occurred in March 2004, with serologically proven infection in four individuals working at the same institute in Beijing.

A total of 8422 cases were reported to the WHO by August 2003, with 916 deaths, giving a case fatality rate of 11%. The fatality rate for those aged ≥60 was 43%. 29 countries were affected in Asia, Europe, and North America, with 83% of the worldwide cases in China and Hong Kong. No deaths occurred in the United States or the UK, with 41 deaths (of 251 cases) in Canada.

Case definition The WHO defined criteria for those presenting with the disease after July 2004:
- Fever > 38 °C *plus*
- One or more symptom of lower respiratory tract illness (cough, difficulty breathing, shortness of breath) *plus*
- Radiographic evidence of lung infiltrate consistent with pneumonia or ARDS, *or* autopsy findings consistent with the pathology of pneumonia *or* ARDS without identifiable cause *plus*
- No alternative diagnosis to explain the illness.

Laboratory case definition
- A person with symptoms or signs suggestive of SARS *plus*
- Positive laboratory findings for SARS-CoV based on one or more of:
  - PCR positive for SARS-CoV
  - Seroconversion by ELISA or IFA
  - Virus isolation.

Testing should only be undertaken in a national or regional reference laboratory, as per WHO recommendations.

Pathophysiology A novel, previously undescribed *coronavirus* (SARS-CoV) is thought to be the causal agent. It is still to be ascertained whether microbiological and other cofactors enhance severity or transmissibility. The complete genetic sequence of the SARS-CoV has now been determined. It is currently thought that animals act as the main reservoir.

SARS is mostly spread by large droplets and person to person contact. There have been no reports of food- or water-borne transmission. However, SARS-CoV is shed in large quantities in stool, and profuse watery diarrhoea is a common symptom. Nosocomial transmission of SARS-CoV has been a striking feature in most outbreaks. The use of aerosol generating procedures (endotracheal intubation, nebulization, bronchoscopy) may amplify transmission.

Incubation period is 2–10 days prior to the onset of the first symptom, which is typically fever.

SARS: clinical features and management

Clinical features The disease is a two-stage illness, commencing with a prodrome of fever (>38°C), with or without rigors, with non-specific systemic symptoms, e.g. malaise, headache, and myalgia.

The respiratory stage of the illness starts 3–7 days after the prodromal phase with dry cough and breathlessness. Progression to respiratory failure needing ventilation is well recognized. Up to 70% of patients develop large volume watery diarrhoea without blood or mucus.

Destruction of lung tissue is thought to result from an excessive immune response to the virus, rather than from the direct effects of virus replication. The peak viral load is at day 10 of infection, with virus shed not only in respiratory secretions, but in faeces and other body fluids.

Children experience a milder form of the disease, with a low death rate.

Investigations The illness is a symptom complex, and the case definition is broad. The diagnosis is made on the basis of the clinical syndrome and the absence of positive bacteriology and virology. SARS is a diagnosis of exclusion.

Recommended investigations in a suspected case include

- Blood tests
    - White blood count is normal or reduced, with a low total lymphocyte count (in 98% in the Hong Kong case series)
    - Leucopenia and thrombocytopenia are also recognized, with raised creatine kinase (CK) and alanine transferase (ALT). A raised lactate dehydrogenase (LDH) is associated with a poorer outcome.
- Chest X-ray ranges from normal to diffuse bilateral interstitial infiltrate. Areas of focal consolidation are also described
- CT may reveal areas of interstitial infiltrate in those with a normal CXR. Spontaneous pneumothorax, pneumomediastinum, subpleural fibrosis, and/or cystic changes can occur in later stages
- SARS-CoV can be detected by RT-PCR (sensitivity 70%, dependent on specimen type and duration of illness). An initial positive result on PCR must be confirmed by another clinical sample, re-extracting and testing the original sample, and using assays that target different parts of the genome. However, identification of seroconversion on a whole virus immunoassay remains the gold standard for the retrospective virological confirmation of the disease. Agreement has been reached between international agencies to share specimens and laboratory data to develop a diagnostic test as soon as possible. Work to standardize PCR and ELISA testing for the SARS virus is ongoing.

Treatment

- There is no specific treatment for SARS other than general supportive care
- Some patients have been treated with oseltamivir and/or intravenous ribavirin
- Steroids lead to reduced fever, improved oxygenation and CXR appearance, but do not alter need for ITU, or the death rate at 3 weeks

- A series from Toronto showed a trend towards worsening outcome in those treated with ribavirin, due to elevated transaminases and haemolysis. There is no *in vitro* data to show any anti-SARS virus activity of ribavirin
- Experimental animal models show reduced viral replication with peglycated interferon alpha, and human studies using interferon and corticosteroids have shown no adverse effects
- Some studies show benefit from therapy with high-dose methyl prednisolone given in the later stages of the illness; however, randomized placebo-controlled trials are awaited
- Vaccinations are being developed.

Hospital admission Nosocomial transmission of SARS-CoV has been a striking feature in most outbreaks. Infected and suspected cases should be managed in negative pressure side rooms. Full protective clothing, including protective eye wear and face masks are recommended for all visitors and health care workers. The use of aerosol generating procedures should be avoided where possible.

Prognosis Older age is associated with a poorer outcome, with diabetes and other co-morbid illness being independent risk factors for death.

Prevention The mainstay of treatment has been in the maintenance of avoidance of exposure and effective infection control measures. Closure of hospitals and schools in affected areas and the use of quarantine measures helped to limit the spread of the disease in a number of countries.

At the height of the epidemic, the WHO and many governments advised against non-essential travel to affected areas. This had a significant economic impact on tourism to these areas. Travel limitation advice ended in July 2003.

Further information

The severe acute respiratory syndrome. Peiris JSM, Yuen KY, *et al*. *NEJM* 2003; **349**: 2431–41

WHO website for continuously updated information: *www.who.int/csr/sars/en*

Mycobacterial respiratory infection

Tuberculosis (TB): epidemiology and pathophysiology

Tuberculosis is the second leading infectious cause of death worldwide (after AIDS), killing around 2 million people per year. This is despite it being a potentially curable disease. Rising rates of HIV and immigration mean that TB remains a large part of the workload for respiratory physicians in some parts of the UK. The disease is a great mimicker, and should often be considered as a differential diagnosis.

Epidemiology The highest incidence is in sub-Saharan Africa (290 cases per 100,000 population). High population density countries in Asia (India, China, Pakistan, and Indonesia) account for half the global burden. The countries comprising the former Soviet Union have rapidly increasing rates, because of economic decline, and failing health services, with around 10% multidrug resistance in this area. Globally, around 11% of TB cases are co-infected with HIV, with this number increasing to 38% in sub-Saharan Africa, and less than 1% in India and China.

In the UK, 37% of TB cases are in Caucasians (usually over the age of 50), with 56% in people born abroad (median age of 30). At least 3% of cases are co-infected with HIV.

Pathophysiology The disease is spread by airborne droplets, containing *Mycobacterium tuberculosis* (MTB). Droplets can remain airborne for hours after expectoration, because of their small size. Infectious droplets are inhaled and become lodged in the distal airways.

MTB is taken up by alveolar macrophages, with either successful containment of the infection, or progression to primary disease (primary progressive TB).

MTB replicates following ingestion by alveolar macrophages, with spread via the lymphatics to hilar lymph nodes. Cell-mediated immunity leads to granuloma formation by activated T lymphocytes and macrophages, which limits further bacterial replication and disease spread. Unless there is a deficiency in cell-mediated immunity, active disease may never occur.

Active disease occurs when the host's immune response is unable to contain MTB replication, occurring most often in the lung parenchyma and hilar lymph nodes. It can occur in any organ, from haematogenous spread. This is most common in young children, and in immunosuppressed adults.

Many factors influence whether or not infection leads to active disease, including age, host immunity, and time since infection. The estimated lifetime risk of clinical disease of a child newly infected with MTB is about 10%.

Most disease in adults is due to reactivation of childhood disease, so-called 'post primary disease', from activation of latent TB lying dormant in the (usually) lung Gohn's focus.

Main risk factors for active TB in the UK:

1. Place and date of birth:
   Caucasian population, increasing prevalence with age (M > F)
   Black immigrants, highest prevalence in the young (M = F)
   Indian subcontinent, highest prevalence in middle age (M = F)
2. HIV/AIDS
3. Poverty—1 in 50 homeless people in London have TB
4. Medical factors—diabetes, renal disease, malignant disease, systemic chemotherapy, steroids and new TNFα antagonists e.g. infliximab. Also smoking and vitamin D deficiency (a relationship between the vitamin D receptor and interleukin-1 levels is postulated).

Smear positive=
Acid-fast bacilli (AFB) seen on sputum smear (Ziehl–Neelson stain), potentially infectious. Patient may need to be isolated.

Culture positive=
AFB not seen on smear. TB grown on culture (may take up to 9 weeks). Much less infectious.

TB: pulmonary disease

Symptoms

Most cases present with pulmonary disease, classically:
- Productive cough
- Haemoptysis
- Breathlessness
- Systemic symptoms—weight loss, night sweats, and malaise
- Chest pain.

Haemoptysis is more common with cavitary disease, and many (2/3rds) will be smear positive. Most haemoptysis is small volume. Massive haemoptysis is rare, and is most common as a consequence of destruction of a lobe, with consequent bronchiectasis formation (possibly with secondary aspergillus infection or mycetoma in a healed TB cavity). This is seen in those untreated in the pre-chemotherapy era. Most haemoptysis will resolve with antituberculous chemotherapy.

Signs are often non-specific.
- Examination may be normal
- Lymphadenopathy (particularly cervical)
- Crackles
- Signs of a pleural effusion
- Signs of consolidation (with extensive disease)
- Signs of weight loss/underlying immunocompromise
- Look for evidence of extrapulmonary disease, e.g. skin, joints, CNS, retina, and spinal disease.

Complications Long-term sequelae of inadequately treated infection include:
- **Bronchiectasis**, bronchial obstruction, and airway stenosis (uncommon) may result from endobronchial disease, though this is much less common in the post-chemotherapy era. It is more common in the presence of extensive parenchymal disease, and is associated with lymph node enlargement with compromise of airway size
- **Pleural disease** is due either to primary progressive disease or reactivation of latent infection. It probably represents an increased immune response—a delayed type hypersensitivity reaction to mycobacterial antigens, rather than a diminished one, which is the case in other forms of TB infection. Culture is more likely from pleural tissue than fluid (where the organism burden is lower). See page 312
- **Pneumothorax** is rare (<1% in the developed world) and results from the rupture of a peripheral cavity. Can lead to the formation of a bronchopleural fistula
- **Draining abscess**
- **Right middle lobe syndrome**—compression of the right middle lobe bronchus by hilar lymph nodes leads to lobar collapse
- The previous treatment with **thoracoplasty** can lead to respiratory failure in later life, due to compromised vital capacity.

TB: extrapulmonary disease

Extrapulmonary disease is seen in about 20% of HIV seronegative patients. This proportion is higher in HIV positive patients.

The tuberculin skin test (see page 232) is more often positive in extrapulmonary disease, as this most commonly represents reactivation disease, and less commonly primary disease. Anergy is more likely in those with poor nutritional status, underlying disease (including HIV), and the elderly.

CNS disease This is the most serious manifestation, and includes meningeal involvement and space-occupying lesions (tuberculoma) that lead to cranial nerve lesions.

The clinical manifestations are due to the presence of MTB, and the host's immune response to it.

TB meningitis presents with headache, fever, altered conscious level, and focal neurological signs, including cranial nerve palsies. Fits are not uncommon.

CSF contains lymphocytes, high protein, and low glucose. PCR of CSF may be useful, but is not 100% sensitive.

Pericardial TB The yield is low from pericardial fluid and biopsy. 85% have a positive tuberculin test. A large effusion may lead to cardiac tamponade, and may need to be drained.

Spinal disease can affect any bone or joint; spine involvement (Pott's disease) is most common in the thoracic spine. Surgery may be needed if there is evidence of cord compression or instability.

GU disease from seeding during haematogenous spread.
Involvement of the renal and genital tracts is uncommon.

In men—may cause prostatitis and epididymitis.

In women—genitourinary TB is a cause of infertility. Sterile pyuria (white and red blood cells in the urine, in the absence of bacterial infection) may indicate TB infection.

Peripheral cold abscess can occur at almost any body site.

Disseminated disease is more common in immunosuppressed individuals. Pulmonary disease is typically a miliary (millet seed) pattern, but pulmonary disease is not universal in disseminated disease. This has a higher mortality than localized disease.

TB: investigations

The diagnosis is usually made in one of three ways: sputum (or other sample, e.g. pus, CSF, urine, a minimum of three samples) *smear, culture*, or the identification of tissue *caseating granulomas*.

- *CXR* classically shows upper lobe infiltrates with cavitation. May be associated with hilar or paratracheal lymphadenopathy

  May show changes consistent with prior TB infection, with fibrous scar tissue and calcification.

  HIV infected patients typically have less florid CXR changes, and are less likely to have cavitary disease. Miliary pattern is more common in later stages of AIDS

- *Sputum Ziehl–Neelson (ZN) stain and culture* is required for definitive diagnosis, and is vital for drug resistance testing. ZN is only 50–80% sensitive
  - Smear negative disease accounts for about 20% of disease transmission; smear positive cases are more infectious
  - Induced sputum is as effective as BAL, especially if the CXR shows changes consistent with active disease (but should not be used for potential MDR-TB, due to the danger to health workers)
  - Conventional culture takes 6 weeks or longer
  - Nucleic acid amplification techniques and DNA finger printing may be used to confirm mycobacteria serotype, and drug susceptibility. May also be useful in elucidating the epidemiology of TB outbreaks
  - Non-mycobacterial TB (opportunistic mycobacteria) tend to be present in much lower concentrations than MTB, and are therefore seen on a smear much less commonly, but many grow much faster, and are therefore seen on culture much earlier

- *Tuberculin skin test* is only useful if grade 3 or 4 (suggesting active disease), or if negative. The skin test must be interpreted with the clinical picture, and with knowledge of the patient's ethnic origin, exposure and BCG vaccination history

- *Bronchoscopy* may be needed to obtain BAL samples if there is a high index of clinical suspicion, but a non-productive cough, or unhelpful sputum culture. In extensive disease, macroscopic bronchoscopic abnormality may be present, with erythematous or ulcerated airways. Granulation tissue or enlarged lymph nodes may be visible. Nodes can perforate or protrude into the bronchial lumen, extruding caseous material into the airway. This is rare in the developed world

- *Biopsy from extrapulmonary* sites, e.g. neck lymph nodes, or mediastinoscopy may be warranted. Bone marrow or liver biopsy— may aid diagnosis in miliary TB. Higher bone marrow culture yield in pancytopenia

- *Gastric washings* reflect TB swallowed overnight. Rarely performed if bronchoscopy is readily available. Used more commonly in children

- *Blood tests* Baseline FBC, renal, and liver function tests. Useful to document normal baseline levels, before starting antituberculous chemotherapy. Consider HIV test

- *Urine* Early morning urine (EMU; if renal disease suspected)

- **CT scan** is more sensitive than CXR, especially for smaller areas of disease. It may show cavitatory disease, and signs of airway disease—the 'tree in bud' appearance, useful for differentiating between active disease, and non-active, old disease. Less commonly needed.

A tuberculoma is an encapsulated focus of reactivated TB. These lesions rarely cavitate, and the differential diagnosis is wide, including malignancy and vasculitis. Diagnosis may only be possible by percutaneous biopsy as, in the absence of a main airway component, cultures may be negative.

Skin tests

- Mantoux
Read at 48 hours.
Intradermal. Use 0.1 ml of 1 in 1000 (= 0.1 ml of 100 TU/ml = 10 Tuberculin Units)
Graded:
<5 mm   negative
5–14 mm positive
>15mm   strongly positive
- Heaf test.
Read at 1 week
100,000 TU/ml (multipuncture)
Graded:
Grade 0 no reaction
Grade 1 4–6 small dots
Grade 2 coalesces, normal skin in centre
Grade 3 coalesces, central skin filled (5–10 mm wide)
Grade 4 solid induration > 10 mm ± vesiculation or ulceration
An excessive response can be treated with topical betnovate (PPD is dead material).

TB: management

Treatment aims to cure disease without relapse, prevent transmission, and prevent emergence of drug resistance.

Long-term treatment with a number of drugs is required as, before treatment is started, TB can remain dormant for long periods, making the emergence of naturally resistant mutants possible.

- Never treat with a single drug
- Never add a single drug to a failing regime
- Send material for bacteriological diagnosis prior to initiating treatment.

The majority of patients can be treated as out-patients.

Smear-positive HIV-negative patients should become smear-negative within 2 weeks of starting treatment (does not apply to MDR-TB). These patients should be isolated either at hospital (if they are admitted) or at home for this time period.

Notification All new cases must be notified (including those diagnosed after death), as this initiates contact tracing. In some districts notification triggers specialist nursing input. The doctor making the diagnosis has a legal responsibility to notify. It also provides epidemiological and surveillance data, enabling treatment and screening services to be planned. A patient can be denotified if the mycobacterium cultured turns out to be an opportunistic mycobacteria, for example.

Drug treatment It is vital to send material for laboratory diagnosis if possible (to allow for subsequent drug susceptibility testing) prior to the initiation of treatment. In practice, if there is a high clinical suspicion of TB, treatment is usually started before full sensitivities are available.

Drug treatment is usually in 2 phases:

Initial intensive phase (designed to kill actively growing bacteria), followed by a *continuation phase* (designed to eliminate residual bacteria).

- The intensive phase (8 weeks) shortens the duration of infectiousness. At least two drugs are needed, e.g. isoniazid (bactericidal), rifampicin (bacteriostatic). The addition of pyrazinamide reduces the treatment time from 9 to 6 months
  Ethambutol added if there is a high likelihood of drug resistance (in practice this is standard therapy for non-Caucasian patients, who are more likely to have come from an area with a high prevalence of resistance)
- The continuation phase is usually with two drugs. Fewer bacteria are present at the start of this phase, and there is therefore a lower chance that drug-resistant mutants will emerge, making drug resistance less of a problem.

Compliance is of major importance.

If the clinical response is not satisfactory, check sputum 2 months before the end of the planned treatment period.

Compliance can be monitored with urine colour testing (turns red with rifampicin) and tablet counts. If concerns re compliance, consider directly observed treatment (DOT).

TB: further management

Directly observed therapy (DOT) aims to increase compliance, by nurse-supervised and -observed daily or weekly tablet swallowing. This has been shown to increase treatment completion, reduce relapses, and reduce development of drug resistance, as the ingestion of each dose is witnessed. This is recommended for patients unlikely to comply, including alcoholics, drug abusers, the homeless, those with serious mental illness, and those with MDR-TB.

Compulsory detention under Sections 37 and 38 of the Public Health Act (England) is allowed for infectious pulmonary TB, but compulsory treatment is not allowed. This is only used in extreme circumstances to protect the public health.

Standard treatment regimes (see page 238)

- The standard regime is for 6 months—four drugs in the initial 2 month phase (rifampicin (R), isoniazid (H), pyrazinamide (Z), and ethambutol (E) (or streptomycin) and 2 drugs in the last four months (rifampicin and isoniazid) in patients with fully sensitive organisms
- If drug sensitivity is unavailable at 2 months, continue the 4 drug regime until it is available (even if this is for more than 2 months)
- The fourth drug (usually ethambutol) can be omitted in those at low risk of isoniazid resistance (non-previously treated, HIV-negative, UK-born Caucasians, with no drug-resistant contacts). There is a higher risk of isoniazid resistance in ethnic minority groups, immigrants, refugees, those who have had previous treatment, and those who are HIV-positive. This depends on local policy and the ethnic make up of the local area. If in doubt, start treatment with 4 drugs
- Other treatment regimes are also effective (e.g. daily for 2 months, then 2 or 3 times weekly for 4 months, or 3 times weekly for the whole 6 months)
- Check baseline renal and liver function in all patients. If normal, and not at high risk of adverse drug reaction, they do not need to be re-checked
- Dosages are weight calculated, and may need to be changed for weight loss or gain
- A 6 month treatment course is effective for all other forms of non-CNS extrapulmonary TB (including lymph node and spinal disease), with the same drugs as for respiratory disease. Surgery may be needed in addition, for spinal disease
- CNS disease needs a 12 month treatment course
- Steroids may be useful for large pleural effusions, pericardial effusions (60 mg/day for constrictive pericarditis), and CNS disease, especially if associated with neurological impairment. Steroids may also be indicated in ureteric disease, and to suppress hypersensitivity reactions to the TB drugs
- Peripheral lymph nodes may enlarge and abscesses may form during treatment; this does not imply failure of treatment, but should prompt a compliance check

- Pyridoxine is not required, unless subjects are at higher risk of pyrazinamide-related peripheral neuropathy—in diabetes, renal failure, HIV, and alcoholics.

Meningitis A 12 month course of rifampicin and isoniazid, with pyrazinamide and a fourth drug for at least the first 2 months, is effective. If pyrazinamide not used, extend treatment period to 18 months. Steroids may be needed for severe disease. Ethambutol should be used with caution in unconscious patients, as visual acuity cannot be tested and there is a small risk of ocular toxicity.

Cerebral tuberculoma without meningitis 12 month regime.

Disseminated TB/miliary TB 6 month regime unless CNS involvement. Exclude CNS disease in miliary TB with CSF examination.

Patient advice to document on starting standard anti-TB chemotherapy:
- Possibility of nausea and abdominal pain
- Persistent vomiting and/or jaundice—stop drugs *immediately* and contact doctor
- Red urine with rifampicin
- Red contact lenses with rifampicin
- Contraception advice, if on the oral contraceptive pill as efficacy reduced
- Visual acuity (Snellen chart) (ethambutol)
- Visual disturbance (ethambutol)—stop drugs *immediately* and contact doctor
- Potential drug interactions.

First-line antituberculosis drugs

Isoniazid (H) bactericidal. Single daily dose, well tolerated. Major side-effect is age-dependent hepatitis. Increased toxicity with alcohol.

Peripheral neuropathy is uncommon; reduce incidence with 10 mg pyridoxine daily (increased risk with diabetes and pregnancy).

Rifampicin (R) bactericidal. Single daily dose, well tolerated.

Increases hepatic microsomal enzymes; therefore increases clearance of hepatic metabolized drugs, including prednisolone. Red discolouration of urine and contact lenses. GI upset.

Pyrazinamide (Z) bactericidal. Single daily dose. GI upset common. Major side-effect is hepatic toxicity. Renal excretion leads to hyperuricaemia.

Ethambutol (E) has some bacteriostatic effect, mostly bacteriostatic at usual doses. Single daily dose, well tolerated. Side-effect—optic neuritis, uncommon. Document visual acuity (Snellen chart) before starting.

Streptomycin bactericidal. Given parenterally. Increased risk of ototoxicity in the fetus and the elderly.

Combined preparations:

Rifinah 150 (contains rifampicin 150 mg and isoniazid 100 mg), **Rifinah 300** (contains rifampicin 300 mg and isoniazid 150 mg).

Rifater (contains 120 mg rifampicin, 50 mg isoniazid, and 300 mg pyrazinamide).

Recommended doses of standard antituberculous drugs

Drug		Daily dose	Intermittent dose
Isoniazid		300 mg	15 mg/kg 3 times weekly
Rifampicin	<50 kg	450 mg	600–900 mg 3 times weekly
	≥50 kg	600 mg	
Pyrazinamide	<50 kg	1.5 g	<50 kg 2.0 g
	≥50 kg	2.0 g	≥50 kg 2.5 g 3× weekly or 3.5 g twice weekly
Ethambutol		15 mg/kg	30 mg/kg 3× weekly or 45 mg/kg twice weekly

For example: a 75 kg adult, commencing quadruple therapy would be given:
- Isoniazid 300 mg
- Rifampicin 600 mg
- Pyrazinamide 2.0 g
- Ethambutol 1.2 g.

If using a combined preparation e.g. Rifater with ethambutol,
- 45 kg adult: rifater 4 tablets and ethambutol 700 mg od
- 60 kg adult: rifater 5 tablets and ethambutol 900 mg od
- 80 kg adult: rifater 6 tablets and ethambutol 1.2 g od.

Interactions of TB drugs

Drug	Increases level of	Decreases level of
Rifampicin	(Level decreased by ketoconazole & PAS)	Warfarin OCP Phenytoin Glucocorticoids Theophyllines Digoxin Methadone Sulphonylureas Cyclosporin
Isoniazid	Phenytoin Carbamezepine Warfarin Diazepam	Azoles, e.g. ketoconazole
Pyrazinamide	Probenecid	

TB: in-patient admission

- This is rarely needed but, if necessary, patients with suspected pulmonary TB should initially be admitted to a side room vented to the outside air (until proven non-infectious)
- Patients with smear-positive non-MDR-TB should be managed as infectious (in a side room, with face mask). This especially applies if they are on a ward with immunosuppressed patients (who may be at higher risk)
- A risk assessment (including the immune status of other ward patients) can be made once the infectiousness and likelihood of drug resistance of the patient are known
- Patients with non-pulmonary TB can be nursed on a general ward (but aerosol generating procedures, e.g. abscess irrigation, may need patient isolation)
- Staff should wear face masks if the patient is potentially infectious
- Barrier nursing is unnecessary for smear-negative non-MDR-TB
- Liaise closely with infection control/microbiology/public health specialists
- If a patient on an open ward is found to have infectious TB, the risk to the other patients is small. Patients whose exposure is considered comparable to that of a household contact should be screened. Only those in the same bay as a coughing infectious case, for at least 8 hours, are considered at risk. Exposure should be documented and the patient and the GP contacted
- Non-MDR-TB HIV-negative patients usually become non-infectious after 2 weeks chemotherapy. Any bacilli seen in smears after that time are likely to be dead
- Patients with HIV and those with TB should not be nursed in close proximity
- All patients with known or suspected MDR-TB should be admitted to negative pressure ventilated side room. Staff should wear protective face masks
- At discharge, a clear plan must be made, including for the administration of all chemotherapy.

Treatment failure/disease relapse

- This is usually due to poor compliance
- Drug resistance may have developed
- Never add a single drug to a failing regime. Add only 2 or 3, ideally those to which the patient has not been previously exposed
- Assume drug resistance to all or some of the drugs in the failed regime
- Repeat cultures and sensitivity testing in this situation. Consider specific molecular tests for rifampicin resistance. If found, then treat as for MDR-TB (see page 249).

TB: treatment follow-up

- CXR is advised at the end of therapy
- Relapse is uncommon in those compliant with standard treatment regimes in the UK (0–3%), therefore long-term follow-up is not recommended
- Relapse after good compliance is usually due to fully sensitive organism; therefore treatment can be with the same regime again
- Relapse due to poor compliance needs a fully supervised regime.

MDR-TB follow-up

Follow for at least 12 months; lifelong for HIV-positive patients.

TB in pregnancy

There is no increased risk of developing clinical disease in pregnancy. Presentation is the same as in non-pregnant individuals, but the diagnosis may be delayed by the non-specific nature of the symptoms in the early stages of disease, with malaise and fatigue being common in the early stages of pregnancy. A CXR is more likely to be delayed.

The tuberculin skin test result is not affected by pregnancy; this applies to HIV positive and negative subjects. A negative skin test should not lead to BCG vaccination, as live vaccines are contraindicated in pregnancy. In this situation, the skin test should be repeated after delivery, and BCG given then, after a second negative test.

TB outcome in pregnancy

- If diagnosed in the first trimester, the disease has the same outcome as for non-pregnant women
- If diagnosed in the second or third trimester, studies give more variable outcomes (some studies show a good fetal outcome, some show higher rates of small-for-dates babies, pre-eclampsia, and spontaneous abortion), but these effects tend to be related to late diagnosis and incomplete drug treatment. Some studies also show a poorer fetal outcome in extrapulmonary disease
- Late diagnosis of pulmonary TB can lead to a fourfold increased obstetric mortality and ninefold increased pre-term labour in some Third World countries.

Treatment in pregnancy

- Isoniazid, rifampicin, and ethambutol are not teratogenic, and can be used safely in pregnancy. The 'standard' short course therapy is recommended (i.e. 6 month treatment)
- Limited pyrazinamide data on the risk of teratogenicity
- Streptomycin may be ototoxic to the fetus
- Active TB must be treated in pregnancy, because of the risk of untreated disease to the mother and fetus
- Reserve drugs may be toxic, and the risk/benefit ratio of each case must be assessed individually if second-line drugs are needed
- Babies of sputum-positive mothers, who have had less than 2 weeks treatment by delivery, should be treated with isoniazid and have a skin test at 6 weeks. If the skin test is negative, the chemoprophylaxis should be stopped and BCG given 1 week later (as BCG is sensitive to isoniazid)
- Congenital infection is very rare (less than 300 reported cases). The child can be infected at delivery (this is rare).

Breast feeding

- Most antituberculous drugs are safe
- Concentrations of drugs reaching breast milk are too low to prevent or treat infection in the infant.

TB chemotherapy with co-morbid disease

Liver disease (see opposite page)
- Drug-induced hepatitis can be fatal
- Pyrazinamide should not be used in patients with known chronic liver disease
- Decompensated liver disease—use a drug regime without rifampicin
- Baseline and regular monitoring of liver function is necessary (weekly LFTs for the first 2 weeks, then at 2 weekly intervals).

Renal failure
- Isoniazid, rifampicin, and pyrazinamide have biliary excretion, so can be given in normal doses in renal disease
- Give pyridoxine in addition to isoniazid in those with severe renal disease, to prevent isoniazid-induced peripheral neuropathy
- Ethambutol can accumulate causing optic neuropathy; therefore use a lower dose
- Dialysis patients should receive drugs after dialysis.

HIV infection
- Regimes are similar for HIV-positive and HIV-negative patients; give standard 4 drug regime. Liaise closely with HIV specialist
- Better outcome with regimes including rifampicin
- Death during tuberculosis chemotherapy is more common in HIV-infected patients, who also have higher relapse rates than non-HIV-infected subjects
- Higher incidence of miliary disease in those with low CD4 counts
- Protease inhibitors and non-nucleoside reverse transcription inhibitors should not be used with rifampicin (they interfere with each other's metabolism)
- Paradoxical worsening of disease (worsening fever, CXR infiltrates, or new manifestations of the disease) at the initiation of HIV treatment are more common in HIV-positive patients. This is probably due to immune reconstitution, and the increased recognition of mycobacterial antigens with improvement of the subject's immune response
- Patients co-infected with TB and HIV should be considered potentially infectious at each admission, until proved otherwise, and should be segregated from others, considering the immune status of other patients and their likely drug resistances, and their potential infectiousness
- In HIV-infected individuals (in whom the HIV diagnosis is new), usual practice is to start tuberculosis chemotherapy before HIV chemotherapy. Antiretroviral therapy is usually started later (but there is no consensus as to when). Liaise closely with HIV specialists.

Diabetes
Increased risk of TB, and the disease may be more extensive. Rifampicin reduces the efficacy of sulphonylureas.

TB drugs in patients with abnormal liver function tests

- Chronic liver disease—regular monitoring of LFTs, weekly for first 2 weeks, then at 2 weekly intervals
  - Virological tests to exclude concomitant viral hepatitis
    AST/ALT rise 2x normal—monitor LFTs weekly for 2 weeks, then 2 weekly until normal.
    AST/ALT rise under 2x normal—repeat LFT at 2 weeks.
    AST/ALT-5x normal or bilirubin rise—cease rifampicin, isoniazid, and pyrazinamide unless patient is unwell. If patient unwell, or sputum still positive, consider admission for parenteral therapy, e.g. streptomyicn and ethambutol with appropriate monitoring.
- Drug re-challenge.

Once LFTs normal:
  - Re-introduce sequentially, in order:
    Isoniazid: at 50 mg/day, sequential increase to 300 mg/day after 2–3 days if no reaction.
    Rifampicin: at 75 mg/day, increase to 300 mg/day after 2–3 days if no reaction, then to maximum dose/kg.
    Pyrazinamide: start at 250 mg/day, increase to 1 g/day after 2–3 days and to maximum dose/kg if no reaction
  - Daily monitoring of LFTs and clinical condition
  - If no further reaction, continue chemotherapy
  - If there is a further reaction, exclude the offending drug, and change to an alternative regime
  - If intolerant of pyrazinamide, use rifampicin and isoniazid for 9 months, with ethambutol for 2 months.

TB: adverse drug reactions

These occur in around 10% of patients, often requiring a change of therapy. Reactions are more common in those on non-standard therapy, and in HIV-positive individuals.

Isoniazid peripheral neuropathy can be prevented by pyridoxine 10 mg daily (recommended in those at highest risk—diabetes, renal failure, alcoholics, HIV-positive).

Rifampicin causes shock, acute renal failure, thrombocytopenia. Withdraw and do not reintroduce the drug. Double maintenance steroid doses at start of treatment (because of enzyme induction).

Ethambutol causes rare optic toxicity; recommend baseline visual acuity assessment with Snellen chart. Use only in those with adequate visual acuity, and those able to report changes in visual acuity or new visual symptoms. Document that the patient has been told to cease the drug **immediately** at the onset of new visual symptoms.

Check baseline renal function before starting ethambutol, and avoid in renal failure.

HIV-positive patients Rifampicin and isoniazid lead to reduced serum concentrations of antifungals. Ketoconazole can inhibit rifampicin absorption. Rifampicin may reduce drug levels of protease inhibitors (as they are metabolized via the cytochrome P450 pathway, which is induced by rifampicin). Rifabutin can cause a severe iritis. Liaise closely with HIV specialist.

Drug resistance occurs in less than 2% of Caucasian cases in the UK, with higher levels in ethnic minority groups.

Isoniazid resistance is seen in up to 6% in patients of African and Indian subcontinent origin.

Increased drug resistance is seen in HIV-positive patients (fourfold increased risk).

- Second-line drugs are generally more toxic and less effective than first-line drugs, and the treatment of drug resistance can therefore often be complex and difficult
- The regime must include at least three drugs to which the organism is known to be susceptible. An injectable drug is often added, as this has shown improved outcomes
- The initial regime will depend on the incidence of drug resistance in the community, and should be altered depending on local drug susceptibility patterns
- In general, always add at least two drugs to which the MTB is susceptible
- Parenteral treatment is usually recommended when there is resistance to two or more drugs.

Isoniazid monoresistance If documented before treatment started, use regime of:
- Rifampicin, pyrazinamide, ethambutol, and streptomycin for 2 months, then rifampicin and ethambutol for 7 months.

If resistance is documented after the start of a standard chemotherapy regime, stop isoniazid.
- Give ethambutol and rifampicin together for 12 months, with pyrazinamide for 2 months.

Pyrazinamide monoresistance is uncommon. Use rifampicin and isoniazid for 9 months, with 2 months initial ethambutol.

Ethambutol monoresistance is uncommon. Use 6 months of rifampicin and isoniazid, with 2 months initial pyrazinamide.

Rifampicin monoresistance is uncommon, but does require regime modification. Use 18 months therapy, with 2 months of pyrazinamide, isoniazid, and ethambutol, followed by isoniazid and ethambutol for a further 16 months.

In most cases, rifampicin resistance is a marker of MDR-TB, and should be treated as such until full sensitivities are known.

Molecular methods allow accurate drug susceptibility testing (at the PHLS reference laboratory).

Combined drug resistance

Streptomycin and isoniazid is the commonest dual resistance. Use a regime as for isoniazid resistance, but with full supervision throughout.

Multiple drug resistant TB (MDR-TB)

Defined as MTB resistant to two or more first-line agents, usually isoniazid and rifampicin.

- Treatment is complex and time-consuming
- MDR-TB is not more infectious than other forms of TB, but the consequences of acquiring it are more serious
- Seek specialist advice; patients should be managed by specialists with experience of managing resistant cases, in hospitals with isolation facilities. Liaise closely with the reference laboratory
- Close monitoring (because of increased drug toxicity) is needed
- Compliance is paramount
- MDR-TB comprised 1.3% of all UK cases in 1998
- Start treatment with 5 or more drugs to which the organism is likely to be susceptible. Continue until sputum cultures are negative. Continue with at least 3 drugs to which TB is sensitive, for a minimum of 9 months, sometimes for 24 months
- Surgery may be indicated.

Contacts of MDR-TB Chemoprophylaxis for contacts should include at least 2 drugs. Base the drug choice on the sensitivities of the index case, for a minimum of 6 months (though there is no data to support this treatment period). If there is extensive resistance, no regime may be suitable, and regular follow-up needed instead.

Risk factors for resistant disease

- Previous anti-TB treatment
- HIV infection
- Contact with drug-resistant disease
- Treatment failure.

Second-line tuberculosis chemotherapy

Drug	Dose	Potential side-effects
Amikacin	15 mg/kg	Tinnitus, ataxia, renal impairment, vertigo
Azithromycin	500 mg od	GI upset
Capreomycin	15 mg/kg	As for amikacin
Ciprofloxacin	750 mg bd	Abdominal upset, headache, drug interactions
Clarithromycin	500 mg bd	GI upset
Ethionamide (or prothionamide)	<50 kg: 375 mg bd ≥50 kg: 500 mg bd	GI upset, hepatitis. Avoid in pregnancy
Kanamycin	15 mg/kg	As for amikacin
Ofloxacin	400 mg bd	Abdominal upset, headache
PAS	10 g od or 5 g bd	GI upset, fever, rash, hepatitis
Rifabutin	300–450 mg od	As for rifampicin. Uveitis with drug interactions, e.g. with macrolides
Streptomycin	15 mg/kg (max dose 1 g od)	As for amikacin
Thiacetazone	150 mg	GI upset, rash, conjunctivitis, vertigo. Avoid if HIV-positive (risk of Stevens–Johnson syndrome)

If the drug choice is limited by drug resistance and intolerance, consider desensitization and reintroduction of the offending drug. Desensitization must be done with concurrent treatment with 2 other drugs (to minimize emergence of resistant strains).

Latent TB infection

Defined as a positive skin test, with a normal CXR and no symptoms. This represents the presence of a small total number of bacteria.

Tuberculin skin test A positive skin test results from the development of cell-mediated immunity against TB. The multiple puncture method (Heaf) is more commonly used than the Mantoux test in the UK.

Potential problems with skin testing:
- Low sensitivity in the immunocompromised, and cross-reactivity with BCG
- The patient has to return to have the test read after 48–72 hours
- Criteria for a positive test depend on the population in which it is being used.

An enzyme linked immunosorbant assay (ELISPOT) with greater sensitivity and specificity has recently been developed.

Latent infection versus active disease

It is important to differentiate between active and latent disease.

Active disease is a positive skin test (usually), abnormal CXR, and symptoms.

Latent infection (small numbers of bacilli present) is a positive skin test, normal CXR, and no symptoms, and is usually treated with chemoprophylaxis (see below).

HIV infection The tuberculin skin test may be falsely negative, and radiological changes may be atypical. Current guidelines recommend close monitoring and no chemoprophylaxis, because of the difficulties in identifying active from latent disease, and because of the risk of emergence of resistant strains. Exposure to smear positive disease should lead to chemoprophylaxis in the absence of clinical disease. Recommended follow-up is at 3 and 12 months for those not receiving chemophrophylaxis (but who were eligible for it).

HIV-positive patients should receive long-term follow-up as part of their ongoing HIV management.

Chemoprophylaxis is given to contacts with strongly positive Heaf reactions, who have no radiological or clinical evidence of active disease. The risk of developing disease after exposure depends on a number of factors, including BCG and HIV status, and whether infection was recent. Younger patients must have had relatively recent infection, and have a longer life expectancy from which to gain the benefits of chemoprophylaxis. Chemoprophylaxis is recommended for:
- Those with recent documented tuberculin conversion
- HIV-infected contacts of smear-positive cases
- Children aged < 16 with a strongly positive Heaf (grade 2–4 if no prior BCG, grade 3–4 if prior BCG).

Drug regimes:
- Rifampicin (R) and isoniazid (H) daily for 3 months (3HR). Best compliance, but slightly higher side-effect profile
- Isoniazid (H) daily for 6 months (6H). Lowest toxicity regime. Has a 60–90% effectiveness in reducing progression of latent infection to clinical disease.

TB and anti-TNFα treatment

Humanized monoclonal anti-TNFα antibody has recently been approved for the treatment of rheumatoid arthritis (RA) and Crohn's disease. Etanercept (Enbrel) is a fusion protein that binds free TNFα using a soluble portion of the TNFα receptor, and is licensed for use in rheumatoid arthritis. Adalimumab (Humira) is a recombinant humanized monoclonal antibody against TNFα, also used in RA. Infliximab (Remicade) is a direct neutralizing antibody.

These drugs cause profound immunosuppression, and concern has been raised about the frequency of tuberculosis seen during their use. Most TB cases have been seen with infliximab (242 at time of publication), with most occurring within three treatment cycles (within a mean of 12 weeks of starting treatment). In RA a 4-fold increased risk of TB has been seen in America with infliximab. 50% of the reported cases have been extrapulmonary disease.

The BTS has recently made recommendations on the management of, and screening for TB in patients due to start anti-TNFα antibody treatment.

- All patients should have a clinical examination, with history of previous TB treatment and exposure carefully documented. All should have a CXR and tuberculin test
- Those with an abnormal CXR consistent with previous TB or those who have a history of extrapulmonary TB, who have received adequate treatment need regular monitoring only
- Those with an abnormal CXR consistent with previous TB or those who have a prior history of extrapulmonary TB, who have NOT had adequate treatment need to have active tuberculosis excluded by appropriate investigations. They should receive chemoprophylaxis before anti-TNFα therapy commences (assuming active disease is not identified)
- If active TB is present, patients should receive a minimum of 2 months anti-TB chemotherapy before starting anti-TNFα therapy
- If the CXR is normal, the tuberculin test may be helpful if the patient is not on immunosuppressants. It is unhelpful if the patient is on immunosuppressants
- If the patient develops TB whilst on anti-TNFα therapy, treat with the full standard course of antituberculous chemotherapy. The anti-TNFα can be continued if indicated
- Close liaison between the prescriber of the TNFα antibody treatment and TB specialists is needed.

TB: screening and contact tracing

Immigrant screening Immigrants are screened, as ethnic minority groups in the UK constitute 50% of TB cases. The incidence of TB is highest in the first few years after arrival to the UK, with return visits to countries with a high background prevalence being a risk factor for acquiring disease. Immigrants with symptoms suggestive of TB, and those who are asymptomatic, with a grade 3 or 4 tuberculin skin test should be referred to the local chest clinic for CXR and assessment. BCG vaccination is recommended for tuberculin-negative immigrants (but not in those who are HIV-positive, because of the risk of generalized BCG infection).

Contact tracing identifies those with TB, and those who are infected, but without evidence of disease. It also identifies those suitable for BCG vaccination.

Close contacts are usually those within the same household, sharing kitchen facilities, and frequent household visitors.

Casual contacts usually include most occupational contacts. Examination is usually only needed if the index case was smear-positive, or if the contacts are at high risk. This also applies if more than 10% of the close contacts have been infected, i.e. the index case is considered highly infectious.

- 10% of TB is diagnosed by contact tracing, with disease occurring in about 1% of contacts
- Smear-negative patients are much less infectious, but contact tracing is still recommended in these patients
- Contacts should be traced for the period the index case has been infectious, or for 3 months prior to the first positive sputum or culture, if the time period is uncertain
- Most disease in contacts is found at the first screening visit
- Subjects should be advised to report suspicious symptoms
- Follow-up is recommended at 3 and 12 months for those not receiving chemoprophylaxis.

Extrapulmonary disease Contact screening is not recommended.

Contact examination This usually involves symptom enquiry, BCG vaccination status, Heaf test, and CXR.

Contacts of smear-positive index case If symptoms are present, and if the contact was not previously vaccinated, those with grade 0 or 1 Heaf should be retested after 6 weeks to allow for tuberculin conversion. If retesting is not possible, give BCG after first negative Heaf.

HIV-infected contacts CXR is indicated, as a negative Heaf test may be due to anergy, and may therefore be a false negative. Heaf testing is not contraindicated in HIV (PPD is dead). BCG is contraindicated (it is a live vaccine).

BCG vaccination is recommended for previously unvaccinated, Heaf grade 0 or 1 contacts under the age of 16. It should only be offered to older potential contacts who have travel, ethnic, or occupational risk.

It has an efficacy of around 70% against TB in children, but difficulties with vaccine supply, and regional policies have meant that not all children in the UK have been vaccinated. It is less effective in adults, and is not used in America.

Adverse events include pain and suppuration at the injection site, and localized lymphadenitis. A short course of rifampicin may be recommended in this situation.

Airplane transmission Transmission rates are low, even on long haul flights. Contract tracing of passengers and crew is only necessary if the index cases was smear-positive and coughing during a flight of at least 8 hours. In this situation, screening is only recommended in those at high risk—immunocompromised travellers and children, or if the index case was unusually infectious.

M. bovis Cattle TB is due to *M. bovis*. Humans are at low risk, as the majority of milk consumed is pasteurized. *M. bovis* is distinguishable from *M. tuberculosis* in the laboratory, though initial diagnosis can be difficult (only distinguishable on culture, not using DNA or RNA testing). Around 40 cases are isolated per year. BCG is live attenuated *M. bovis*.

Future developments
- New TB vaccine, to boost the immune response to BCG
- ELISPOT test for diagnosis, using MTB specific antigen—ESAT-6 and CFP10
- Nebulized gamma interferon used as additional treatment in MDR-TB in those failing multiple agent chemotherapy in the United States.

Further information

Chemotherapy and management of tuberculosis in the UK: recommendations 1998. Drug doses and regimes as recommended in this document. *Thorax* 1998; **53**: 536–48

Control and prevention of tuberculosis in the UK: Code of practice 2000. *Thorax* 2000; **55**: 887–901

Non-tuberculous mycobacteria (NTM)

NTM may also be called atypical mycobacteria, opportunistic mycobacteria, environmental mycobacteria, mycobacteria other than tuberculosis (MOTT).

Aetiology

- Found in the environment: in soil, water (including tap water), dust, milk, animals, and birds
- Many different species. The four most important are *Mycobacterium avium complex (MAC)*, *Mycobacterium kansasii*, *Mycobacterium malmoense*, and *Mycobacterium xenopi*
- They are low-grade pathogens in humans
- Most commonly cause pulmonary infections in middle-aged and older adults, and in those with pre-existing lung disease, such as bronchiectasis, emphysema, or old healed TB, or in immunodeficiency
- *Disseminated infection* may occur, especially in the immunocompromised
- *Lymphadenitis* typically occurs in children aged 1–5. This presents with enlarged, non-tender, cervical lymph nodes and a normal CXR. The node should be surgically resected. Antibiotic treatment is only required if there is recurrence. Large nodes may need antituberculous chemotherapy to shrink the node prior to resection
- *Local invasion* may occur from skin lesion (e.g. M. marinum, M. ulcerans, M. fortuitum, M. abscessus, M. chelonae, M. avium complex).

Clinical features
The symptoms are generally non-specific, hence the difficulty in diagnosis.

- Sub-acute illness with weight loss, productive cough, dyspnoea, fever, and occasionally haemoptysis
- May present in a patient with known underlying lung disease, such as COPD, in whom disease progression is atypical
- Colonization of abnormal lung may not cause symptoms, but can progress to cause disease later
- May be similar to symptoms caused by *Mycobacterium tuberculosis*.

Investigations

- *CXR* can be indistinguishable from that of MTB, with upper zone infiltrate with cavitation. Airway nodularity and associated bronchiectasis are recognized. The CXR may be difficult to interpret in the presence of pre-existing lung disease. It is impossible to identify which atypical mycobacterium is causing infection from the CXR appearance
- *Sputum samples* Microbiology for ZN stain, culture, and further testing. If there is growth of an atypical acid-fast bacillus:
  - *Where was the isolate from?* Culture from lung biopsy, BAL, pleural fluid, or blood culture is more significant than culture from sputum
  - *What is the isolate and what is the degree of growth?*
  - *How many samples have been positive?*

- A single isolate from a non-sterile site may not be significant. Contamination can occur, especially from bronchoscopes when BAL is performed. Multiple isolates (>2) from non-sterile sites are needed to establish disease, or >1 from a sterile site, especially if there is supportive histopathology. Liaise with microbiologists to help to determine the significance of a positive result
- May need *lung biopsy* to help differentiate
- *No skin test* is available.

Diagnosis Pulmonary disease is likely if:
- CXR is suggestive and 3 or more positive sputum cultures are obtained 1 week apart, with or without symptoms
- or 1 positive culture from a sterile site, such as pleural fluid or biopsy
- or 2 positive cultures from bronchoalveolar lavage on separate occasions.

In the UK, pulmonary infection is most commonly caused by *Mycobacterium kansasii*, *Mycobacterium avium* complex, *Mycobacterium malmoense*, and *Mycobacterium xenopi*.

NTM: management

- The decision to treat is based on the likelihood of active infection
- No need to notify or contact trace as there is low-risk of cross-infection
- De-notify if the MTB grown turns out to be an atypical mycobacterium, and change treatment accordingly
- Treatment considerations according to BTS guidelines:
  - *M. kansasii*—progresses without treatment. Treat with rifampicin and ethambutol for a minimum of 9 months. A longer treatment period is required if immunocompromise (2 years or until sputum is clear of infection for 12 months). Good response to treatment. Indefinite treatment if non-compliant. 100% response rate, >90% 5 year cure, with <10% relapse with full compliance
  - *M. avium* complex (MAC)—may be asymptomatic. Can be antibiotic resistant. Treat with triple therapy: rifampicin with ethambutol with or without isoniazid for 2 yrs. 50% response rate and 20% relapse rate. Clarithromycin may be effective
  - *M. malmoense*—treat with ethambutol and rifampicin for 18–24 months
  - *M. xenopi*—often resistant. Disease may progress despite treatment. Treat with ethambutol, isoniazid and rifampicin for at least 2 years
  - *M. malmoense*, and *M. xenopi*—90% response rate, and 10% relapse rate at 2 yrs.

It is recognized that laboratory antibiotic sensitivities and resistance may not correlate with the clinical therapeutic response. Antibiotic choice is best judged on clinical response.

HIV positive patients

- *Mycobacterium avium* complex is the cause of infection in 90% of cases
- Infections may occur late in the disease, when CD4 count <50
- Infections may develop during the first 2 months of highly active anti-retroviral treatment (HAART)
- Disease is rarely confined to the lungs. Lymphadenitis and disseminated infection are recognized
- Lung disease causes similar symptoms to those seen in the non-immunocompromised
- CXR shows diffuse interstitial, reticulonodular, or alveolar infiltrates
- A single isolate may represent colonization
- If an organism is repeatedly isolated, in the presence of symptoms and/or an abnormal CXR, start treatment
- Lifelong antibiotic treatment is recommended for pulmonary or disseminated disease, with a 3–4 drug regimen
- Disseminated MAC incidence is decreased by antibiotic prophylaxis (with azithromycin weekly), and HAART restoring immunocompetence
- There are potential drug interactions between rifampicin, macrolides, and protease inhibitors and NNRTIs.

Further Information

Management of opportunistic mycobacterial infections. *Thorax* 2000; **55**: 210–18

Fungal respiratory diseases

Aspergillus lung disease: classification

Types of disease *Aspergillus fumigatus* and other Aspergillus moulds are ubiquitous fungi that can be isolated from the air in most houses, and this increases with increasing indoor humidity. Inhalation can produce a range of different diseases, some of which are related to each other, and some of which are not. The finding of fungal hyphae (rather than just spores) in the sputum should provoke an assessment.

Classification

1) *IgE-mediated allergic asthma* from inhaled Aspergillus spores. One of many common antigens provoking airway inflammation and bronchospasm

2) *Exuberant IgE and IgG reaction* to Aspergillus in the airways of (usually) asthmatics provoking mucous plugging with distal consolidation that may flit from area to area. This is one of the causes of pulmonary eosinophilia

3) *Allergic bronchopulmonary aspergillosis* (APBA). A probable evolution and progression of (2) in (usually) asthmatics with inflammatory damage to the airways and resultant bronchiectasis (but no actual invasion of Aspergillus into the airway walls)

4) *Invasive aspergillus pneumonia* due to invasion of Aspergillus into lung tissue secondary to immunosuppression. This can be a multisystem disorder with Aspergillus invading almost any part of the body

5) *Semi-invasive aspergillosis*, a much lower grade process than (4), usually seen in older individuals with no apparent immunosuppression, and usually some underlying chronic lung disease

6) *Aspergilloma*, where Aspergillus lives and grows as a separate ball of fungus in a pre-existing lung cavity. There is usually an inflammatory response to limited hyphae invasion into the tissue walls of the cavity

7) *Extrinsic allergic alveolitis* due to an immune inflammatory reaction to inhalation of large numbers of spores (see page 458).

The presentation and clinical setting of these various Aspergillus-related disorders are clearly different and thus detailed separately.

1) Atopic allergy to fungal spores

Approximately 10% of asthmatics are skin prick positive to Aspergillus species, compared to about 70% positive to house dust mite. It is assumed that this allergy contributes to allergic inflammation in the airways but, in the few relevant studies, symptoms have not correlated with exposure. Particularly high exposure will result from working with mouldy vegetable matter such as compost heaps.

2) Asthma and positive IgG precipitins to Aspergillus

Definition Asthmatics with IgE responses to Aspergillus can also develop IgG antibodies (precipitins). Why this happens is not clear. Aspergillus hyphae can *sometimes* be isolated from the sputum and it has been suggested that Aspergillus spores are able to germinate and grow in the mucous within the airways. This may explain the mucous plugging and flitting areas of pulmonary consolidation.

Clinical features and investigations

Associated features may include:
- Serum IgE > 1000 ng/ml
- Blood eosinophilia > 500/mm^3
- Skin prick +ve to Aspergillus
- IgG precipitins to Aspergillus
- Long history of asthma, perhaps recently deteriorated.

Therefore suspect this development in:
A patient with long-term asthma whose control deteriorates, with CXR changes, IgE & IgG to Aspergillus, eosinophilia, and perhaps hyphae in the sputum.

Management may only require an increase in inhaled steroids. However, there is a suggestion that courses of oral steroids are particularly effective and may prevent progression to bronchiectasis (see next section). Steroids limit the host's immunological response but do not seem to lead to Aspergillus invasion of the tissues. Poorly documented evidence of improvement with antifungal agents such as itraconazole.

3) Bronchopulmonary aspergillosis

Definition This condition is probably an extension of (2), where the inflammatory response to the Aspergillus in the airways provokes a more exuberant response, with damage to the bronchial walls and bronchiectasis. Some authors reserve the use of the term ABPA for when bronchiectasis is present, others may include (2), and subdivide into ABPA-S (seropositive only), and ABPA-CB (central bronchiectasis).

The prevalence of ABPA in asthmatic populations has varied considerably between studies, and clearly will depend on whether the definition includes bronchiectasis or not. It probably occurs in about 1–2% of asthmatics. A related condition occurs in patients with cystic fibrosis where it appears about 7% have evidence of colonization and potential ongoing damage.

Pathophysiology The factors promoting the evolution from atopic asthmatic to ABPA are not known. A particular HLA association has been shown, with the suggestion that a CD4/Th2 response to a particular Aspergillus antigen (Asp f1 antigen) with release of IL-4 and IL-5 may be critical. Proteolytic enzymes are released by Aspergillus as part of its exophytic feeding strategy and these enzymes may damage airway mucosa. However, most believe that the damage results from *host defence mechanisms*. Hyphae (rather than just spores) may be visible in the mucus and grown from sputum, but there does not appear to be actual invasion of the bronchial mucosa. This immune inflammatory activity produces mucoid impaction in the airways, eosinophilic pneumonitis, and bronchocentric granuloma formation.

Main criteria for diagnosis (the first four are the most important)
- Long history of asthma
- Skin prick/IgE +ve to *Aspergillus fumigatus*
- IgG precipitins to *Aspergillus fumigatus*
- Central (proximal) bronchiectasis
- Blood/sputum eosinophilia
- Total serum IgE > 1000 mg/ml
- Lung infiltrates—flitting.

Clinical features
- Long-standing asthma, recent deterioration
- Recurrent episodes of mucous plugging
- Fever/malaise
- Expectoration of dark mucous plugs, sometimes as casts of the airways
- Eosinophilia (sputum and blood)
- Occasional haemoptysis.

The major complication is poorly controlled asthma that requires repeated courses of oral steroids.

Investigations
- *Spirometry*—degree of airways obstruction
- *Skin prick sensitivity* to Aspergillus (IgE)
- *Sputum*—Aspergillus hyphae and eosinophils

- *Blood*
  - IgG precipitins
  - IgE RAST to Aspergillus
  - Total serum IgE
  - Eosinophil count (suppressed if on steroids)
- *CXR*
  - Flitting infiltrates
  - Bronchiectasis, mucous impaction (gloved finger shadows)
- *CT* Central (proximal) bronchiectasis with upper lobe predominance.

Management The management is essentially that of severe chronic asthma but with generous use of courses of oral steroids. Several studies have shown courses of itraconazole (200 mg bd for 4 months) are well tolerated, reduce steroid requirements, and improve exercise tolerance. There appears to be a sustained effect after the itraconazole is stopped, suggesting at least temporary eradication of the Aspergillus. Response and relapse can be monitored with IgG precipitins to Aspergillus. Itraconazole can cause liver dysfunction, so LFTs need monitoring.

Differential diagnosis This list revolves mainly around the pulmonary infiltrates and eosinophilia.
- Acute/chronic eosinophilic pneumonia
- Churg–Strauss syndrome
- Various parasites (e.g. filariasis, ascaris) (Löffler's syndrome)
- Drug-induced eosinophilic pneumonia.

4) Invasive aspergillosis

Definition The term 'invasive aspergillosis' is reserved for the situation where Aspergillus hyphae actually invade tissue. This usually occurs in the setting of severe immune suppression, particularly neutropenia with steroid use. The port of entry is probably the lungs, but spread can be to almost any area of the body. The species most commonly seen are *Aspergillus fumigatus, flavus, terreus,* and *niger.*

Pathogenesis Alveolar macrophages probably normally destroy Aspergillus spores. Macrophage failure may allow more spores to germinate and any subsequent invasion with hyphae seems to require neutrophils to arrest it. Inadequate neutrophil function allows invasion across tissue planes, into vessels, with infarction and further spread throughout the body. There is some evidence that CMV may inactivate macrophages, thus allowing spores to germinate. It is assumed that the fungal digestive proteases do the damage rather than the host's limited immunological responses.

Clinical features

Typical setting

Fever, chest pain, cough, haemoptysis, dyspnoea, and pulmonary infiltrate in a neutropenic patient failing to respond to broad spectrum antibiotics.

Risk factors
- following chemotherapy, particularly neutropenia
- bone marrow suppression for allogeneic stem cell transplants
- advanced HIV infection
- immune suppression following transplant
- infliximab (or other anti-TNFα) therapy.

Spread can occur anywhere with the following well recognized:
- Sinuses (paranasal) and spread into the brain
- Endocarditis
- Eyes
- Skin (papular, ranging to ulcerative, lesions).

Careful examination and particular investigations may be needed to detect spread to these areas

Investigations
- *Isolate aspergillus hyphae* from respiratory tract by:
  sputum
  expressed sputum (3% saline via nebulizer)
  bronchoalveolar lavage
  transbronchial biopsy
  (hyphae may be present when not the primary cause of the infiltrate)
- *Biopsies* from other sites (most convincing when acute-angle branching, septated non-pigmented hyphae are seen)

- Circulating levels of *galactomannan*, an exoantigen of Aspergillus (commercial EIA kit not universally available, and not found so useful by all groups on account of low sensitivity and false positivity due to certain antibiotics, piperacillin and tazobactam)
- *CXR/CT* halo sign. This is a crescent of air appearing at the edge of an area of consolidation. It usually occurs when the neutrophil count is rising, and probably represents a gradual containment of the infection into a cavity, not unlike an aspergilloma.

Ultimately it is the clinical picture that dominates the diagnosis.

Management
- Intravenous amphotericin B (only about 35% response rate)
- Intravenous lipid-based amphotericin (less nephrotoxic, but very expensive)
- Intraconazole IV: 200 mg bd for 2 days, then 200 mg od for 12 days
- Voriconazole (recently available, little experience but probably better than itraconazole, very expensive)
- Caspofungin (recently available, little experience, very expensive).

Some centres use oral itraconazole as prophylaxis when commencing substantial immune suppression.

Differential diagnosis
The differential will be the large number of other opportunistic infections seen in immunosuppressed patients.

5) Semi-invasive aspergillosis

(also known as chronic necrotizing aspergillosis, or chronic pulmonary aspergillosis)

Definition This entity is poorly defined but it is clear that a low grade, chronic, invasion of Aspergillus into airway walls and surrounding lung can occur. In the original descriptions, some cause of mild immuno-incompetence was present, such as diabetes, steroid therapy, chronic lung disease, poor nutrition, etc. Previous asthma is not usually present, as in ABPA.

Pathogenesis It is assumed that this form of aspergillosis results from lowered immunity in those without a tendency to make Th2, eosinophilic, responses to antigens. There is infiltration of hyphae into lung tissue, ranging from minor patchy consolidation to multiple cavities. There is little, if any, angio-invasion. It is assumed that the fungal digestive proteases gradually do the damage rather than the host's immunological response.

Clinical features

Suspect semi-invasive aspergillosis when:

- Middle-aged
- Reason for mild immunosuppression
- A pre-existing chronic lung disease
- Fever
- Productive cough
- Patchy, indolent, CXR changes.

Investigations

- Sputum samples may allow isolation of hyphae
- CT will show an airway-centred type of picture with 'tree in bud' appearance. With increasing severity this gives way to denser areas and small cavities that occasionally may contain a fungus ball
- Likely to have IgG precipitins to Aspergillus, but not always.

Management On the assumption that mild immune suppression is the dominant cause, steroids are not usually recommended for fear of further immune suppression. This is in contrast to ABPA where the damage is due to the host's immune defence mechanisms. Oral antifungals, such as itraconazole, are recommended. Fluconazole has been used with apparent success in case series only.

6) Aspergilloma/mycetoma

Definition The term aspergilloma is used to describe a ball of fungal hyphae within a cavity in the lung. It is assumed that this is colonization of a prior cavity, rather than arrested invasion. Aspergillomas can occur in other organs, including the pleural space.

Pathogenesis Cavities can occur in the lung following a variety of insults such as tuberculosis, sarcoid, ordinary pneumonia/lung abscess, treated tumours, and cystic fibrosis. Fungal spores entering the cavity germinate and survive in a relatively protected environment. The ball consists of hyphae, inflammatory cells, fibrin, and debris. Around the cavity is an intense inflammatory response, often with considerable extra vascularization from bronchial arteries and occasional fungal hyphae.

Clinical features Aspergillomas are often asymptomatic. Up to 75% will present with haemoptysis, assumed to come from damaged vessels, on the inner surface of the cavity wall, via a communication with a bronchus. Sometimes there are systemic symptoms, malaise and fever, as well as chest pain. Superadded infection may provoke exacerbations.

Investigations
- *CXR* apical cavity with ball within, that changes position if CXR is performed decubitus
- *CT* obvious cavity with fungus ball, and possible invasion into surrounding lung (uncommon)
- *Sputum culture*
- *Aspergillus IgG precipitins.* Often higher levels than seen in other Aspergillus diseases.

Management
- May not require treatment
- Systemic symptoms of fever and malaise may be hard to ascribe to a mycetoma and require a therapeutic trial of itraconazole
- The most significant complication is life-threatening haemoptysis. The emergency management of haemoptysis is described on page 25
- Itraconazole will not eradicate the fungus, but seems to reduce cavity size and lessen the tendency to haemoptysis. It is assumed that it kills any fungus in the walls and inhibits growth in the cavity. The place of newer agents such as voriconazole is not known.

General approach to chronic haemoptysis
- Tranexamic acid (must be taken during clot formation as binds to fibrin to prevent action of endogenous fibrinolytics)
- Treat associated bacterial infections.

Specific to aspergilloma
- Itraconazole
- Arterial embolization
- Surgical resection.

- Bronchial arteriograms should reveal a leash of vessels supplying part of the cavity wall that can be embolized, even if not actively bleeding. Short-term success rate is good; long-term, less good
- Surgery can be difficult, as mycetomas may be stuck to the chest wall. Problems of seeding the pleural space are seen less often than in the past, probably due to better antifungal agents
- Older approaches involving intracavity injections of amphotericin are rarely used now, although a recent case series of 40 patients seemed promising.

Overview of Aspergillus lung disease

The essential differences between the Aspergillus lung diseases depends on whether the damage to the lung is mediated by host defence mechanisms (atopic asthma, flitting consolidation, ABPA, possibly aspergilloma) or by the fungus's own digestive proteolytic enzymes (invasive aspergillosis, semi-invasive, aspergilloma). These two disease states are clearly different but there probably exists a continuum between each of the subdivisions within each group, and the dominant mechanism in aspergilloma is not entirely clear. Therefore, it is likely that patients with mixed and transitional features will be encountered.

Future developments

- New antifungals—voraconazole, posaconazole, ravuconazole, caspofungin
- Antifungal action of older drugs—flucytosine, rifampicin, fluconazole
- Place of early surgery
- Place of prophylaxis
- Value of galactomannan in diagnosis.

Further information

Aspergillus Trust (for patients), *www.aspergillustrust.org*

Pneumocystis pneumonia (PCP): diagnosis

Definition Pneumocystis pneumonia (PCP) is the clinical syndrome of pneumonia resulting from infection with the fungus *Pneumocystis jiroveci* (previously termed *Pneumocystis carinii*). *Pneumocystis jiroveci* is widespread in the environment and most people are infected by the age of 2 years; PCP is thought, however, to follow new infection rather than reactivation of latent infection.

Causes Risk factors for PCP include: HIV infection (particularly with CD4 count $< 200 \times 10^6/l$), treatment with chemotherapy (especially fludarabine), corticosteroids, or other immunosuppressive agents, and malnutrition in children. PCP is much less common following the routine use of septrin prophylaxis in HIV and post-transplantation, although cases still occur, e.g. in patients presenting with advanced HIV or in those non-compliant with prophylaxis. The threshold steroid dose for predisposition to PCP is unclear, and may depend on the underlying condition, e.g. PCP may develop in patients with haematological malignancy taking as little as 5 mg prednisolone daily. PCP often presents as steroid doses are tapered.

Clinical features Gradual onset of dry cough and exertional breathlessness, sometimes with retrosternal tightness. Fever and tachypnoea may occur; chest examination is typically normal. May present with pneumothorax. Extrapulmonary disease is very rare.

Investigations

- **CXR** pattern is classically of bilateral perihilar infiltrates that progress to alveolar shadowing. Less common patterns include small, nodular infiltrates, or focal consolidation. CXR is normal in about 10%. Pleural effusions are very rare. CT is not routinely required except in cases of a normal CXR, when it may demonstrate a bilateral ground-glass pattern
- **Hypoxia** is common. Desaturation on exercise may suggest the diagnosis in at-risk individuals with normal saturations at rest
- **White blood count** is usually normal. Serum lactate dehydrogenase is typically raised (sensitive but non-specific)
- **Induced sputum** (see page 701) has a diagnostic yield of about 60% in HIV infection, but is much less sensitive when performed in the setting of non-HIV immunocompromise, where the organism burden is lower. It should not be performed on the open ward or out-patient department
- **Bronchoscopy with BAL** is the diagnostic investigation of choice in non-HIV-infected patients and in patients with HIV in whom induced sputum analysis is non-diagnostic. BAL with silver or immunofluorescent staining has a specificity of nearly 100% and sensitivity of 80–90%. This sensitivity is lower in non-HIV-infected immunocompromised patients, reflecting their lower pathogen loads

- *Transbronchial lung biopsy* has a slightly higher sensitivity (around 95%) but is associated with an increased risk of complications, so is reserved for cases where BAL is non-diagnostic. Surgical lung biopsy may be required for diagnosis in a minority of HIV-negative patients.

PCP: treatment

Antimicrobial

- Liaise with infectious diseases or HIV specialist
- High-dose co-trimoxazole (trimethoprim and sulphamethoxazole) remains the drug of choice. Administer 120 mg/kg daily in 4 divided doses PO or IV (dilute 480 mg ampoules in at least 75 ml 5% dextrose; infuse over 60 min). Use IV route initially and then PO during clinical improvement; PO may be used initially in mild cases. Side-effects (e.g. rash, nausea, vomiting, blood disorders) are common, particularly in HIV-infected patients. Consider routine use of anti-emetics
- Second-line choices if intolerant or unresponsive to co-trimoxazole include: intravenous pentamidine, clindamycin and primaquine, dapsone and trimethoprim, atovaquone, trimetrexate
- All treatments should be for 2–3 weeks
- If PCP is strongly suspected and the patient is unwell, treatment can be started immediately, as BAL *Pneumocystis* stains remain positive for up to 2 weeks. Empirical treatment is also required in the occasional situation where the diagnosis is suspected but bronchoscopy is non-diagnostic or not tolerated
- In cases of HIV presenting with PCP, subsequent early introduction of HAART may rarely be associated with acute respiratory failure, perhaps due to an aggressive inflammatory response to residual *Pneumocystis*; consider steroid trial or temporarily withholding further HAART.

Steroids

- High-dose steroids (prednisolone 40–80 mg daily PO, or IV hydrocortisone) are recommended for patients in respiratory failure. Treat at high-dose for 5 days; taper dose over 1–2 weeks.

Supportive therapy

- Hypoxia is common: administer supplementary high-flow oxygen, and consider use of CPAP. Mechanical ventilation, if considered appropriate, may be required; make this decision prior to initiating CPAP.

Outcome

- Mortality < 10% in the setting of HIV, but around 30% in patients with cancer. Mortality from PCP requiring mechanical ventilation in HIV-infected patients is about 60%, although may be significantly higher in patients with low CD4-counts
- Relapse rate in AIDS is high (60% in one year), so secondary prophylaxis with co-trimoxazole is recommended. Primary prophylaxis is offered to HIV-positive patients with CD4 count < 200×10^6/l. The indications for prophylaxis in non-HIV patients are less well-defined; consider prophylaxis for patients who are likely to receive high doses of prednisolone for prolonged periods.

Future developments

- The effect of co-infection with CMV on the outcome of PCP in HIV-infected patients is unclear. In patients with severe PCP treated with steroids, the presence of CMV in BAL fluid is associated with a worse outcome; the role of anti-CMV therapy such as gancyclovir in such cases is unknown

- The use of PCR to detect *Pneumocystis* may further increase diagnostic sensitivity, although in a proportion of cases detection using PCR is not accompanied by evidence of clinical infection, and appears to represent colonization. It is unclear if asymptomatic carriage precedes infection in such patients, and the consequences of carriage in immunocompetent individuals are also unknown.

Further information

New insights into transmission, diagnosis, and drug treatment of *Pneumocystis carinii* pneumonia. Kovacs JA, et al. *JAMA* 2001; **286**: 2450–60

The pulmonary physician in critical care. Illustrative case 5: HIV associated pneumonia. Boyton RJ et al. *Thorax* 2003; **58**: 721–5

Endemic mycoses 1

Several types of dimorphic fungi are known to commonly cause pulmonary disease in endemic regions, particularly in North America: **histoplasmosis, blastomycosis, coccidioidomycosis, and paracoccidioidomycosis**. Endemic fungi can rarely present in non-endemic areas, and diagnosis is often delayed because of their non-specific and varied clinical features, and the failure to obtain a detailed travel history. Fungal infection may mimic other diseases such as tuberculosis and lung cancer, often leading to inappropriate investigations and treatment. Fungal infections can also cause granulomata on lung biopsy, which sometimes results in diagnostic confusion (e.g. with sarcoidosis).

Infection in immunocompetent individuals is usually either asymptomatic or mild and self-limiting, although severe infection may rarely occur in apparently immunocompetent individuals. Outbreaks of disease may occur as well as sporadic cases. Unlike invasive candidosis and aspergillosis, where neutrophils are the key host defence mechanism, T cell-mediated immunity is essential for defence against the endemic mycoses. Patients with impaired T cell-mediated immunity (e.g. AIDS, lymphoma, steroid use) are therefore at particular risk of developing severe or disseminated infection.

Histoplasmosis

Epidemiology *Histoplasma capsulatum* is found in bird and bat dropping contaminated soil in the midwest and south-east USA, particularly the Ohio and Mississippi valleys, as well as in Mexico and parts of South America. The mycelial form is inhaled and subsequently develops into the yeast form ('dimorphism') within the lung, before spread via the lymphatics and the activation of T cell-mediated immunity with granuloma development.

Clinical features Manifestations of infection are highly variable:
- *Asymptomatic* infection occurs in the majority of cases. CXR may be normal or demonstrate single or multiple nodules, which may calcify in a characteristic 'target lesion' pattern. Lymphadenopathy may occur with eggshell calcification
- *Acute* symptoms may follow heavy or recurrent exposure (e.g. pigeon fanciers, cavers). Range from a self-limiting 'flu-like' illness of fever, cough, and malaise to fulminant disease with respiratory failure. CXR may be normal or show consolidation, bilateral alveolar shadowing, multiple small nodules, and sometimes lymphadenopathy
- *Chronic*, progressive lung disease occurs particularly in patients with underlying COPD; lung cavitation is common, sometimes leading to an incorrect diagnosis of tuberculosis or cancer
- *Disseminated* disease may affect the immunocompromised (particularly AIDS) and the elderly. Presentation may be acute or chronic, and manifestations include fever, weight loss, and diffuse lung involvement, although almost any organ system may be affected; other features may include hepatosplenomegaly, gastrointestinal symptoms, headache and meningism, cytopenias, endocarditis, and adrenal failure

- Other, unusual manifestations include broncholithiasis, mediastinal fibrosis (with compression of large airways, oesophagus, or superior vena cava), or isolated extrapulmonary disease (e.g. arthritis, pericarditis, erythema nodosum, erythema multiforme).

Diagnosis

- Smears or culture of infected material, e.g. sputum or BAL fluid (for chronic pulmonary disease, insensitive for acute disease), blood, urine, or bone marrow (for disseminated disease). May take several weeks
- Serology in acute disease—typically negative at presentation, and becomes positive after several weeks. A variety of serological tests are in use, including:
  - Complement fixation, designed to detect antibodies to *Histoplasma* mycelial antigen or *Histoplasma* yeast antigen. A positive result (serum titre ≥ 1 : 16 for mycelial antigen, ≥ 1 : 32 for yeast antigen) for either antigen, in a compatible clinical setting, is considered diagnostic of active disease
  - Immunodiffusion may distinguish active disease from previous exposure, but is less sensitive than complement fixation, and a negative result does not exclude the diagnosis
- Serum or urine *Histoplasma* polysaccharide antigen test—useful for diagnosis of disseminated disease and also pulmonary disease. Positive in 85–95% cases in AIDS patients. Antigenuria is seen in 90%, and antigenaemia in < 50% of non-AIDS patients.

Treatment

- Infection in immunocompetent individuals is typically self-limiting, and symptoms usually resolve within 2–4 weeks without treatment
- Indications for antifungal treatment are:
  - Persistent symptoms (usually lasting > 1 month)
  - Progressive disseminated disease
  - Heavy exposure leading to ARDS
  - Infection in the setting of immunocompromise
- Oral itraconazole is appropriate for persistent symptoms in mild/moderate disease and for disseminated disease, including patients with AIDS who have mild disease. Treat for 6–12 weeks in acute histoplasmosis, and for 1–2 years in chronic disease. In the setting of AIDS, treatment should be lifelong or until CD4 count > 200 for at least 6 months after starting HAART. Check itraconazole drug interactions and monitor liver function (ideally monthly) if taking for > 1 month. Hypokalaemia may be associated with long-term use
- Intravenous amphotericin B should be used to treat severe infection in the setting of ARDS or immunocompromise.

Endemic mycoses 2: blastomycosis

Epidemiology Infection with *Blastomyces dermatitidis* follows the inhalation of spores from contaminated soil, and clinical infection may follow outdoor activities. Blastomycosis is endemic in a distribution similar to that of histoplasmosis in the USA, although extending further north: it is endemic in the south-east USA, and the Mississippi, Ohio, and St. Lawrence river valleys. Blastomycosis also occurs in Africa, India, and the Middle East. It is significantly less common than histoplasmosis.

Clinical features Clinical presentation is variable, and may mimic other diseases such as bacterial pneumonia, tuberculosis, and lung cancer. Clinical manifestations include:

- *Asymptomatic* in at least 50% of those infected
- *Acute* presentation is typically with fever, cough, productive of mucopurulent sputum, and sometimes pleuritic chest pain; misdiagnosis as bacterial pneumonia is common. Acute presentation of fulminant respiratory disease with ARDS may occur. Other acute presentations include a 'flu-like' illness with fever, myalgia, arthralgia, and erythema nodosum
- *Chronic* presentation may occur with fever, productive cough, and weight loss
- *Disseminated* disease occurs in a minority of patients (especially in the immunocompromised), and most commonly involves the lungs, skin, bone, joints, and CNS.

CXR Airspace infiltrates are the most common finding, but a very wide range of appearances are seen, including nodular pattern, lobar consolidation, diffuse infiltrates, or large, peripheral masses (often with air bronchograms). Lymphadenopathy and pleural effusions may rarely occur.

Diagnosis

- Diagnosis is by the staining or culture of infected material. A pyogenic inflammatory response to the fungus is common (unlike in histoplasmosis), and facilitates diagnosis
- Culture of sputum has a high yield and is diagnostic in most cases of acute pulmonary disease. Multiple specimens may be required, however. A drawback of sputum culture is that several weeks may be required before the fungus is identified. Cytological examination of sputum may provide a rapid diagnosis if the examiner is trained appropriately and alerted to the possible diagnosis
- Bronchoscopy has a similar diagnostic yield to sputum culture (92% in one study), and is recommended for patients with negative sputum results; note that lidocaine may inhibit the fungal growth and minimal concentrations should be used

- More invasive procedures such as surgical lung biopsy or thoracoscopy are only rarely needed. Histological specimens require particular stains (e.g. silver stain) to facilitate identification of the fungus
- Currently available serological tests lack sensitivity and are rarely helpful.

Treatment is usually with itraconazole for at least 6 months. Observation without treatment is not generally recommended, although this is controversial and symptoms are usually self-limiting in immunocompetent individuals. Amphotericin B should be used to treat very ill patients.

Endemic mycoses 3

Coccidioidomycosis

Coccidioidomycosis is endemic in parts of south-west USA (Arizona, California, Texas, New Mexico, Utah, Nevada), northern Mexico, and Central and South America. Infection follows inhalation of *Coccidioides immitis* spores from soil. Manifestations of infection are variable, including:

- *Asymptomatic* infection, which appears to be common in endemic regions
- *Acute* pulmonary disease. Presents in a similar manner to bacterial pneumonia, with fever, cough, pleuritic chest pain, and often skin rash (e.g. erythema nodosum or erythema multiforme). Eosinophilia may be present. CXR appearance is variable, and may show areas of consolidation, lymphadenopathy, pleural effusion, or be normal. The disease is self-limiting in most cases; a minority progress to ARDS or chronic disease
- *Chronic* pulmonary disease. Uncommon, may be asymptomatic. CXR typically shows single or multiple nodules that may cavitate; upper lobe infiltrates similar to those seen in tuberculosis may develop
- *Disseminated* disease. Rare, occurs particularly in the immunocompromised. Presentation may be acute or chronic. Pulmonary disease occurs in association with involvement of the skin, bones, joints, genitourinary system, or CNS.

Diagnosis is with stains or culture of infected tissues. Sputum cultures are often positive in cavitating disease. BAL fluid culture and lung biopsies may also be diagnostic. Serological tests are also available.

Treatment is not required in the majority of patients, who have mild, self-limiting disease. Fluconazole is the antifungal of choice, when required.

Paracoccidioidomycosis

- Paracoccidioidomycosis is endemic in parts of Central and South America and Mexico
- Typically presents as chronic pulmonary disease, although acute disseminated disease may occur in the immunocompromised
- Diagnosis is made on culture of sputum or BAL fluid, or following staining of lung biopsy samples
- Treatment is with itraconazole, and long courses of up to 6 months may be needed.

Other fungi: cryptococcosis

Epidemiology

- *Cryptococcus neoformans* is found worldwide in bird droppings. Following inhalation, yeasts propagate within the alveoli without usually causing symptoms. Migration to the central nervous system may then occur, and meningoencephalitis is the most common clinical manifestation of infection
- Patients with impaired cell-mediated immunity (e.g. AIDS, steroid use, lymphoma) are particularly vulnerable to cryptococcal infection.

Clinical features

- Clinically evident cryptococcal lung disease is rare but well-described, even in HIV-negative patients. Symptoms are non-specific, including fever and cough, and presentations may be acute or chronic. The CXR appearance is very variable, ranging from a single mass or multiple nodules to interstitial or pleural involvement
- Pulmonary involvement is often associated with meningitis, and clinical signs of meningism are characteristically absent. CT head (to exclude a space-occupying lesion) followed by lumbar puncture should therefore be considered in all patients with pulmonary cryptococcal disease.

Diagnosis Diagnostic techniques include:

- India ink stain on CSF, or latex agglutination test for capsular antigen in BAL or pleural fluid, blood, or CSF
- Stains and culture of sputum, blood, urine, or BAL fluid. Positive culture from sputum may indicate colonization rather than active disease, and should be interpreted in the clinical context
- Serum cryptococcal antigen test is extremely sensitive and specific for the diagnosis.

Treatment of cryptococcal infection in the immunocompromised is with amphotericin B IV and flucytosine IV for 2–3 weeks, followed by fluconazole. The natural history of disease in immunocompetent patients is poorly understood, and observation alone is often recommended; disseminated disease may occur, however, and some experts advise treatment with fluconazole.

Candidal pneumonia

- *Candida* occurs as part of the normal human flora, and is found in the gastrointestinal tract and on the skin. Invasive disease may occur in the immunocompromised, particularly in neutropenic patients. Prophylaxis with fluconazole is used following bone marrow transplantation
- *Candida* is often isolated from respiratory secretions, but very rarely causes respiratory disease. Seeding of the lungs leading to infiltrates or enlarging nodules may occur with disseminated candidal infection
- Risk factors for candidaemia include immunocompromise, central venous lines, parenteral nutrition, and gastrointestinal surgery. In lung transplant recipients a positive donor tracheal culture for *Candida* is a marker for post-transplant candidal infection
- The clinical and radiological features of pulmonary involvement are non-specific. Extrapulmonary manifestations of infection are common, e.g. skin, eye, hepatic, or CNS involvement. Candidaemia is typically associated with a high fever
- Definitive diagnosis of pulmonary disease requires identification of tissue invasion by *Candida* on TBB or surgical lung biopsy
- Treat with amphotericin B 0.7 mg/kg/day IV, or fluconazole 400 mg/day PO, and remove any central lines
- Candidaemia carries a mortality of 30–40%.

Parasitic lung disease

A wide variety of parasitic organisms may infect the lungs, although clinical disease is rare in the UK. In general, parasites may cause lung disease by two different mechanisms:

- Hypersensitivity reactions, e.g. Löffler's syndrome and eosinophilic lung disease, most commonly from helminths such as ascariasis, toxocara, and liver flukes
- Direct infection and invasion, e.g. amoebic disease, pulmonary hydatid disease.

Some of the more important examples are noted below.

Pulmonary hydatid disease

- Hydatidosis is the commonest parasitic lung disease worldwide
- Human infection follows ingestion of parasite eggs, with the adult worm found in dogs, sheep, goats, horses, camels, and moose; infection is common in sheep-raising regions, particularly Central Europe and the Mediterranean, as well as Alaska and Arctic Canada
- Two main forms:
  - *Echinococcus granulosus*, which causes cystic hydatid disease as the larvae grow in the lungs. Common. Symptoms include cough (sometimes productive of cyst contents, 'hydatidoptysis'), haemoptysis, and chest pain. CXR shows rounded cysts, sometimes with calcified walls, most commonly in lower lobes; CT may show 'daughter cysts'. Cyst rupture may occur, with wheeze, eosinophilia, and bronchial or pleural spread
  - *Echinococcus multilocularis*, which leads to alveolar hydatid disease following tissue invasion. Rare. Lung masses are less clearly delineated on CT than in cystic disease
- Diagnose from serology or sputum analysis. Serology is insensitive for the diagnosis of pulmonary disease (around 50%). Demonstration of liver cysts supports the diagnosis. Avoid needle aspiration of cysts, which may result in hypersensitivity or dissemination
- Treatment is with surgical excision in most cases. Medical treatment with albendazole if the patient is unfit for surgery or following cyst rupture and dissemination.

Amoebic pulmonary disease

- Intestinal and liver infection is common, with lung involvement in a minority
- Lung disease can develop either directly from the liver or via the bloodstream or lymphatics
- Pulmonary manifestations include right lower lobe consolidation, empyema, lung abscess, or hepatobronchial fistulae (resulting in large volumes of brown or 'anchovy' sputum). May be associated pericardial disease
- Diagnose using serology or following identification of trophozoites in stool, sputum, or pleural fluid
- Treatment is with metronidazole plus iodoquinol or diloxanide.

Pulmonary ascariasis

- Distributed worldwide
- Lung involvement occurs during maturation of *Ascaris lumbricoides*, and is typically manifest as a hypersensitivity reaction with cough, wheeze, fever, CXR infiltrates, and peripheral eosinophilia
- Examination of stool for eggs may confirm the diagnosis
- Usually resolves spontaneously after 1–2 weeks. Consider treatment with mebendazole for gastrointestinal infection.

Strongyloidiasis

- Caused by *Strongyloides stercoralis*, found in Central and South America and Africa
- Pulmonary involvement may lead to a Löffler-type syndrome with wheeze, skin rash, eosinophilia and CXR infiltrate. In the setting of immunocompromise, disseminated infection may occur leading to the 'hyperinfection syndrome'. ARDS may develop, and secondary bacterial sepsis is common
- Diagnose using serology or following microbiological analysis of stool or duodenal fluid
- Treatment is with thiabendazole.

Toxocara canis

- Caused by *Toxocara canis*, distributed worldwide. Dogs are the primary host
- Ingestion of eggs from contaminated soil may result in visceral larva migrans. Migration of larvae through the lungs results in an immune response, with wheeze, cough, and eosinophilia
- Diagnosis may be made from serology
- Treatment often not required; steroids may be beneficial in severe cases.

Dirofilariasis

- Found in USA, Japan, South America
- Infection is caused by *Dirofilaria immitis* following mosquito transfer from animals, especially dogs. Worms lodge in the pulmonary arteries and elicit an inflammatory response, leading to a necrotic nodule
- Presentation is classically asymptomatic with a single peripheral nodule on CXR, mimicking cancer. Patients may present with cough, chest pain, and haemoptysis, presumably due to pulmonary infarction
- Definitive diagnosis requires lung biopsy. Serology lacks sensitivity and specificity
- Treatment is not usually needed.

Schistosomiasis

- Found in the Middle East, South America, South-east Asia, Africa, and the Caribbean
- *Schistosoma* species are carried by snails, and infection follows skin penetration, often during swimming
- Pulmonary involvement may reflect acute tissue migration, causing cough, wheeze, and CXR infiltrates, or chronic infection, leading to interstitial infiltrates, pulmonary hypertension, or AV fistulae
- Diagnosis from observation of ova in sputum, BAL, urine, or stool, or from lung biopsy
- Treatment is with praziquantel.

Paragonimiasis

- Caused by *Paragonimus westermani*, distributed in West Africa, the Far East, India, and Central and South America
- Following ingestion, flukes migrate to the lung or pleura. Clinical features may be acute or chronic, and include chest pain, pneumothorax, pleural effusion, Löffler's syndrome, and recurrent haemoptysis. Serum eosinophilia is common
- Diagnose with serology or observation of eggs in sputum, TBB, BAL, or pleural fluid
- Treatment is with praziquantel.

Tropical pulmonary eosinophilia

- Follows infection with *Wuchereria bancrofti* or *Brugia malayi* in the tropics
- Pulmonary involvement is common and represents a hypersensitivity reaction to the organism, with cough, wheeze, CXR infiltrates, and raised serum IgE
- Treatment is with diethylcarbamazine.

Pneumothorax

Clinical features and investigations

Definition A pneumothorax is air in the pleural space. May occur with apparently normal lungs (primary pneumothorax) or in the presence of underlying lung disease (secondary pneumothorax). May occur spontaneously or following trauma.

Epidemiology

- Annual incidence of primary pneumothorax is around 9 per 100,000
- Primary pneumothoraces occur most commonly in tall, thin men aged between 20 and 40. They are less common in women (male:female 5:1)—consider the possibility of underlying lung disease (e.g. lymphangioleiomyomatosis, catamenial pneumothorax)
- Cigarette smoking is a major risk factor for pneumothorax, increasing the risk by a factor of 22 in men and 9 in women. The mechanism is unclear; a smoking-induced influx of inflammatory cells may both break down elastic lung fibres (causing bulla formation) and cause small airways obstruction (increasing alveolar pressure and the likelihood of interstitial air leak)
- May rarely be familial.

Causes and pathophysiology

Primary

- Pathogenesis is poorly understood; they are presumed to occur following an air leak from apical bullae, although small airway inflammation is often also present and may contribute by increasing airways resistance.

Secondary

- Underlying diseases include: COPD (60% of cases), asthma, interstitial lung disease, necrotizing pneumonia, tuberculosis, PCP, cystic fibrosis, Langerhans' cell histiocytosis, lymphangioleiomyomatosis, Marfan's syndrome, oesophageal rupture, lung cancer, catamenial pneumothorax, and pulmonary infarction
- Pneumothorax may be the first presentation of the underlying disease.

Clinical features

- Classically presents with acute onset of pleuritic chest pain and/or breathlessness. Breathlessness is often minimal in young patients and is more severe in secondary pneumothorax
- Signs of pneumothorax include tachycardia, reduced expansion, hyper-resonant percussion note, and quiet breath sounds on the pneumothorax side. These are frequently absent in small pneumothoraces. Hamman's sign refers to a 'click' on auscultation in time with the heart sounds, due to movement of pleural surfaces with a left-sided pneumothorax
- May feel 'bubbles' and 'crackles' under the skin of the torso and neck if there is subcutaneous emphysema
- Presents in ventilated patients with acute clinical deterioration and hypoxia or increasing inflation pressures.

Investigations

- **CXR** is the diagnostic test in most cases, revealing a visible lung edge and absent lung markings peripherally. Blunting of the ipsilateral costophrenic angle due to bleeding into the pleural space is common. Pneumothoraces are difficult to visualize on supine films: look for a sharply delineated heart border, hemidiaphragm depression, and increased lucency on the affected side
- Width of the rim of air surrounding the lung on CXR may be used to classify pneumothoraces into small (rim of air < 2 cm) and large (≥ 2 cm). A 2 cm rim of air approximately equates to a 50% pneumothorax in volume
- Tiny pneumothoraces that are not apparent on PA CXR may be visible on lateral chest or lateral decubitus radiographs
- CXR appearance may also show features of underlying lung disease, although this can be difficult to assess in the presence of a large pneumothorax
- **CT chest** may be required to differentiate pneumothorax from bullous disease, and is useful in diagnosing unsuspected pneumothorax following trauma and in looking for evidence of underlying lung disease
- **ABGs** frequently show hypoxia and sometimes hypercapnia in secondary pneumothorax.

Prognosis

- Average of 30% (range 16–54% in studies) of primary pneumothoraces recur, most within 2 years. Continued smoking increases the risk of recurrence. Risk of recurrence increases with each subsequent pneumothorax: risk of recurrence is around 30% after a first pneumothorax, about 40% after a second, and > 50% after a third
- Mortality of secondary pneumothorax 10%
- Recurrence of secondary pneumothorax occurs in 39–47%, and is associated with age, pulmonary fibrosis, and emphysema. Recurrence rates may be as high as 80% in patients with Langerhans' cell histiocytosis or lymphangioleiomyomatosis.

Further information

Spontaneous pneumothorax. Sahn SA, Heffner JE. *NEJM* 2000, **342**(12): 868–74

Initial management

There is considerable variation amongst clinicians regarding optimal pneumothorax management. The treatment algorithms presented on pages 294–5 follow the BTS guidelines.

General management points

- Management is determined by the degree of breathlessness and hypoxia, evidence of haemodynamic compromise, the presence and severity of any underlying lung disease, and to some extent the pneumothorax size
- Severe breathlessness out of proportion to pneumothorax size may be a feature of impending tension pneumothorax
- Secondary pneumothorax has a significant mortality (10%), and should be managed more aggressively. Treat also the underlying disease.

Aspiration

- Procedure described on page 679
- Halt the procedure if painful, or if the patient coughs excessively; do not aspirate > 2.5 l of air, as this suggests a large air-leak and aspiration is likely to fail
- Ideal timing of repeat CXR following aspiration is unknown; it may be advisable to wait several hours before performing the CXR, in order to detect slow air leaks
- Aspiration is successful if the lung is fully or nearly re-expanded on CXR
- If initial aspiration of a primary pneumothorax fails, repeat aspiration should be considered (unless ≥ 2.5 l has already been aspirated). At least one-third of patients will respond to second aspiration, although the optimal timing of repeat aspiration is unclear.

Chest drainage

- Procedure described on page 688
- Associated with significant morbidity and even mortality, and not required in the majority of patients with primary spontaneous pneumothorax
- Small (10–14F) drains are sufficient in most cases; consider large-bore (24–28F) drain in secondary pneumothorax with large air leak, severe subcutaneous emphysema, or in mechanically ventilated patients
- Never clamp a bubbling chest drain (risk of tension pneumothorax)
- When air leak appears to have ceased, clamping of the drain for several hours followed by repeat CXR may detect very slow or intermittent air leaks, thereby avoiding inappropriate drain removal; this is controversial, however, and should only be considered on a specialist ward with experienced nursing staff. Addition of washing-up liquid to water in underwater seal bottle aids visualization of bubbling in very slow air leaks
- If drain water level does not swing with respiration, the drain is kinked (check underneath dressing, as tube enters skin), blocked, clamped, or incorrectly positioned (drainage holes not in pleural space; check CXR)
- Heimlich flutter valves (or thoracic vents) are an alternative to underwater bottle drainage, and are being used increasingly in some

centres. They allow greater patient mobilization, and sometimes out-patient management of pneumothorax.

Oxygen
- All hospitalized patients should receive high flow (10 l/min) inspired oxygen (unless CO_2 retention is a problem). This reduces the partial pressure of nitrogen in blood, encouraging removal of air from the pleural space and speeding up resolution of the pneumothorax.

Persistent air leak
- Defined as continued bubbling of chest drain 48 hours after insertion
- Consider drain suction (−10 to −20 cm H_2O), insertion of large-bore drain, and/or thoracic surgical referral
- Check that persistent bubbling is not the result of 'outside' air being sucked down the drain, e.g. following drain displacement such that a hole lies outside the pleural cavity, or, if enlargement of the drain track occurs, allowing outside air to enter and then be released down the drain.

Discharge
- Prior to discharge, discuss flying and diving (see page 292), and advise to return to hospital immediately if breathlessness worsens. Document this in medical notes.

Further management

Out-patient follow-up
- Repeat CXR to ensure resolution of pneumothorax and normal appearance of underlying lungs
- Discuss risk of recurrence and emphasize smoking cessation, if appropriate
- Ascent to altitude with a pneumothorax is potentially hazardous. Guidelines recommend that patients should not fly for at least 6 weeks from the resolution of pneumothorax on CXR or surgical treatment. This time interval is arbitrary, however, and patients should understand that there is a high initial risk of recurrence that falls with time, and they may wish to avoid flying for a longer period, e.g. 1 year
- Advise never to dive in the future, unless patient has undergone a definitive surgical procedure.

Surgical management

Indications for cardiothoracic surgical referral:
- Second ipsilateral pneumothorax
- First contralateral pneumothorax
- Bilateral spontaneous pneumothorax
- Persistent air leak (>5–7 days of drainage)
- Spontaneous haemothorax
- Professions at risk (e.g. pilots, divers) after first pneumothorax.

Note that these are guidelines only, and patient choice will also influence the decision for surgical intervention.

Surgical treatments aim to repair the apical hole or bleb and close the pleural space. Options:
- *Video-assisted thoracoscopic surgery (VATS)* Recurrence rates are higher than for open thoracotomy (4% vs. 1.5%), although less invasive procedure and probably shorter hospital stay. Pleural abrasion (rather than talc poudrage) is usually favoured for closure of the pleural space. Often the procedure of choice in young patients with primary pneumothorax
- *Open thoracotomy* Apical bleb resected, pleural space closed by pleural abrasion or parietal pleurectomy. Effective procedure with a recurrence rate <1%, but probably prolonged recovery rates compared to VATS
- *Transaxillary minithoracotomy* uses a relatively small axillary incision and may be a less invasive alternative to open thoracotomy.

Chemical pleurodesis
- Talc or tetracycline most commonly used; procedure described on page 692
- Can be performed via intercostal drain or at VATS
- Failure rates around 10–20%, and some concern about the long-term safety of intrapleural talc; therefore not recommended in younger patients

- Consider pleurodesis via intercostal drain only as a last resort in older patients with recurrent pneumothorax in whom surgery would be high-risk (e.g. patients with severe COPD)
- Likelihood of successful pleurodesis in the setting of an incompletely re-expanded lung with a persistent air leak remains uncertain, although it may be attempted if surgery is not an option.

Treatment algorithm for primary pneumothorax

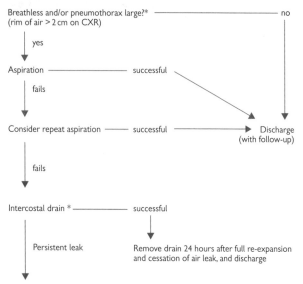

Breathless and/or pneumothorax large?* ———————————— no
(rim of air > 2 cm on CXR)

↓ yes

Aspiration ——————————— successful

↓ fails

Consider repeat aspiration ——— successful ——————→ Discharge
(with follow-up)

↓ fails

Intercostal drain * ——————— successful

Persistent leak → Remove drain 24 hours after full re-expansion
and cessation of air leak, and discharge

↓

Consider drain suction
Thoracic surgical referral after 7 days of air leak

* Some disagreement exists regarding this point: in the setting of a relatively asymptomatic patient
with a large pneumothorax, the risk of intervention may outweigh the risk of the pneumothorax,
and conservative management may be considered.

Treatment algorithm for secondary pneumothorax

Consider in-patient observation without aspiration in relatively asymptomatic patients with tiny (<1 cm) pneumothoraces.

Further information

BTS Guidelines for the management of spontaneous pneumothorax. M Henry, T Arnold *et al.* *Thorax* 2003; **58** (suppl. II): ii39–ii52

Specific situations

Tension pneumothorax

- Pneumothorax acts as a one-way valve, with air entering the pleural space on each inspiration and unable to escape on expiration. The progressive increase in pleural pressure compresses both lungs and mediastinum and inhibits venous return to the heart, leading to hypotension and potentially cardiac arrest
- Occurrence is not related to pneumothorax size, and tension can occur with very small pneumothoraces in the context of air trapping in the lung from obstructive lung disease
- Typically presents with acute respiratory distress, agitation, hypotension, raised jugular venous pressure, and tracheal deviation away from the pneumothorax side. Reduced air entry on affected side
- May present with cardiac arrest (pulseless electrical activity), or with acute deterioration in ventilated patients
- If suspected, give high-flow oxygen and insert large-bore cannula into second intercostal space in midclavicular line on side of pneumothorax. Do not wait for a CXR if cardiac arrest has occurred or the diagnosis is clinically certain. Hiss of escaping air confirms diagnosis. Aspirate air until the patient is less distressed and then, leaving cannula in place, insert chest drain in midaxillary line.

Iatrogenic pneumothorax

- Causes include transbronchial biopsy, transthoracic needle lung biopsy, subclavian line insertion, mechanical ventilation, pleural aspiration, pleural biopsy, external cardiac massage, and percutaneous liver biopsy
- Presentation may be delayed, even several days after procedure
- Most cases do not require intervention and improve with observation, although aspiration is sometimes required
- Drainage is seldom needed, although is more commonly required in patients with COPD. The exception is mechanically ventilated patients, who will require an intercostal drain in the majority of cases.

Traumatic pneumothorax

- Up to half may not be clinically apparent or visible on CXR; chest CT is required for diagnosis
- Majority of patients require intercostal drain
- Consider VATS early if persistent air leak.

Subcutaneous (or 'surgical') emphysema

- Occurs as air tracks below skin under pressure from the pleural space
- May result from large air-leaks, particularly in the presence of underlying lung disease such as COPD. Also may occur if chest drain is blocked or displaced so that holes lie subcutaneously
- Harmless in majority of cases, although rarely may result in significant respiratory compromise from upper airway compression
- Treat with high-flow (10 l/min) inspired oxygen (unless CO_2 retention a problem). Check that the drain is patent (swinging, bubbling)

- Management if unwell: oxygen, large-bore chest drain on suction. If the airway is compromised, consider anaesthetizing and incising areas of affected skin and 'milking' out subcutaneous air; subcutaneous drains are sometimes used, and in rare cases tracheostomy is required.

Pneumothorax in HIV

- Most commonly occurs as a result of PCP. Empirical treatment of PCP is advised (see page 272)
- Use of nebulized pentamidine may increase the risk of pneumothorax
- Consider early intercostal drainage and surgical referral.

Pneumothorax in cystic fibrosis

- Associated with severe underlying lung disease
- Subsequent ipsilateral and contralateral pneumothorax common
- Manage as for secondary pneumothorax, although intercostal drainage frequently required
- Give course of intravenous antibiotics
- In cases of persistent air leak despite suction, discuss management with cardiothoracic surgical team at local transplant centre. Partial pleurectomy is effective in preventing recurrence. Pleurodesis renders later transplant technically more difficult, but it is not an absolute contraindication to transplantation.

Catamenial pneumothorax

- Pneumothorax occurring at the same time as menstruation
- Usually recurrent
- Pathogenesis is unknown; possibilities include pleural endometriosis or transfer of air into pleural spaces through a diaphragmatic defect from the peritoneal cavity at menstruation
- Treatment options: VATS, pleurodesis, ovulation-suppressing drugs.

Re-expansion pulmonary oedema

- Occurs in up to 14% of cases following treatment, and causes breathlessness and cough with evidence of oedema in the re-expanded lung (and sometimes both lungs) on CXR
- More common in young patients with large primary pneumothoraces, and may be associated with late presentations to hospital
- May be precipitated by early use of suction (<48 hours)
- Self-resolving in most cases, although may rarely be fatal.

Pleural effusions

Clinical features and imaging

A pleural effusion results from the accumulation of abnormal volumes (>10–20 ml) of fluid in the pleural space. Pleural effusions are common and are associated with many different diseases: see Chapter 6 for a step-by-step approach to the diagnosis of a patient with a pleural effusion, differential diagnosis of transudates and exudates, and details of pleural fluid analysis.

Clinical features

- May be asymptomatic, or associated with breathlessness, dry cough, pleuritic chest pain (suggesting pleural inflammation), chest 'heaviness', and sometimes pain referred to the shoulder or abdomen
- Signs on examination include reduced chest expansion, reduced tactile vocal fremitus, a stony dull percussion note, quiet breath sounds, and sometimes a patch of bronchial breathing above the fluid level. A friction rub may be heard with pleural inflammation.

Imaging

CXR

- Sequential blunting of posterior, lateral, and then anterior costophrenic angles are seen on radiographs as effusions increase in size
- PA CXR will usually detect effusion volumes of 200 ml or more; lateral CXR is more sensitive and may detect as little as 50 ml pleural fluid
- Classical CXR appearance is of basal opacity obscuring hemidiaphragm, with concave upper border. Massive effusion may result in a 'white-out' of the hemithorax, with mediastinal displacement away from the effusion; lack of mediastinal shift in such cases raises the possibility of associated volume loss due to bronchial obstruction from a primary lung cancer
- Other CXR appearances include rounded or lentiform shadowing in loculated interlobar effusions, and diffuse shadowing throughout the hemithorax on supine films
- CXR appearance may suggest the underlying diagnosis, e.g. bilateral effusions with cardiomegaly in cardiac failure; massive effusions are most commonly due to malignancy.

Ultrasound is extremely sensitive at detecting fluid volumes of 100 ml or more, and is useful for distinguishing pleural fluid from pleural masses or thickening, and for demonstrating loculation.

CT chest with pleural contrast is useful in distinguishing benign and malignant pleural disease: nodular, mediastinal, or circumferential pleural thickening are all highly specific for malignant disease. CT may also reveal evidence of extrapleural disease, e.g. lymphadenopathy or parenchymal change, which may suggest a diagnosis such as cancer or tuberculosis. Role of *MRI* is unclear; it may have increasing role in distinguishing benign from malignant pleural disease.

Pleural thickening

- Pleural fibrosis and thickening may follow previous episodes of pleural inflammation. Causes include previous empyema, tuberculous pleuritis, rheumatoid pleuritis, haemothorax, thoracotomy, and asbestos exposure (diffuse pleural thickening, page 320)
- May be asymptomatic or cause breathlessness
- CXR features include blunting of the costophrenic angle or apices, sometimes with associated calcification
- Ultrasound or CT may be required to distinguish from a pleural effusion
- Treatment is difficult and usually unnecessary; decortication may be considered.

Malignant pleural effusion: causes and investigations

Epidemiology Commonest cause of exudative pleural effusion in patients older than 60 years. About 40,000 cases of malignant effusion each year in the UK.

Causes Most malignant effusions are metastatic, with lung and breast the most common primary sites:

Primary site	Approximate frequency (%)
Lung	37
Breast	16
Lymphoma	10
Mesothelioma	10
Genitourinary tract	9
Gastrointestinal tract	7
Unknown primary	10

Other, rarer tumours include sarcoma, melanoma, leukaemia, and myeloma; almost any malignant tumour may spread to the pleural cavity. *Mesothelioma* is an important cause of malignant effusions and is discussed on page 324.

Clinical features Breathlessness is the main symptom; chest pain, cough, weight loss, and anorexia may also be present. A small proportion of patients are asymptomatic. Effusions may be unilateral or bilateral, and are frequently large volume.

Differential diagnosis Consider other potential causes of pleural effusion in patients known to have cancer, e.g. due to pneumonia, pulmonary embolism, radiotherapy, pericardial disease, or drugs.

Investigations A strategy for investigating the patient with an undiagnosed pleural effusion is detailed on page 32. Key investigations in patients suspected to have a malignant effusion are:

1. Pleural fluid cytology Sensitivity for malignancy is about 60%; yield is increased by analysis of a second, but not a third sample. Immunostaining of malignant cells may provide clues as to the likely primary site. Visualization of monoclonal cells in fluid on flow cytometry may support a diagnosis of lymphoma.

2. CT chest with pleural contrast Nodular, mediastinal, or circumferential pleural thickening on CT are highly specific for malignant disease. May also demonstrate extrapleural disease, e.g. lymphadenopathy.

3. Pleural biopsy histology Required in cytology-negative cases. Options:
- *CT-guided* cutting needle biopsy has been demonstrated to be a more effective diagnostic test for malignant pleural disease than Abrams' pleural biopsy (sensitivity 87% in CT-guided biopsy group vs. 47% in Abrams' group)
- *Ultrasound-guided* needle biopsies are also effective and relatively straightforward to perform
- *Thoracoscopy* is an extremely useful investigation allowing direct visualization of the pleural space with a high sensitivity (90%) for biopsies. Therapeutic talc poudrage (talc is 'puffed' directly on to the pleural surfaces) may be performed at same time, with a pleurodesis success rate > 80%. Can be performed under general anaesthesia, although well tolerated with sedation and local anaesthesia. Complications (such as empyema) are rare.

Serum tumour markers (CEA, CA19-9, CA15-3, CA125, PSA) may be helpful in the investigation of patients with malignant effusion of unknown primary, although their diagnostic and prognostic value are limited.

Prognosis Median survival 3–12 months from diagnosis; shortest in lung cancer, longest in mesothelioma and ovarian cancer. Pleural fluid pH < 7.3 tends to be associated with shorter survival (median survival 2.1 months) and decreased success of pleurodesis.

Further information

BTS guidelines for the management of malignant pleural effusions. Antunes G, *et al*. *Thorax* 2003; **58** (suppl. II): ii 29–38

Standard pleural biopsy versus CT-guided cutting-needle biopsy for diagnosis of malignant disease in pleural effusions: a randomised controlled trial. Maskell NA, *et al*. *Lancet* 2003; **361**: 1326–31

Malignant pleural effusion: management

Key points influencing the management of malignant effusions are:
- Symptoms, performance status, and wishes of the patient
- Sensitivity of the primary tumour to chemotherapy, e.g. small cell lung carcinoma, lymphoma, ovarian and breast carcinoma may respond to chemotherapy, although in some cases pleural effusions remain problematic and require additional treatment
- Extent of lung re-expansion following effusion drainage.

Treatment options

Observation and follow-up if asymptomatic.

Therapeutic pleural aspiration of 1–1.5 l pleural fluid to improve breathlessness. Can be performed at the bed-side as a day-case procedure, avoiding hospital admission. Useful in the palliation of breathlessness in patients with a poor prognosis, and in rare cases where effusion reaccumulates very slowly. Most effusions recur within 1 month of aspiration, and these patients should be considered for pleurodesis; repeated aspiration may be inconvenient and uncomfortable for the patient, and carries a risk of complications such as empyema, pneumothorax, and tumour seeding (in mesothelioma).

If the breathlessness does not improve following fluid aspiration, then there is little to be gained by repeated aspiration and other causes of breathlessness should be considered, e.g. lymphangitis carcinomatosa, pulmonary embolism.

Intercostal chest drainage and pleurodesis The aim of pleurodesis is to seal the visceral pleura to the parietal pleura with adhesions to prevent pleural fluid accumulating. The success of pleurodesis depends on the degree of apposition of the visceral and parietal pleura, which depends on the degree of lung re-expansion following drainage of the effusion. 'Trapped lung' occurs when tumour encases the visceral pleura and prevents lung expansion. Lung expansion may also be inhibited by a proximal airway obstruction or by a persistent air leak (e.g. after tearing of a friable, tumour-infiltrated lung on re-expansion). Trapped lung may also be caused by non-malignant, fibrotic processes, e.g. rheumatoid pleuritis, haemothorax, tuberculosis.

The patient should be admitted and the effusion drained with an intercostal tube. If lung fully re-expands on CXR, proceed to pleurodesis (see page 691). If lung fails to re-expand fully (trapped lung; CXR shows a pneumothorax or hydropneumothorax), consider chest drain suction, which may encourage lung expansion and allow pleurodesis.

Treatment options for trapped lung or failed pleurodesis:
- *Pleurodesis* may be successful despite only partial lung re-expansion and should still be considered. It may be repeated if unsuccessful initially
- *Repeated therapeutic pleural aspiration*
- *Intrapleural fibrinolytics* (e.g. streptokinase 250,000 IU) may be of benefit in the management of multiloculated effusions resistant to drainage and

pleurodesis, encouraging free fluid drainage and in some cases enabling successful pleurodesis. Haemorrhage is a theoretical complication, although appears to be uncommon

- *Thoracoscopy* enables the disruption of pleural adhesions and may have a role in facilitating pleurodesis in select patients with trapped lung
- *Long-term indwelling pleural catheter* may be beneficial in patients with trapped lung and frequent accumulation of symptomatic effusions, and avoids the need for recurrent pleural aspiration. The most frequent complications are tumour seeding around the drain site and pleural space infection. Can be inserted as a day-case procedure. Needs additional out-patient support (e.g. trained district nurse or respiratory specialist nurse), although most patients perform the drainage themselves after education
- *Pleuroperitoneal shunts* are effective in patients with trapped lung or failed pleurodesis, in the absence of multiple loculations. Shunting of fluid may occur spontaneously, at high pressures, or may require manipulation of a percutaneous pump chamber, inserted at thoracoscopy or mini-thoracotomy. Main problem is shunt occlusion, which occurs in at least 10% of cases and necessitates shunt removal. Malignant spread may also occur
- *Surgical parietal pleurectomy* may be performed as a VATS (video-assisted thorascopic surgery). The procedure is effective in the management of refractory malignant effusions. May be useful in a minority of patients with good performance status and prognosis. Not suitable for patients with heavily diseased visceral pleura and trapped lung; consider in patients who have failed pleurodesis
- *Palliative care team* involvement should also be considered.

Parapneumonic effusion and empyema: definition and clinical features

Definition and pathophysiology Pleural effusions occur in up to 40% of patients with pneumonia. An initial sterile exudate (simple parapneumonic effusion) may in some cases progress to a complicated parapneumonic effusion and eventually empyema:

Simple parapneumonic effusion	Exudative stage
	Clear, sterile fluid with normal pH, glucose, LDH
	Frequently resolves with antibiotics alone
	Drainage not usually required
Complicated parapneumonic effusion	Fibrinopurulent stage
	Fibrin deposited and septations occur
	Fluid infected but not yet purulent; appears clear or cloudy/turbid
	pH< 7.2, glucose < 2.2 mmol/l and LDH > 1000 IU/l
	Gram stain/culture may be positive
	Drainage required
Empyema	Pus in pleural space
	May be free-flowing or multiloculated
	Gram stain/culture may be positive
	Drainage required
	Eventually, fibroblast growth may result in development of thick pleural peel (organizing stage). Treatment at this stage is difficult and decortication may be required

Pleural infection may also occur in the absence of a preceding pneumonic illness ('primary empyema').

Clinical features

Common

- Consider the diagnosis particularly in cases of 'slow to respond' pneumonia, pleural effusion with fever, or in high-risk groups with non-specific symptoms such as weight loss
- Similar to clinical presentation of pneumonia: fever, sputum production, chest pain, breathlessness
- Anaerobic empyema may present less acutely, often with weight loss and without fever.

Rare
- Infected pleural fluid may spontaneously drain through the chest wall ('*empyema necessitatis*') or into the lung, leading to a bronchopleural fistula and severe pneumonia
- History of atypical chest pain, vomiting, or oesophageal instrumentation suggests possible underlying oesophageal rupture (measure pleural fluid amylase)
- History of a recent sore throat may suggest Lemierre's syndrome (acute oropharyngeal infection with *Fusobacterium* species leads to septic thrombophlebitis of the internal jugular vein and subsequent metastatic infection and abscess formation, commonly in the lungs and pleura; consider ultrasound of internal jugular vein if suspected); see page 202.

Risk factors for developing empyema include diabetes, alcohol abuse, gastro-oesophageal reflux, and intravenous drug abuse. Anaerobic infection is associated particularly with aspiration or poor dental hygiene. Empyema may rarely occur following bronchial obstruction from a tumour or foreign body. Many patients, however, have no apparent risk factors.

Differential diagnosis includes malignancy, tuberculosis (when the pleural fluid is usually lymphocytic), and rheumatoid pleuritis.

Parapneumonic effusion and empyema: bacteriology and investigations

Bacteriology

- **Community-acquired** infection (% of cases):
  - *S. milleri* (28%)
  - Anaerobes (19%)
  - *S. pneumoniae* (14%)
  - Staphylococci (12%)
  - Other less common organisms include other Streptococci, Enterobacteria, *H. influenza*, Pseudomonas, TB, and Nocardia. Legionella may very rarely cause empyema.
- **Hospital-acquired** infection (% of cases):
  - MRSA (27%)
  - Staphylococci (22%)
  - Enterobacteria (20%)
  - Enterococcus (12%)
  - Others include Streptococci, Pseudomonas, and anaerobes.

Gram-negative organisms may occur in mixed growths with other Gram-negatives or with anaerobes.

Investigations

- **Diagnostic pleural tap** is essential if pleural infection is suspected. Frankly purulent or turbid/cloudy pleural fluid, organisms on pleural fluid Gram stain or culture, or pleural fluid pH < 7.2 are all indications for chest tube drainage. 40% of pleural infections are culture-negative. Identification of anaerobes is improved following inoculation of blood culture bottles with pleural fluid
- **Ultrasound** typically shows echogenic effusion that may be septated, and is useful in guiding pleural tap in patients with small or loculated effusions or following an unsuccessful 'blind' tap. Very small effusions (<10 mm maximal thickness on ultrasound) probably do not require tapping and can be observed
- **Contrast-enhanced CT** may be useful both in supporting the diagnosis and visualizing the distribution of fluid. Empyema is associated with pleural enhancement and increased attenuation of extrapleural subcostal fat. The displacement of adjacent lung by empyema may help to distinguish from a parenchymal lung abscess. Empyemas frequently appear lenticular and may exhibit the 'split pleura' sign of enhancing, separated visceral and parietal pleura. Absence of pleural thickening on CT is unusual in empyema. CT may also sometimes identify a proximal endobronchial obstructing lesion
- **Blood cultures** positive in only 13% of cases, but in these cases they are often the only positive microbiology
- **Bronchoscopy** is only indicated if a bronchial obstructing lesion is suspected.

Parapneumonic effusion and empyema: management and outcome

Management

1. Antibiotics All patients with pleural infection should be treated with antibiotics; refer to local hospital prescribing guidelines. Typical choices:

- *Community-acquired* empyema—second-generation cephalosporin (e.g. cefuroxime) plus metronidazole as anaerobic cover. Ciprofloxacin and clindamycin together may be appropriate. Add macrolide if Legionella is suspected
- *Hospital-acquired* empyema—cover Gram-positive and Gram-negative organisms and anaerobes. MRSA infection is common. Consult with microbiology team. One option is meropenem and vancomycin.

Rationalize with culture and sensitivity results (although note that anaerobes are frequently difficult to culture and may coexist with other organisms). Avoid aminoglycosides, which penetrate the pleural space poorly.

Switch to oral antibiotics when apyrexial and improving clinically. Augmentin is a useful single agent with anaerobic cover (not if penicillin allergic). Optimal duration of antibiotic treatment unclear, although likely to be at least 3 weeks.

2. Chest tube drainage

Indications for chest tube drainage

- Frankly purulent or turbid/cloudy pleural fluid
- Organisms on pleural fluid Gram stain or culture
- Pleural fluid pH < 7.2.

Consider earlier chest tube drainage in the elderly and patients with co-morbidity, and loculated effusions, as these are associated with a worse outcome.

Drain insertion should ideally be carried out under ultrasound or CT guidance, as effusions are frequently loculated. Ideal chest tube size remains subject to debate. Small (10–14 French) flexible tubes are more comfortable and have been demonstrated to be as effective as large drains in the management of empyema. Usually apply suction (– 20 cm water) and flush regularly (e.g. 30 ml normal saline every 6 hours) to prevent occlusion. Consider drain removal when clinical improvement occurs. If there is no indication for drainage, give antibiotics and monitor closely. If slow to improve or deteriorate, re-sample the effusion and consider chest drain.

3. Intrapleural fibrinolytics Current evidence suggests that intrapleural streptokinase has no effect on mortality, need for surgery, or hospital stay, and the routine use of fibrinolytics is therefore not recommended.

4. Nutritional support Dietician review, consider supplementary nasogastric feeding. Intravenous feeding may be required.

5. Surgery Consult with thoracic surgeon if there are ongoing features of sepsis and residual pleural collection after 7 days despite tube drainage and treatment with antibiotics. Surgical techniques include:

- *Video-assisted thoracoscopic surgery (VATS)* allows the breakdown of adhesions and drainage of residual collection, but it is frequently unsuccessful in chronic empyema with very thickened visceral pleura
- *Thoracotomy and decortication* Removal of fibrinous and infected tissue from the pleural space, a major surgical procedure
- *Open thoracic drainage* Resection of segments of several ribs adjacent to the empyema and insertion of large-bore drains into the cavity: a more minor procedure that can be performed under local anaesthesia, but results in open chest wound for long period (typically around 5 months).

Difficulties in management

Chest drainage ceases despite residual pleural collection

- Attempt to flush drain with normal saline
- Ensure that drain is not kinked at skin insertion site or lying subcutaneously
- Consider CT to assess extent of residual collection and drain position
- Remove drain if persistently blocked
- Consider further image-guided chest drain(s), surgery.

Failure to clinically improve despite antibiotics and chest drain

- Review microbiology results and ensure appropriate antibiotics
- CT to assess extent of residual collection and drain position
- Surgical referral
- Options if unfit for surgery:
  - Further image-guided small-bore drains into loculated effusions
  - Large-bore drain
  - Surgical rib resection and open drainage under local anaesthesia.

Outcome About 15% of patients require surgery. Empyema one-year mortality is about 15%. Increased age, renal impairment, low serum albumin, hypotension, and hospital-acquired infection are associated with a poor outcome. CXR may remain abnormal despite successful treatment of empyema, with evidence of calcification or pleural scarring or thickening.

Further information

BTS Guidelines for the management of pleural infection. Davies CWH, *et al. Thorax* 2003; **58** (suppl. II): ii18–28

Tuberculous pleural effusion

Definition and epidemiology Tuberculous pleural effusion usually develops from a delayed hypersensitivity reaction to mycobacteria released into the pleural space. It is a common manifestation of primary tuberculosis in regions with a high prevalence, affecting children and young adults; it may also be associated with reactivation of tuberculosis in older individuals. May occur more commonly in the setting of HIV co-infection.

Rarely, tuberculosis may present as pseudochylothorax or tuberculous empyema.

Clinical features

- Clinical features are similar to those of pulmonary tuberculosis, i.e. fever, sweats, weight loss, and dyspnoea, although it may present acutely with pleuritic chest pain and fever, mimicking pneumonia
- Effusions are typically small-moderate in volume, although can be massive.

Investigations

- Associated parenchymal infiltrate on **CXR** in less than one-third of cases
- **Tuberculin skin tests** positive in two-thirds of cases
- **Pleural fluid** lymphocytosis, exudative effusion, pH and glucose moderately depressed, mesothelial cells rare. Pleural fluid acid-fast bacilli (AFB) smears are positive in around 5–10% of cases; pleural fluid cultures are positive in 25% of cases and take 2–6 weeks
- Blind **Abrams' pleural biopsy** alone has a sensitivity of 75%, but this increases to nearly 90% when histology and culture of both the fluid and biopsy are analysed
- **Thoracoscopic biopsies** have a sensitivity of nearly 100%
- Measurement of **adenosine deaminase** (an enzyme released by macrophages after phagocytosis of mycobacteria) in pleural fluid may be of benefit in regions where tuberculosis is highly prevalent; a raised value is very sensitive for pleural tuberculosis, but is non-specific and may also occur in empyema and malignancy
- **PCR** for mycobacterial DNA in the pleural fluid may be useful diagnostically, but is not widely available
- **Induced sputum** for acid-fast bacilli may have a diagnostic role in high-risk patients with lymphocytic effusions, even in the absence of parenchymal disease on CXR.

Treatment and outcome

- Tuberculous pleural effusions resolve spontaneously in the majority of cases, but two-thirds of untreated patients go on to develop pulmonary tuberculosis within 5 years and so treatment is recommended
- Treatment is the same as for pulmonary tuberculosis (page 234)
- Pleural fluid volumes may increase during effective treatment, and therapeutic thoracentesis is often required
- Steroids may reduce fluid volumes but do not affect long-term outcome
- Pleural thickening and calcification are common long-term consequences of tuberculous pleural effusion.

Other causes

Pleural effusion due to pulmonary embolism

- Fourth commonest cause of pleural effusion in the USA
- Consider in all patients with undiagnosed pleural effusion, particularly if there is a history of pleuritic chest pain or of breathlessness/hypoxia out of proportion to the size of the effusion
- Frequently complicates other disease processes, e.g. occurs in one-fifth of patients with cardiac failure and pleural effusions
- Effusions are usually small (<one-third of hemithorax) and unilateral, although may be bilateral
- Pleural fluid analysis is non-diagnostic; appearance varies from clear to bloody, 80% are exudates and 20% transudates. Bloodstained pleural fluid is not a contraindication to anticoagulation
- Imaging investigations, such as CTPA of the chest, are required to make the diagnosis; these should be performed prior to thoracentesis if pulmonary embolism is strongly suspected.

Rheumatoid arthritis-associated pleural effusion

- Pulmonary changes may be the first manifestation of rheumatoid arthritis
- Rheumatoid pleurisy is more common in men (70% are in men)
- Pleural fluid may be yellow-green, serous, turbid, or bloody
- May be unilateral or bilateral
- Pleural fluid glucose level is frequently low (<1.6 mmol/l), and progressively falls in chronic effusions
- Pleural fluid pH is commonly reduced (<7.3)
- Low pleural fluid complement levels (C4 <0.04 g/l) may also favour the diagnosis
- Elevated pleural fluid rheumatoid factor titre is found, but it is not more diagnostically helpful than serum rheumatoid factor
- Typically persist for months to years, although duration may be several weeks
- Some cases may respond to treatment with steroids.

Haemothorax

- Haemothorax is defined as a pleural effusion with a haematocrit >50% of peripheral blood haematocrit
- Causes include trauma, iatrogenic, malignancy, pulmonary infarction, benign asbestos-related pleural effusion, pneumonia, post-cardiac injury syndrome, pneumothorax, thoracic endometriosis, and aortic rupture
- Massive haemothorax defined as >1500 cm^3 of blood in hemithorax, and is most commonly due to trauma. Traumatic haemothorax is said to require a chest drain and sometimes thoracotomy; all cases should be discussed immediately with the cardiothoracic surgical team
- Large volumes of residual blood in the pleural space will clot and may lead to pleural thickening, empyema or trapped lung. Tube drainage is difficult and thoracoscopy or thoracotomy with decortication are often needed. However, undrained cases can resolve without intervention.

Pleural effusion after coronary artery bypass grafting
- Small, typically left-sided pleural effusions occur in the majority of patients post-CABG, and most resolve spontaneously
- Larger (>25% of hemithorax) effusions can be subdivided:
  - Pleural effusions occurring **within 30 days** of surgery. Classically bloody and eosinophilic exudate, with high LDH; probably related to post-operative bleeding into pleural space
  - Pleural effusions **more than 30 days** after surgery. Typically clear and lymphocytic exudate; cause unknown, perhaps immunological or a form of postcardiac injury syndrome
- Main symptom in each case is breathlessness; chest pain and fever are unusual
- Management consists of repeated therapeutic thoracentesis to alleviate breathlessness. Recurrent effusions after one year are rare and may be difficult to treat; NSAIDs, prednisolone, or thoracoscopy and pleurodesis may be considered
- Differential diagnosis of pleural effusion post-CABG includes: pulmonary embolism, cardiac failure, pleural infection, post-cardiac injury syndrome, chylothorax.

Pleural effusions after coronary artery bypass graft surgery. R. W. Light. *Curr Opin Pulm Med* 2002; **8**: 308–11

Pleural effusion following asbestos exposure
The main differential diagnosis is between benign asbestos pleural effusion (page 320) and mesothelioma (page 324).

Pleural effusion in immunocompromised patients
- Differential diagnosis includes cardiac failure and fluid overload, pulmonary embolism, parapneumonic, drug-related, PCP, other infections (fungal, Nocardia), or related to the underlying disease (e.g. leukaemic infiltrates, lymphoma, chylothorax, myeloma)
- Commonest causes of pleural effusion in HIV infection are Kaposi's sarcoma, parapneumonic effusion, tuberculosis, PCP, and lymphoma.

Chapter 27

Asbestos and the lung

Asbestos

Asbestos consists of a family of naturally occurring hydrated silicate fibres that may be subdivided into two groups:
- Curly *serpentine* fibres, of which chrysotile (white) is the only fibre currently in commercial use
- Straight, needle-like *amphiboles*, which comprise crocidolite (blue), amosite (brown), anthophyllite, tremolite, and actinolite.

Fibres differ in their lung clearance kinetics and pathogenic potential; amphibole fibres clear more slowly from the lung and are more carcinogenic than chrysotile. Whilst asbestos usage in developed countries is restricted, the use of chrysotile asbestos in developing economies continues to rise.

Mechanisms of exposure

Occupational exposure accounts for the majority of cases of asbestos-related disease and includes:
- Mining, milling, and transport of asbestos
- Use of asbestos products, e.g. in construction and demolition, floor tiling, insulation, fireproofing, textiles, friction materials (brake linings), ship building, pipefitting, electrical repair, boiler fitting and lagging, carpentry, plumbing, and welding.

Domestic exposure may include:
- Relatives of asbestos workers exposed to 'carry home' asbestos in hair or clothes
- Following remodelling or renovation in contaminated buildings
- Local geological exposure from natural deposits, e.g. areas of central and south-east Turkey, north-west Greece, and Corsica
- Urban environment.

A complete occupational history is essential if asbestos-related disease is suspected, and should include the method of exposure with dates and names of employers. This information may be of medicolegal importance and ideally should be elicited during the first consultation.

Asbestos-related lung disease comprises:
- Benign asbestos-related pleural disease
  - Pleural plaques
  - Benign asbestos-related pleural effusion
  - Diffuse pleural thickening
  - Rounded atelectasis
- Asbestosis
- Mesothelioma
- Lung cancer.

Other diseases linked to asbestos exposure include pericarditis, pericardial mesothelioma, peritoneal mesothelioma, head and neck cancers, and gastrointestinal cancers.

Asbestos-related disease typically exhibits a long latency period of 20–40 years from exposure. Peak industrial asbestos use in the UK occurred in the early 1970s, and asbestos-related disease is likely to remain common for at least the next 20 years. The incidence of mesothelioma is forecast to peak in 2020, and mesothelioma may account for 1% of all deaths of men born in the 1940s in the UK.

All deaths should be notified to the coroner if asbestos-related disease is suspected or proven.

Benign asbestos-related pleural disease

Pleural plaques
- Most common manifestation of asbestos exposure
- Discrete areas of white or yellow thickening on the parietal pleura; may calcify
- Frequently bilateral and symmetrical; occur particularly on the posterolateral chest wall, over the mediastinal pleura, and on the dome of the diaphragm
- Develop 20 to 30 years after exposure; incidence increases with longer duration of exposure; found in up to 50% of asbestos-exposed workers, and may also occur after low-dose exposures
- Usually asymptomatic, although if extensive may be associated with mild breathlessness due to pleural restriction
- Effect on pulmonary function is uncertain: most studies have failed to demonstrate abnormal lung function, although otherwise unexplained mild airways obstruction has been described in some populations of asbestos workers with pleural plaques—the mechanism of this is unclear
- HRCT is more sensitive than CXR in detecting pleural plaques
- There is no evidence that plaques are pre-malignant
- Discuss compensation with the patient (page 328).

Benign asbestos-related pleural effusions
- Relatively early manifestation of asbestos pleural disease; usually occurs within 10 years of exposure
- Development is considered to be dose-dependent, although can occur after minimal exposure
- Typically small and unilateral, and may be asymptomatic or occasionally associated with pleuritic pain, fever, and dyspnoea
- Usually resolve spontaneously over a few months, although some recur
- The pleural effusion is an exudate, often bloodstained, with no characteristic findings on pleural fluid analysis
- Diagnosis depends on a history of asbestos exposure and the exclusion of other causes, including mesothelioma
- Benign asbestos pleurisy may precede the development of diffuse pleural thickening; there is no clear association with mesothelioma
- Treat symptomatically, with pleural aspiration for breathlessness and NSAIDs for pain.

Diffuse pleural thickening (DPT)
- Consists of extensive fibrosis of the visceral pleura with areas of adhesion with the parietal pleura and consequent obliteration of the pleural space
- Unlike pleural plaques, its margins are ill-defined and it may involve the costophrenic angles, apices, and interlobar fissures
- Development appears to be dose-related and may follow recurrent asbestos pleurisy

- On CXR, it may be defined as a smooth, uninterrupted pleural opacity extending over at least a quarter of the chest wall, with or without obliteration of the costophrenic angles; on CT, the pleural density extends more than 8 cm craniocaudally, 5 cm laterally, and is more than 3 mm thick
- Symptoms are relatively common and comprise exertional breathlessness and chest pain, which can be chronic and severe
- May lead to significant restrictive pulmonary function impairment, especially if the costophrenic angle is obliterated; hypercapnic respiratory failure has been described
- Pleural biopsy may be required to distinguish it from mesothelioma
- Treatment is difficult; decortication often fails to result in clinical or functional improvement
- Patient may be eligible for compensation (see page 328).

Rounded atelectasis

(also known as folded lung, Blesovsky syndrome, or shrinking pleuritis with atelectasis)

- Develops as contracting visceral pleural fibrosis ensnares and then twists the underlying lung, resulting in the distinctive radiological appearance of a rounded or oval pleural-based mass of 2.5–5 cm in diameter
- CT is often diagnostic, demonstrating a 'comet tail' of vessels and bronchi converging toward the lesion, adjacent thickened pleura, and volume loss in the affected lobe
- An atypical appearance may require biopsy to exclude malignant disease
- Typically asymptomatic, although breathlessness or dry cough may occur
- Usually stable or slowly progressive, and no specific treatment is required
- Surgical decortication may improve symptoms but frequently results in reduced lung volumes and is not generally recommended.

Further information

Rudd R.M. New developments in asbestos-related pleural disease. *Thorax* 1996; **51**: 210–16

Asbestosis

Definition Chronic interstitial fibrosis resulting from asbestos inhalation.

Causes Factors affecting disease development include:
- *Degree and length of asbestos exposure*—a clear dose-response relationship exists; usually seen in workers with many years of high exposure although may follow a very high exposure of short duration, resulting in a shorter latency period
- *Fibre type*—amphibole fibres are probably more fibrogenic than chrysotile, although most exposures are mixed fibre types
- *Cigarette smoking* increases the severity and rate of progression of asbestosis.

Latency period from first exposure to clinical disease is usually at least 15–20 years, and may be >40 years.

Clinical features Insidious onset of breathlessness, dry cough. Bibasal late-inspiratory crackles, clubbing in 40% of cases. May progress to respiratory failure, cor pulmonale.

Differential diagnosis includes other causes of interstitial fibrosis, particularly usual interstitial pneumonitis (UIP).

Investigations
- *CXR* Bilateral symmetrical reticulonodular pattern, primarily affecting the lower lobes peripherally, which may extend upwards to involve the mid and upper zones; may progress to honeycomb lung. Associated pleural thickening or plaques may be seen. Classification is based on size, thickness, and profusion of opacities. CXR insensitive to early disease; may be normal in 15–20% of symptomatic, biopsy-proven asbestosis
- *HRCT* is more sensitive than CXR and is abnormal in 10–30% of cases with a normal CXR. Features include basal 'ground-glass' opacities (seen early in the disease), parenchymal bands, subpleural curvilinear lines and opacities, interlobular septal thickening, and signs of fibrosis (traction bronchiectasis, loss of lobular architecture, honeycombing in advanced disease)
- *PFTs* are classically restrictive with reduced lung volumes and transfer factor, although obstructive or mixed patterns may also occur
- Positive *gallium scan* may be seen with normal CXR; correlates poorly with lung function.

In general, CXR and HRCT show only very limited correlation with physiological disease severity.

Diagnosis Gold standard is pathological demonstration of fibrosis with mineralogical quantification of asbestos bodies; in practice histology is rarely required and a diagnosis can be made on the basis of a history of significant asbestos exposure with appropriate delay between exposure and disease, and radiographic evidence of fibrosis.

Treatment
- No pharmacological treatment is of proven benefit
- Supportive management, including supplementary oxygen as required, influenza and pneumococcal immunization, smoking cessation, compensation if exposure was occupational (page 328).

Prognosis varies widely. After removal from exposure, progression occurs in 5–40% of patients over 10 years; progression is faster following greater exposure. Fewer CXR opacities after exposure are associated with better prognosis. Increased risk of developing lung cancer.

Mesothelioma: diagnosis

Definition Malignant tumour of the pleura or peritoneum usually resulting from asbestos exposure.

Causes Asbestos is the major single cause and there is a history of occupational asbestos exposure in up to 90% of cases. All types of asbestos can cause mesothelioma—amphibole is the most potent, but also evidence for chrysotile. Mean latent interval between first exposure and death is around 40 years; cases with latency <15 years are rare. Not dose-related (unlike asbestosis or bronchogenic cancers)—and no evidence for a threshold asbestos dose below which there is no risk, although the risk at low exposure levels is small. No significant association with smoking.

Other causes include non-asbestos fibres such as erionite, which is found in rocks in Cappadocia, Turkey—mesothelioma accounts for up to a quarter of all adult deaths in local villages. Evidence for simian virus 40 (contaminated polio vaccine in 1950s/60s) is limited. 'Spontaneous' mesothelioma in children is described.

Clinical features

- Chest pain (typically dull ache, 'boring', diffuse, occasionally pleuritic), breathlessness; a small proportion are asymptomatic. Profuse sweating may occur
- Consider in any patient with a pleural effusion or pleural thickening, particularly if chest pain is present
- Rarely may present with persistent chest pain and a normal CXR
- Clubbing may occur but is rare
- Chest wall invasion may be seen (especially at thoracentesis sites)
- Bilateral pleural involvement is unusual at presentation
- Paraneoplastic syndromes are described, e.g. disseminated intravascular coagulation

Differential diagnosis includes benign asbestos pleural effusion, diffuse pleural thickening, and adenocarcinoma involving the pleura.

Investigations

1. Pleural fluid aspiration typically reveals an exudative, straw-coloured or bloody effusion. Cytological analysis rarely provides the diagnosis (sensitivity 32%), although it may be useful in excluding other pathology, e.g. adenocarcinoma. Pleural fluid glucose and pH may be low in extensive tumours. Mesothelioma may track through the chest wall along thoracocentesis sites; avoid repeated pleural aspiration if the diagnosis is suspected, and 'tattoo' aspiration sites with indelible ink to guide subsequent prophylactic radiotherapy.

2. Imaging. CXR and CT features include:

- Moderate to large pleural effusion, usually with pleural nodularity and enhancement following pleural contrast and involvement of mediastinal pleura
- Pleural mass or thickening without free fluid
- Entrapment of lung resulting in small hemithorax

- Local invasion of chest wall, ribs, heart, mediastinum, hilar nodes, and diaphragm; transdiaphragmatic spread and invasion of contralateral pleura
- Associated pleural plaques or interstitial fibrosis in a minority of cases.

The role of MRI is unclear—it may provide additional information in some cases, e.g. chest wall invasion, although is rarely required.

3. Biopsy. The diagnosis should be confirmed histologically except when the patient is too unwell or too frail for biopsy. Ultrasound- or CT-guided cutting needle biopsy and thoracoscopic biopsy of pleural masses have a high diagnostic yield and should be used in preference to blind (Abrams') biopsy techniques. Early use of thoracoscopy may both provide a diagnosis and enable treatment of large effusions with talc pleurodesis, thereby avoiding repeated non-diagnostic procedures with attendant problems of needle-track spread.

Histological subtypes

- Epithelioid (50% of cases; may be confused with adenocarcinoma; better prognosis)
- Sarcomatoid (or fibrous)
- Mixed (biphasic).

Variety of stains may be useful in distinguishing from adenocarcinoma or benign pleural disease.

Staging No widely accepted staging system. Proposed schemes include Stage I–IV scheme and TNM classification. Poor prognostic features include transdiaphragmatic muscle invasion and involvement of mediastinal lymph nodes.

Further information

BTS Statement on malignant mesothelioma in the United Kingdom. *Thorax* 2001; **56**: 250–65

Mesothelioma: treatment and outcome

Treatment

Management of pleural effusions Talc pleurodesis is the treatment of choice, and early pleurodesis is preferable to repeated pleural aspirations. This can be achieved either medically or at thoracoscopy, depending on local resources. Pleurodesis is not possible if the lung does not re-expand following drainage of pleural fluid ('trapped lung'), and the resulting recurrent pleural effusions are difficult to manage; indwelling pleurex catheters allow fluid drainage without needle aspiration and are useful in this situation. The value of pleuroperitoneal shunts remains uncertain.

Radiotherapy Prophylactic radiotherapy greatly reduces chest wall invasion by tumour following pleural aspiration or biopsy: three daily fractions reduced the risk of tracking from 40% to 0 in a randomized study of 40 patients. Recurrence may follow delayed prophylactic radiotherapy, so it is usually administered within 4 weeks. Palliative radiotherapy provides pain relief in a proportion of patients, but is less useful in the treatment of breathlessness or SVCO.

Surgery There are no randomized-controlled trials to investigate the outcomes of radical surgery. It should be considered only in centres with experience and if there is a firm diagnosis of epithelioid mesothelioma, the patient is otherwise fit, and there is no radiological evidence of lymph node involvement. Avoid chemical pleurodesis in such cases. Trimodality therapy (extrapleuropneumonectomy followed by radiotherapy and chemotherapy) may have a role; trials are pending.

Chemotherapy The role of chemotherapy is currently unclear and is the subject of several trials, including a BTS/MRC trial assessing triple therapy. Patients should have the option of discussing chemotherapy with an appropriate specialist.

New approaches include gene therapy and immunotherapy. The new drug pemetrexed has been shown to prolong survival and may become standard therapy.

General management Early involvement of a pain relief and palliative care service is required. Ensure adequate analgesia; nerve blocks and cordotomy may be needed. Breathlessness may be multifactorial, e.g. pleural effusion, lung compression, chest wall restriction, pericardial involvement, pain, anxiety. Liaise with GP, specialist nurse, palliative care teams. Remind GP that all deaths have to be reported to the coroner. Discuss compensation issues (page 328).

Clinical course Median survival is poor, varying 8 to 14 months in different studies. Typically progresses by local extension, but distant metastases are common (50% at autopsy) although occur late and are rarely clinically apparent.

Peritoneal mesothelioma is rarer than pleural mesothelioma, and may be associated with more prolonged asbestos exposure. Remains intra-abdominal in most cases. Clinical features include abdominal discomfort, weight loss, and ascites. Fine needle aspiration of omental masses may provide a diagnosis, although laparoscopy is often required. Prognosis is worse than for pleural mesothelioma, with median survival 7.4 months. No treatment is of proven benefit.

Compensation for asbestos-related diseases

Identification of asbestos exposure is essential for the patient to be able to claim compensation. Patients are not eligible for compensation if their exposure occurred whilst they were self-employed. There are two principal sources of compensation:

1. From the Government: apply to the **Benefits Agency** (Department of Social Security) for industrial injuries disablement benefit, using form BI100PN. Available for the following diseases:

- Diffuse pleural thickening.
- Asbestosis.
- Lung cancer associated with diffuse pleural thickening or asbestosis.
- Mesothelioma.

There must be a clear history of asbestos exposure at work. Compensation is not available for pleural plaques alone. If successful, may then apply for a single payment from the government under the Pneumoconiosis, etc. (Worker's Compensation) Act 1979. The value of compensation reflects the degree of disability from which the patient is considered to suffer and their age at diagnosis. Next-of-kin may also claim within 6 months posthumously. The War Pensions Scheme may provide compensation for disease resulting from asbestos exposure with HM forces (form WPA1).

2. From the Courts: **Common law** compensation directly from a previous employer. Can be claimed from the employer's insurer, even if the employer is now out of existence. Advise patient to seek advice as soon as possible from a solicitor with relevant experience. Claims must be initiated within 3 years of the individual's first awareness of their asbestos-related disease, including pleural plaques; attempts to initiate claims after 3 years may be statute barred. Inform the patient of this and document the conversation in the medical notes. Awards for anxiety relating to pleural plaques are typically in the region of £3500 to £6000, and following this the patient may make later claims if they develop a more serious consequence of asbestos exposure, e.g. mesothelioma. Alternatively, patients with plaques may accept 'once and for all' compensation (typically around £8000 to £15,000) and forego their right to further claims in the event of mesothelioma developing. Awards for asbestosis range from £15,000 to £50,000, depending on symptoms and the degree of disability; such patients may also accept a 'once and for all' award. Typical awards for mesothelioma are £45,000–£50,000 and additional amounts may be claimed for care and future loss of wages; total compensation may exceed £100,000. Successful claims have also been made for mesothelioma occurring in relatives who were exposed to asbestos whilst washing work clothes.

Further information

DSS Benefits Agency enquiry line 0800 882200 or 0800 2792322. Advice on available benefits and completing claim applications. Leaflets SD5 'Ill or Disabled Because of Work' and NI12 'If you have an Industrial Disease' may be helpful. Website *www.dwp.gov.uk/index.asp* contains further information on the Pneumoconiosis etc. (Worker's Compensation) Act 1979, as well as many useful contacts and links

London Hazards Centre. *http://www.lhc.org.uk/members/pubs/books/asbestos/asb_toc.htm*

Occupational and Environmental Diseases Association offers support and advice to patients and their relatives including information on solicitors and the process of compensation. PO Box 26, Enfield, Middlesex EN1 2NT. Telephone 020 8360 8490. Website *www.oeda.demon.co.uk*

Sleep apnoea

Obstructive sleep apnoea (OSA)

Definition and epidemiology OSA, or obstructive sleep apnoea/hypopnoea (OSAH) are currently the preferred terms for the problem of dynamic upper airway obstruction during sleep.

- OSA is part of a spectrum, with trivial snoring at one end and repetitive complete obstruction throughout the night (such that the patient cannot sleep and breathe at the same time) at the other
- Along this spectrum is a point at which the degree of obstruction, and recovery, fragments sleep enough to cause daytime symptoms
- Distinction should be made between the sleep study findings alone (i.e. presence of sleep apnoea episodes), and an abnormal sleep study *plus* the presence of symptoms (i.e. *obstructive sleep apnoea syndrome*, OSAS).

Thresholds defining 'abnormality' are arbitrary (e.g. 10 seconds to define an apnoea). Numerical definitions of OSA, based on counting individual events during a sleep study, are not very helpful. The current definition of the clinical syndrome should be:

Upper airway narrowing, provoked by sleep, causing sufficient sleep fragmentation to result in significant daytime symptoms, usually excessive sleepiness.

- Prevalence depends on the chosen thresholds for defining both an abnormality on the sleep study and significant symptoms
- 0.5–1% of adult men in the UK (and about a fifth as many women) have OSA syndrome sufficient to be candidates for treatment with nasal continuous positive airway pressure (CPAP) treatment
- Prevalence figure depends on levels of obesity and will be higher in the USA, and probably in the UK in the future
- The prevalence in women is thought to be lower due to the different fat distribution. Upper body obesity (and thus neck obesity) is more a male pattern
- OSA is the third most common serious respiratory condition after asthma and COPD. In some respiratory units it has now become the commonest reason for specialist referral.

Pathophysiology and associated conditions Control of the upper airway musculature is complex; upper airway patency depends on dilator muscle activity. All postural muscles relax during sleep (including pharyngeal dilators); some narrowing of the upper airway is normal. Excessive narrowing with the onset of sleep is due to the following factors:

Causes of a small pharyngeal size awake (such that normal muscle relaxation with sleep is enough to provoke critical narrowing).

- Fatty infiltration of pharyngeal tissues and external pressure from increased neck fat and/or muscle bulk
- Large tonsils
- Subtle 'abnormalities' of craniofacial shape, e.g. minor micrognathia or retrognathia
- Extra submucosal tissue, e.g. myxoedema, mucopolysaccharidoses.

*Causes of excessive narrowing of the airway occurring with muscle
relaxation at sleep onset*

- Mass loading from an obese or muscular neck may simply 'overwhelm' residual dilator action, as well as reduce the starting size
- Neuromuscular diseases with pharyngeal involvement may lead to greater loss of dilator muscle tone, e.g. stroke, myotonic dystrophy, Duchenne dystrophy, motor neurone disease
- Muscle relaxants, such as sedatives and alcohol
- Increasing age.

OSA is found more commonly in certain conditions, such as acromegaly and Marfan's, but the reasons are not well understood. It is unclear whether there need to be any other factors (such as unstable ventilatory control, or pharyngeal mucosal abnormalities) to provoke OSA. Most associated abnormalities that have been described are likely to be *secondary* to long periods of snoring and OSA, rather than primary causal factors.

In severe OSA, repetitive collapse of the upper airway, with arousal required to re-activate the pharyngeal dilators, occur approximately every minute throughout the sleeping period (60 events per hour, or over 400 per night); they are usually attended by hypoxia and hypercapnia that are corrected during the inter-apnoeic hyperventilatory period. Obstructive events short of complete obstruction also provoke arousal, as it is usually the compensatory reflex increase in inspiratory effort, rather than the blood gas deterioration, that wakens the brain. In this situation the drops in oxygen saturation may be very much less and, in younger thinner individuals, almost imperceptible on oximetry tracings. This is because the compensation afforded by the increased inspiratory effort may be adequate, and the bigger oxygen stores in the lungs of the less obese will buffer any brief hypoventilation.

- Recurrent arousals lead to highly fragmented and unrefreshing sleep
- Excessive daytime sleepiness results
- The correlation between the sleep fragmentation and the resultant degree of sleepiness is not tight, with some patients being sleepy with low levels of fragmentation, and vice versa
- This is thought to result partly from interindividual differences in sensitivity to the effects of sleep fragmentation
- With every arousal there is a rise in blood pressure, often over 50 mmHg. It is unclear if these BP rises do any damage to the cardiovascular system. There is also a carry-over of hypertension (average of 3 mmHg) into the waking hours that falls after treatment at one month
- There is true nocturia, mechanism unclear: there may be raised atrial natriuretic peptide (ANP) levels from increased central blood volume, brought about by the subatmospheric intrathoracic pressures during the obstructed breathing: or it may be simply a reflection of highly fragmented sleep preventing the normal reduction in urine flow associated with sleep.

OSA: clinical features

Chapter 11 (page 71) covers many of the essential features in the history and discusses the differential diagnosis of excessive daytime sleepiness.

Most patients present with:
- Excessive sleepiness, measured using the Epworth Sleepiness Scale; >9 is considered abnormally sleepy
- Loud snoring, and apnoeic episodes recognized by the bed partner
- The patient recognizes that he wakes up choking from time to time
- Poor concentration
- Unrefreshing sleep and waking unrefreshed
- Nocturia (true nocturia with reversal of the usual day/night ratio).

Less often there will be:
- Nocturnal sweating
- Reduced libido
- Oesophageal reflux
- Increasingly common are patients arriving with spouses worried by the apnoeic pauses they have observed.

Sleepiness
- Sometimes difficult to assess: failure by the patient to recognize the problem, or denial due to concerns over driving and licensing
- The Epworth scale (page 75) assesses *tendency to fall asleep*, rather than *perceived sleepiness*, as some patients may regard their situation as normal
- It is important to separate the symptom of tiredness from sleepiness (page 72), the latter being much more typical of OSA, although sometimes complained of (rather than sleepiness) by women with OSA.

Examination and investigations
The examination (often unrewarding) and the investigations are detailed in Chapter 11 (page 74). Look for the presence of additional lower airways obstruction, with associated CO_2 retention, so-called 'overlap syndrome'. CO_2 retention in pure OSA is very uncommon (except in the very, very obese). It appears that the additive effect of some lower airways obstruction (often not enough in its own right to precipitate CO_2 retention) is required, which perhaps limits the inter-apnoeic hyperventilation and thus gradually encouraging tolerance to raised levels of CO_2.

The majority of patients with significant OSA are male, tend to have a combination of upper body obesity (neck circumference > 17 in), and a relatively undersized or set back mandible.

Sleep study
The sleep study assesses if there is anything likely to be the cause of the patient's symptoms. The considerable grey area between normality and abnormality means that sometimes it is unclear whether the symptoms can be blamed on the sleep study findings. There is also considerable night

to night variation in sleep study indices that further blurs the distinction between normality and abnormality. In this situation it may be necessary to undertake a therapeutic trial of nasal CPAP and let the patient decide if the benefits of treatment outweigh the disadvantages.

Normal oximetry. Normal baseline and a few dips.

Severe OSA. Large numbers of regular dips, saw-tooth shaped (faster rise in SaO_2 than the fall).

OSA: types of sleep study

- Overnight oximetry alone
- More than just oximetry, with other channels such as snoring, body movement, heart rate, oronasal airflow, chest and abdominal movements, leg movements: so called 'limited' sleep studies, or 'respiratory PSG'
- Full polysomnography, with EEG, EOG, and EMG, to stage sleep electrophysiologically, in addition to the channels listed above.

There is no evidence that diagnosis of OSA needs full polysomnography (PSG, with EEG, etc.) and it is not indicated for most patients. Oximetry will identify most cases, allowing onward referral for CPAP treatment. False positive oximetry occurs with Cheyne–Stokes breathing (heart failure, post-stroke), and when there is a low baseline SaO_2 (COPD allows the SaO_2 to oscillate considerably, with only small changes in PaO_2 due to the increasing steepness of the Hb dissociation curve at lower SaO_2). False negatives, discussed earlier, can occur with younger and thinner patients.

With appropriate expertise, and a recognition of its limitations, oximetry alone is a very valuable tool in the diagnosis and management of OSA.

Limited sleep studies (respiratory PSG) are the usual routine investigation. Different units have expertise in interpreting different sorts of sleep studies. Experience is more important than the particular sleep study equipment used. Any system should assess the degree of sleep fragmentation and the degree of upper airway narrowing: this can be done using many different direct and indirect techniques.

Management

Not all patients need treatment. The evidence for significant treatment benefits rests on *symptoms*, which drive treatment, rather than the degree of OSA on a sleep study. Treatment decisions require a close dialogue between physician and patient.

Key features in making a treatment choice

- How sleepy is the patient, does it affect quality of life, is it critical to the patient's livelihood (e.g. HGV driving), are they motivated to do anything about it?
- Has the patient underestimated the impact of their sleepiness, or misled the doctor because of concerns over driving issues?
- Is there any evidence of the 'overlap' syndrome, where additional lower airways obstruction has contributed to pushing the patient into type II ventilatory failure? If so, is this a stable state, or part of an acute decline with a respiratory acidosis?
- Is obesity the dominant risk factor, or is there a surgically remediable component (e.g. tonsillar hypertrophy)?

There is no RCT evidence that severe CVD, e.g. nocturnal angina, poorly controlled hypertension, or heart failure, should influence the decision to treat. Many, however, would lower the threshold for treatment.

Simple approaches
- Weight loss
- Reduce evening alcohol consumption
- Try to sleep decubitus rather than supine.

For snorers and mild OSA
- Mandibular advancement devices, assuming adequate dentition
- Pharyngeal surgery as a last resort (poor outcome data).

For significant OSA
- Nasal continuous positive airway pressure therapy (CPAP)
- Bariatric surgery (e.g. gastroplasty or gastric bypass operations)
- Tracheostomy (rarely indicated)
- Mandibular/maxillary advancement surgery in highly selected cases.

Severe OSA with CO_2 retention
- May require a period of non-invasive positive pressure ventilation (NIPPV) prior to CPAP if acidotic
- Compensated CO_2 retention may reverse with CPAP alone.

If there are large tonsils then their removal may be appropriate, although this seems to be much more successful in children than in adults. In reality pharyngeal surgery is a poor option for either snoring or OSA; what little evidence there is suggests that the outcomes are little better than placebo. There is no place for alerting agents (such as modafinil) in the routine management of sleepiness in OSA. It is unclear if these drugs help; they may reduce the perception of sleepiness more than the sleepiness itself, and have only been studied in the residual sleepiness sometimes found in patients even when treated successfully with nasal CPAP.

Mandibular advancement devices
- Worn in the mouth at night, holding the lower jaw forward: similar to 'jaw thrust' in an unconscious patient
- Many designs, but essentially one-half clips to the upper teeth and one-half to the lower, and connected together with the lower jaw mis-aligned forward by 5 to 10 mm
- Some give adjustable forward displacement, some are fixed
- They need to be customized to match the patient's dentition, which usually requires the services of a dentist
- Control snoring and OSA at the milder end of the spectrum
- Side-effects include teeth pain and jaw ache, which often lessen with time
- Long-term use may be associated with movement of the teeth and alterations to the bite
- The initial cost (£200) is similar to that of a CPAP machine (£250) and they usually only last about a year.

OSA: nasal CPAP

Nasal CPAP consists of a blower/pressure generator that sits by the patient's bed and is connected to a mask by a length of large-bore tubing. The masks are usually just nasal, but nose and mouth masks are also used. The blower raises the pressure at which the patient is breathing (to about 10 cm H_2O) and splints open the pharynx, preventing its collapse, the sleep fragmentation, and the consequent daytime sleepiness. *Nasal CPAP is a highly effective therapy with resolution of the sleepiness and large gains in quality of life.* It is a sufficiently curious and initially uncomfortable therapy to require a *careful induction programme*. Without this, the take-up and compliance rates are poor. Most centres have found that a dedicated CPAP nurse or technician is required. Many centres use special patient education aids, such as video presentations, and provide helplines manned by previous patients established on CPAP. The best method of establishing a patient on CPAP, and deriving the required mask pressure, is not known and many different approaches appear to work. Recent innovations include CPAP machines that automatically hunt for the required pressure, and do not require a formal overnight titration with a technician present. New mask designs appear at regular intervals with a slow improvement in their comfort and fit (important to prevent air leaks). Patients require subsequent long-term follow-up to maintain their CPAP equipment and attend to problems.

The commonest problems encountered include

- Mouth leaks lead to increased air through the nose and out of the mouth, with excessive drying of the mucosa, nasal congestion, rhinitis, and sneezing. Use either a chin support to close the mouth, or the addition of a heated humidifier
- Pain and ulceration of the skin on the nasal bridge. Try different masks or patient 'interfaces'
- Claustrophobia. This usually settles, may require a different interface
- Temporary nasal congestion, usually during a cold. Try nasal decongestants for these short periods only, such as zylometazoline (Otrivine).

Alternative diagnoses

Most patients who snore, are sleepy, and have an abnormal sleep study will have ordinary obstructive sleep apnoea and respond to nasal CPAP. Sometimes, differentiating obstructive sleep apnoea from central apnoeas (page 344) can be difficult because some patients with Cheyne–Stokes breathing, for example, may have a few obstructed breaths at the end of each apnoeic cycle, even though the problem is primarily central. Poor response to CPAP should at least prompt a reappraisal of the diagnosis. Not all obstructive sleep apnoea is due to pharyngeal collapse; a very small number of patients have laryngeal closure. This can occur with:

- Shy–Drager syndrome (multisystem atrophy). This causes laryngeal abductor weakness with laryngeal closure during sleep, with stridulous obstruction rather than the usual noise of snoring
- Rheumatoid arthritis can damage the larynx with resultant OSA

- Arnold–Chiari malformation can compress the brainstem and interfere with the control of the larynx and pharynx, as well as the control of ventilation, with mixed findings on the sleep study
- These forms of obstruction also respond to nasal CPAP therapy as the larynx is also 'blown open' by raising airway pressure.

Sleep onset periodic ventilation. Short bursts of dipping, otherwise normal.

Cheyne–Stokes ventilation. Prolonged periods of dipping, often sinusoidal rather than saw-tooth.

OSA: driving advice to patients

In UK law one is responsible for one's vigilance levels while driving. We know when we are sleepy and should stop driving. Driving while sleepy has been likened to driving whilst drunk and a prison sentence can result from sleep-related accidents on the road. No one should drive while they are sleepy, and the same applies to pathological causes of sleepiness.

Advice to all patients with OSA. Do not drive while sleepy; stop and have a nap. On diagnosis they should notify the DVLA who will send them a questionnaire. If they admit to excessive daytime sleepiness their licence is revoked. If treated, and the sleepiness has resolved, then the licence is not revoked. It is the doctor's duty to tell the patient of the diagnosis, and of the requirement to inform the DVLA.

The doctor can advise the patient whether they should stop driving entirely (wise if the patient is very sleepy and/or drives a heavy goods vehicle or public service vehicle—class 2 licence holders), or to continue driving only with extreme caution for short distances. The advice given to the patient should be recorded in the notes.

Driving can be restarted as soon as the sleepiness has resolved and *been confirmed by medical opinion*, but in the case of class 2 licence holders the success of the treatment must be *verified by a specialist clinic*. This means a normal ESS and evidence of adequate nasal CPAP usage from the hour meters built into most nasal CPAP machines. A minimum usage has not been defined, but three hours per night on average is often the arbitrary threshold used. Non-usage for even one night can lead to a return of sleepiness so patients have to continue to act responsibly.

OSA in children

Adult respiratory physicians interested in sleep apnoea may be asked to investigate children with OSA due to poor sleep services for children.

- Mainly due to enlarged tonsils and adenoids; varying degrees of OSA are present in up to 4% of children around the age of five; prevalence tails off as tonsils atrophy
- These children present with snoring, restless sleep, and different daytime symptoms to those of adults. Obvious sleepiness is less common
- Sleep-deprived children tend to become hyperactive with reduced attention spans, and be labelled as difficult or disruptive
- Symptoms will fluctuate with the size of the tonsils and this depends on the presence of upper respiratory infections
- Mild intermittent sleep disturbance may not matter, but every night sleep fragmentation for months interferes with development in a variety of ways
- The clinical decision is mainly whether to recommend removal of tonsils, or a wait and see policy, remembering that there is a significant morbidity from adenotonsillectomy, and even the occasional death A halfway house is the use of nasal steroids, which can reduce tonsillar size sufficiently to improve symptoms until natural tonsillar atrophy occurs.

REM sleep hypoventilation in scoliosis. Substantial dips, in bursts, compatible with the occurrence of REM periods.

Moderate OSA with many <4% dips in SaO_2.

OSA: future developments

The old view that sleep apnoea requires polysomnography to diagnose is rapidly being replaced with a more pragmatic and evidence-based approach using simpler equipment. Simpler ways to establish patients on CPAP are also evolving that will bring down costs further. Obesity surgery is improving and in appropriate cases may become the treatment of choice. Appetite suppressants are being developed that will greatly reduce the prevalence of obesity and hence OSA. Pharmacological agents are being tried that attempt to prevent the loss of tone in the pharyngeal dilators during sleep, mainly serotonergic agents, although progress in this area is slow. New pharyngeal operations are being devised all the time, but none have been very effective when investigated properly: randomized controlled trials with objective outcome data are badly needed in this area.

Further information

Obstructive sleep apnoea. Malhotra A and White DP. *Lancet* 2002; **360**: 237–45

Patients association, Sleep Apnoea Trust, *www.sleep-apnoea-trust.org*

SIGN/BTS guidelines (2003), *sign.ac.uk/guidelines/published/numlist.html number 73*

Cochrane database on CPAP (2001), *White J et al.* Continuous positive airways pressure for obstructive sleep apnoea (Cochrane Review). In: *The Cochrane Library*, Issue 3, 2003. Oxford: Update Software. Available on the Web, full version only with subscription, *www.cochrane.org*

American commercial website showing all the CPAP equipment, *www.cpapman.com*

Main American Sleep Information website, *www.sleephomepages.org*

American website with patient information on a variety of sleep disorders (simple), *www.nlm.nih.gov/medlineplus/tutorials/sleepdisorders/nr249101.html*

Nocturnal hypoxia in COPD. Low baseline SaO$_2$, with more dramatic falls (often quite prolonged) during periods compatible with the occurence of REM.

Overlap syndrome—OSA and COPD. Low baseline SaO$_2$. Some periods with typical saw-tooth dipping; other periods with prolonged falls in SaO$_2$.

Central sleep apnoea (CSA) and nocturnal hypoventilation

Definition and epidemiology 'Central sleep apnoea/hypopnoea', or 'hypoventilation', or 'periodic breathing' are said to occur when there is no evidence of upper airway obstruction as the cause for the reduced ventilation during sleep. Compared to OSA it is much less common.

- **'Central sleep apnoea'** tends to be used as a term when there are actual apnoeas, and referred to as Cheyne–Stokes breathing when there is regular symmetrical waxing and waning, usually in the context of left heart failure
- **'Periodic breathing'** is an alternative and can be used to describe regular fluctuations in breathing, with or without actual apnoeas
- The description **'nocturnal hypoventilation'** tends to be used when the hypoventilation and hypoxaemic dips are not particularly periodic in nature. However these terms are imprecise and sometimes mixed indiscriminately.

Pathophysiology

Central sleep apnoea, or hypoventilation, or periodic breathing, can occur in a number of settings with different aetiologies (see also Chapter 5, page 28). At one end of a spectrum is pure loss of ventilatory drive, and at the other is pure loss of the ability to expand the chest adequately, with dependence on accessory muscles of respiration. Many clinical presentations are mixtures of these two.

Patients with *reduced ventilatory drive* (e.g. following brainstem damage) can often maintain adequate, or near adequate, ventilation whilst awake as there is a non-metabolic 'awake' ventilatory drive equivalent to about 4 or 5 l/min. During non-REM sleep, this awake drive is lost and ventilation becomes dependent on PaO_2 and $PaCO_2$. During REM sleep, an 'awake like' drive sometimes returns partially and ventilation can improve again (seen in congenital forms of absent drive where REM sleep can temporarily restore SaO_2 levels).

In patients with *impaired mechanical ability to ventilate*, accessory muscles of respiration become critically supportive (e.g. in many neuromuscular disorders and obstructive/restrictive respiratory conditions). However, during non-REM sleep, this reflex recruitment of accessory muscles is attenuated and hypoventilation follows. During REM-sleep the physiological paralysis of all postural muscles (REM atonia) can remove all compensatory mechanisms, leaving only the diaphragm working, and produce profound hypoventilation or apnoea.

Chronic hypoventilation, often secondary to poor respiratory function (e.g. as evidenced by CO_2 retention in some patients with COPD or chest wall restrictive disorders), can eventually force resetting of ventilatory control mechanisms. This is an acquired blunting of ventilatory drive and leads to sleep-related changes in ventilation, similar to those in the paragraphs above.

Unstable ventilatory control can lead to regular oscillations in ventilation, e.g. as occurs in heart failure and altitude. During REM sleep it is normal to have fluctuations in ventilation, sometimes with complete apnoeas.

Sometimes sleep studies can be misinterpreted and apnoeas, really of obstructive origin, are mistakenly labelled as central. For example, if inspiratory muscles are very weak, their poor efforts during obstructive apnoeas may be missed.

Causes and clinical features of CSA/hypoventilation 1

Although there are many different causes, there are only four relatively common clinical scenarios (but with overlap):

1) Absent or reduced ventilatory drive

Brainstem involvement from a stroke, tumours, syringobulbia, surgical damage, post-polio syndrome. Presents clinically with unexplained ventilatory failure, usually much worse during sleep when the 'awake' drive is lost.

May be recognized early, with cyanosis, morning confusion, and ankle oedema;

May be recognized late, with loss of consciousness and an emergency admission to ITU for ventilation.

Lung function is often normal, with no evidence of respiratory muscle weakness indicating normal innervation from the *voluntary* motor system. Arnold–Chiari malformation with brainstem compression can present like this, but there is usually involvement of surrounding structures such as the lower cranial motor nuclei supplying the larynx and pharynx (with associated obstructive sleep apnoea, page 338).

> These patients will have no apparent neuromuscular or respiratory cause for their hypoventilation, but may have a previous history of brainstem stroke (or other form of brain damage). The congenital form presents shortly after birth when the amount of REM sleep reduces and is replaced by non-REM.

Post-polio syndrome is:
• Ill defined syndrome with declines in function usually decades after the initial illness
• Return of weakness in previously affected areas (mechanism unclear)
• Late development of ventilatory failure is more likely if:
  • Inspiratory muscles were affected in the original illness
  • Additional scoliosis due to paravertebral muscle involvement.

This may be due to premature ageing of the upper and lower motor neurons due to their 'over use'. This could follow the original destruction of some of the anterior horn cells to the inspiratory muscles, and the subsequent reinnervation by surviving neurons which then have to continuously supply more neurons than they were 'designed' for.

2) Weak or mechanically disadvantaged inspiratory muscles, with/without secondary reduction of awake ventilatory drive

Neuromuscular inspiratory muscle weakness will produce diurnal ventilatory failure in its own right, particularly when the vital capacity falls below a litre.

With increasing inspiratory muscle weakness, other accessory inspiratory muscles are recruited to maintain ventilation. When this is lost during non-REM and REM sleep, ventilation will fall much more than in normal subjects. Whilst metabolic ventilatory drive is reasonably preserved, this will result in recurrent arousals to 'rescue' the ventilation and consequent marked sleep disturbance.

As ventilatory drive becomes progressively reduced, following the hypoventilation forced on the system by the weak muscles, then extra sleep hypoventilation (from loss of 'awake' drive) is tolerated and profound hypoxaemia is observed until there is finally an arousal that recovers the SaO_2.

The above patients should have a history of a progressive neuromuscular disorder.

Chest wall restrictive diseases, such as scoliosis or post-thoracoplasty patients (page 341), can behave in a similar way with gradual onset of ventilatory failure, particularly when vital capacity < 1 litre. The muscles are not weak, but operating at severe mechanical disadvantage.

The same situation occurs in *COPD*, when muscles are overloaded and accessory muscles provide important support, but this too is reduced with non-REM sleep and lost during REM sleep. Again, any secondary reduction in ventilatory drive amplifies the sleep-related falls in SaO_2.

- Chest wall restrictive patients should have an obvious restrictive disorder with reduced VC to a litre or below
- Increasing degrees of COPD will produce increasing degrees of sleep hypoventilation (page 343)
- If the awake SaO_2 is already low the sleep-related falls in ventilation will produce dramatic dips in SaO_2
- COPD and OSA together (overlap syndrome) provoke profound nocturnal hypoxic dipping (page 343), and probably a more rapid progression to diurnal hypoventilation with CO_2 retention, due to extra blunting of ventilatory drive (see page 334).

The diaphragm is the only respiratory muscle working during REM sleep, as all other postural muscles are profoundly hypotonic.
- If the diaphragm is paralysed, then REM sleep is a particularly vulnerable time as there are *no* muscles of respiration left working, producing particularly profound falls in SaO_2 during this period
- Patients with bilateral diaphragm weakness can present early with no obvious weakness elsewhere. Diaphragm weakness is best detected with the patient supine. Inspiration, particularly on sniffing, will provoke a paradoxical indrawing of the abdominal wall. The vital capacity will also fall on lying down, increasingly with greater degrees of paralysis (often a >30% fall in VC with complete paralysis).

In a progressive neuromuscular disorder, such as motor neurone disease, then the above patterns will be variable between individuals, but will gradually worsen. Predominant diaphragm weakness, as occurs sometimes in motor neurone disease, spinal muscular atrophy, and particularly acid maltase deficiency, can lead to ventilatory failure at a time when the patient is still ambulant.

Causes and clinical features of CSA/hypoventilation 2

3) Cheyne–Stokes breathing associated with LVF (page 339)

The raised left atrial pressure in left heart failure increases ventilatory drive through stimulation of J receptors. This is in addition to ventilatory stimulation due to any hypoxaemia from pulmonary oedema.

- This ventilatory stimulation lowers the awake $PaCO_2$ producing a respiratory alkalosis
- In addition the use of diuretics may produce a mild metabolic alkalosis, especially if there is hypokalaemia
- This extra J receptor ventilatory stimulation appears to reduce at sleep onset. This, together with the loss of the awake ventilatory drive, allows central hypoventilation or apnoea to occur
- This hypoventilation or apnoea will continue until the $PaCO_2$ builds up to drive ventilation again, or until the attendant hypoxaemia causes arousal
- The return of ventilation itself may provoke arousal too. The arousal itself then injects increased ventilatory drive, reducing the $PaCO_2$ again
- Sleep returns, and once again the low $PaCO_2$ and alkalosis cause hypoventilation or apnoea.

Thus a cycle is maintained that involves a fluctuating sleep state with arousals, and usually a fluctuating SaO_2. As with OSA, the patient may be completely unaware of these arousals. The delayed circulatory time of left heart failure may compound this instability by introducing a time delay between any change in $PaCO_2$ in the blood leaving the lungs and its arrival at the carotid body or central chemoreceptors.

4) Cheyne–Stokes breathing associated with altitude

The acute hypoxia following ascent to altitude provokes increased ventilation. The degree is variable between individuals and hence the degree of hypocapnia and respiratory alkalosis varies (see page 570). With sleep onset, with a lessening of the hypoxic drive, and removal of the awake drive, an uncompensated alkalosis will allow hypoventilation and even apnoea—similar to the situation described above for Cheyne–Stokes breathing. Again ventilation will restart either when the $PaCO_2$ rises to a critical level, or the hypoxia provokes arousal. Sleep is fragmented with complaints of insomnia, but the cause of this is rarely recognized by the sufferer.

Skiing in Colorado, altitude 2400–3400 m, ~10,000 ft, is high enough to provoke significant periodic breathing in about a fifth of individuals. It seems that this fifth are the ones with the highest hypoxic ventilatory response. This gives them the largest respiratory alkalosis and hence the greatest tendency to sleep onset hypoventilation. In addition the tendency to arouse with the resultant extra hypoxaemia may be greater too, thus provoking large increases in ventilation on arousal and greater sleep disturbance. As the kidney excretes extra bicarbonate, and produces a compensatory metabolic acidosis over a few days, the periodic breathing lessens.

Two *pharmacological approaches* have been taken to reduce this sleep-related periodic breathing.

- Pre-acclimatization with acetazolamide prior to ascent. This produces a mild metabolic acidosis and maintains the ventilatory drive at sleep onset, thus blocking the hypoventilation. Randomized controlled trials show the efficacy of this approach with doses between 250 mg and 500 mg a day, one to three days prior to ascent
- Hypnotics, such as temazepam, can reduce the degree of periodic breathing by reducing the tendency to arousal with each return of ventilation, and thus damping the system. Randomized trials suggest benefit for the early part of the night with an overall improvement in nocturnal hypoxaemia.

See also pages 570–1.

CSA/hypoventilation: investigations

Simple pulmonary function tests will characterize weakness of inspiratory muscles. Supine vital capacity is the best predictor of ventilatory failure as it incorporates diaphragm weakness that is masked during erect testing. Blood gases will reveal actual diurnal type II ventilatory failure and, if the base excess is raised with a normal $PaCO_2$ (therefore a mild metabolic alkalosis), then this may indicate nocturnal hypoventilation and incipient ventilatory failure.

Sleep Study—examples on pages 339, 341, 343.

Sleep studies in patients with suspected nocturnal hypoventilation or central sleep apnoea are required to confirm the diagnosis and to assess the degree of nocturnal hypoxaemia. Limited sleep studies will reveal falls in SaO_2 in association with hypoventilation but no evidence of obstruction, and in particular no snoring. Oximetry tracings alone will show a variety of patterns, often resembling OSA. The pattern in neuromuscular weakness will vary from oscillations all the time (due to recurrent arousal) to just REM sleep-related dips in SaO_2. The same will be true for chest wall restrictive disorders and COPD with only REM dips occurring initially, and more extensive hypoxaemia developing once there is an element of CO_2 retention and diurnal hypoxaemia.

- In OSA there is a slow fall in SaO_2 as oxygen is gradually removed from the lung stores, followed by a rapid rise engendered by the first deep inspiration as the apnoea breaks (so-called saw tooth pattern), page 335
- In Cheyne–Stokes of left heart failure the oscillations in SaO_2 are often more sinusoidal than in OSA as the pattern of breathing is usually more a symmetrical waxing and waning of ventilation, page 339. However, if each central apnoea is terminated by an arousal, rather than a smooth return of ventilation, then the pattern will look more like OSA.

In COPD the degree of hypoxaemia seen on the sleep study will depend very much on the awake SaO_2. Because of the shape of the haemoglobin dissociation curve, a low awake SaO_2 makes it much easier for the SaO_2 to fall further with a certain reduction in ventilation. Thus during non-REM, with removal of the awake drive, there will be a fairly stable reduction in SaO_2, but during REM sleep there will be further more dramatic dips. It is important not to diagnose OSA from just an oximetry tracing on the basis of SaO_2 oscillations in the presence of a low baseline SaO_2 and COPD. In this situation a fuller sleep study is required to provide evidence of additional upper airway obstruction. The combination of hypoxic COPD and OSA can produce particularly dramatic traces.

Management Intervention in central sleep apnoea or hypoventilation or periodic breathing, depends on symptoms. ***Better control of heart failure*** may improve Cheyne–Stokes breathing but often does not. Further treatment will be required for two reasons: either to prevent the cyclical breathing and restore sleep quality, or to globally improve ventilation overnight and reset the respiratory control mechanisms such that the daytime respiratory failure reverses.

In situations where the hypoxia is playing a part in the pathogenesis (e.g. heart failure) then ***raising FiO_2*** can help. There is limited literature on other forms of treatment for the Cheyne–Stokes of heart failure, although **acetazolamide** and **benzodiazepines** have been tried. Recently, the unstable breathing in heart failure has been treated with either **CPAP or a servo ventilator**. Whether these provide better relief of symptoms than oxygen is not yet clear but preliminary evidence suggests they do. There is some data to suggest that the recurrent arousal in Cheynes–Stokes may raise catecholamine levels and provoke deterioration of left ventricular function. Thus measures to reduce the arousals may improve cardiac function as well as improve daytime vigilance.

Sedatives are contraindicated with a raised PaCO$_2$, and extra oxygen may increase the hypercapnia. In these situations, then **overnight non-invasive ventilation**, via either nose or face mask, may be appropriate. In slowly progressive neuromuscular disorders, with either sleep fragmentation or diurnal type II respiratory failure (or both), the symptomatic and physiological response can be dramatic. The use of non-invasive ventilation in more rapidly progressive disorders is fraught with difficulties and is very much a specialist decision. Increasing dependence on equipment, not designed to be immediately life-sustaining, being a particular issue. In scoliosis there is rarely any question that treatment is appropriate and again responses are dramatic.

Future developments
- Treatment of LVF (acute and chronic, no evidence yet for the latter) with overnight CPAP or non-invasive ventilation
- Introduction of overnight ventilation earlier in the course of a progressive neuromuscular disorder (such as Duchenne dystrophy) to reduce symptoms and possibly prolong life
- Use of overnight ventilation on patients with stable COPD and hypercapnia. This may reduce exacerbations, hospital admissions, and prolong life. The evidence is inadequate yet to justify its wide use in this patient group.

Further information
Sleep-disordered breathing in heart failure: characteristics and implications. Lanfranchi PA, Somers VK. *Respir Physiol Neurobiol.* 2003 Jul 16; **136**(2–3): 153–65

Pathophysiology of central sleep apnea syndrome. Wuyam B *et al. Sleep.* 2000 Jun 15; **23** (suppl. 4): S213–9

Chapter 29

Bronchiectasis

Epidemiology, pathophysiology, and causes

Definition Irreversible abnormal dilatation of one or more bronchi, with chronic airway inflammation. Associated chronic sputum production, recurrent chest infections, and airflow obstruction.

Epidemiology The prevalence of bronchiectasis is unknown, but is probably falling, due to vaccinations and the improved and earlier treatment of childhood infections. However the advent of HRCT scanning may now lead to the diagnosis of more subtle (and possibly subclinical) disease.

Pathophysiology An initial (usually infectious) insult is needed to damage the airways. Disordered anatomy leads to secretion stagnation and secondary infection, causing ongoing inflammation, and further airway damage. Major airways and bronchioles are involved, with mucosal oedema, inflammation, and ulceration. Terminal bronchioles become obstructed with secretions, leading to volume loss. A chronic host inflammatory response ensues, with free radical formation and the production of neutrophil elastase, further contributing to the inflammatory process. Bronchial neovascularization occurs with hypertrophy and tortuosity of the bronchial arteries (which are at systemic pressure), and may lead to intermittent haemoptyses.

Aetiology The causes of bronchiectasis are many and varied. In general, the aetiology is either a one-off infectious insult, or an underlying immune deficiency. The rationale behind determining the aetiology of the condition is alteration in management, if, for example, the underlying cause is found to be cystic fibrosis or an immune deficiency. The cause is idiopathic in around 50% of cases and these are likely to be due to an (as yet unidentified) impairment in host defence.

- The most important cause to exclude is cystic fibrosis (see page 361). Even relatively mild bronchiectasis, diagnosed in middle age can be due to CF. The diagnosis can alter management, with:
  - Involvement of the multidisciplinary CF team
  - Attention to other potential problems, e.g. gastrointestinal disease, sinus disease, diabetes
  - Inheritance (relevant to the rest of the family)
  - Fertility issues.

Consider genotyping for CF if:
  - Predominantly upper lobe disease
  - *Haemophilus influenzae* or *Pseudomonas aeruginosa* colonization
  - Malnutrition ± malabsorption, diabetes
  - Family history of cystic fibrosis or bronchiectasis
  - Associated subfertility or infertility

A normal chloride sweat test does not exclude CF, as some mutations are associated with normal sweat chloride levels. The test is also difficult and subject to a number of technical errors. Only 90% of CF sufferers have a recognizable gene defect (there are over 1000 CFTR mutations).

Causes of bronchiectasis

Genetic	Cystic fibrosis
Congenital	Pulmonary sequestration
Post-infective	Tuberculosis
	Whooping cough (if infection in a localized area)
	Severe pneumonia
	Non-tuberculous mycobacteria (NTM)—there is some debate as to whether the bronchiectasis seen in association with NTM (classically in elderly females) is caused by, or secondarily infected by NTM
Immune deficiency	Primary—hypogammaglobulinaemia
	Secondary—HIV, CLL, nephrotic syndrome
	(Excessive immune response—ABPA)
Mucociliary clearance abnormalities	
	Primary ciliary dyskinesia (see page 566)
	Kartagener's syndrome
	Young's syndrome (bronchiectasis, sinusitis, and azoospermia—i.e. clinical features identical to those of CF)
Toxic insults	Aspiration
	Inhalation (toxic gases, chemicals)
Mechanical insults	Foreign body aspiration
	Extrinsic lymph node compression
	Intrinsic (intraluminal) obstructing tumour
Associations	Bronchiectasis is associated with a number of systemic diseases, so cough & sputum production in these conditions should trigger referral to determine the cause:
	Rheumatoid arthritis (up to 35% of RA patients have bronchiectasis)
	Connective tissue diseases, e.g. Sjögren's syndrome, SLE
	Ulcerative colitis and Crohn's disease (see page 518)
	Chronic sinusitis
	Yellow nail syndrome
	Marfan's syndrome

Clinical features and diagnosis

Suspect bronchiectasis in a patient with recurrent episodes of 'bronchitis' over several years prior to presentation.

The clinical picture is one of:

- *Symptoms*
  - Cough
  - Chronic sputum production (typically tenacious, purulent, and daily)
  - Intermittent haemoptyses
  - Breathlessness
  - Intermittent pleuritic pain (usually in association with infections)
  - Lethargy/malaise.
- *Signs*
  - Coarse inspiratory and expiratory crackles on auscultation
  - Airflow obstruction with wheeze.

Diagnosis is usually made clinically, with high resolution CT chest confirmation.

Investigations are aimed at:

- Confirming the diagnosis
- Identifying a treatable underlying cause for the bronchiectasis (possible in about 40%)
- Optimizing management, to prevent exacerbations and further lung damage.

Essential investigations

- *CXR* sensitivity is only 50%, classically shows 'ring shadows' and 'tramlines'—indicating thickened airways, and the 'gloved finger' appearance—consolidation around thickened and dilated airways
- *HRCT chest* is 97% sensitive in detecting disease. Expiratory scans may be useful to demonstrate post-obstructive air trapping, indicative of small airways disease. Typically shows airway dilatation to the lung periphery, bronchial wall thickening, and airway appearing larger than its accompanying vessel (signet ring sign). If the bronchiectasis is localized to a single lobe, CT is useful to determine whether a central obstructing lesion is present. Contiguous 3 mm slices are needed to exclude a central airway lesion if there is associated haemoptysis. Symptoms correlate with wall thickening and mucous plugging on CT scan. *Traction bronchiectasis* seen in UIP is airway dilatation secondary to airway distortion, seen with chronic, severe interstitial fibrosis
- **Sputum microbiology** Standard M, C & S (including for atypical organisms), acid-fast bacilli, and Aspergillus

- *Pulmonary function tests* with reversibility testing
- *Immunoglobulins A, M, E, G* (including IgG subclasses, if total IgG is low)
- *Aspergillus precipitins* See page 262.

Second-line investigations

- *CF genotyping* (see page 362)
- *Autoantibodies* (ANA, RhF, dsDNA) if associated arthritis/ connective tissue disease
- *Vaccination response* to tetanus, *Haemophilus influenzae*, and pnemococcal antibodies, *if underlying immunosuppression suspected*
- *Skin tests/RAST* to identify specific sensitizers (usually Aspergillus)
- *Detailed immunological investigation* (including neutrophil and lymphocyte function studies)
- *Bronchoscopy* to exclude a foreign body if suggested by CT; obtain microbiological samples if unusual clinical presentation, or failure to respond to standard antibiotics
- *Nasal brushings/biopsy* (in tertiary centre) to assess ciliary beat frequency with video microscopy
- *Saccharin test* The time for saccharin to be tasted in the mouth after deposition of a 0.5 mm particle on the inferior turbinate of the nose. Normal is less than 30 minutes. A poor man's cilial function test
- *Alpha1-antitrypsin levels* if deficiency is suspected
- *Barium swallow/oesophageal imaging* if recurrent aspiration suspected.

General management

The main aims of management are:
- Treatment of any underlying medical condition
- Prevention of exacerbations and progression of underlying disease by physiotherapy. The options for airway clearance include:
  - Postural or autogenic drainage
  - Active cycle of breathing technique—this involves breathing control with forced expiration (huffing) using variable thoracic expansion
  - Cough augmentation—using flutter valves/cough insufflator/high-frequency oscillation
  - Exercise regimes—important to prevent general deconditioning
  - The physiotherapist is also vital during admission for exacerbations to help clear tenacious sputum
- To reduce bacterial load and prevent secondary airway inflammation and damage, with antimicrobial chemotherapy
- To give supportive treatment—treatment of associated airflow obstruction
- To optimize nutrition
- To refer for surgery if necessary—localized resection of affected area
- To refer for transplantation if indicated.

Antimicrobial chemotherapy

- This may be intermittent for exacerbations only (for mild disease), or long term for more severe disease. Antibiotics may be oral, nebulized, or intravenous
- Regular sputum surveillance will ensure the likely colonizing organism is known
- *In vivo* sensitivity may be different to *in vitro* sensitivitiy
- Patients need higher antibiotic dose, and for longer time period (usually 2 weeks minimum) than people without bronchiectasis
- Antibiotic treatment choice depends on the severity of underlying disease
- Treatment response is usually assessed by a fall in sputum volume and change to mucoid from purulent or mucopurulent sputum, with an improvement in systemic symptoms, spirometry, and CRP
- Pseudomonas colonized patients have more frequent exacerbations, worse CT scan appearances, and a faster decline in lung function.

Progressive bacterial colonization Different bacteria colonize the airways at different stages of the disease, and their attempted eradication and suppression is vital to the treatment of bronchiectasis. The usual order of colonization is:
- *Staphylococcus aureus*
- *Haemophilus influenzae*
- *Moraxella catarrhalis*
- *Pseudomonas* species.

Exacerbation treatment An exacerbation is usually a clinical diagnosis, with an increase in sputum volume and tenacity, with discolouration. It may be associated with chest pain, haemoptysis and wheeze, and systemic upset—fevers, lethargy, and anorexia. The CRP may be elevated.

Treatment depends on the potential pathogens and resident flora. Nebulized bronchodilators and regular physiotherapy (as an in- or out-patient) may also be needed.

Exacerbation of mild bronchiectasis

- Antibiotics for exacerbations only (tailored to the colonizing organism)
- 2-week course of oral ciprofloxacin at 750 mg bd if *Pseudomonas aeruginosa* colonized
- If early relapse, with a return to purulent sputum within 6–8 weeks, consider:

  Long term oral antibiotics, e.g. amoxicillin 500 mg bd or doxycycline 100 mg od. If treatment failure, change to appropriate intravenous antibiotics, until clinical improvement.

Exacerbation of more severe bronchiectasis
Chronic suppressive antibiotics aim to prevent progression of disease, by reducing bacterial load and preventing ongoing inflammation, thereby reducing morbidity and improving quality of life.

- Antibiotics are usually given for at least 2 days after the sputum has cleared—often for 2 weeks
- If oral antibiotics fail, intravenous treatment is required. This may mean in-patient admission, or could involve long-line insertion, patient education in self-administration of intravenous antibiotics, and involvement of a home care team.

First isolate of Pseudomonas aeruginosa (see also page 366)

- Initial treatment is often aggressive with a 4–6 week course of oral ciprofloxacin 500–750 mg bd, and concurrent nebulized aminoglycoside, such as colomycin 1–2 mega units bd
- If this fails and the patient still has Pseudomonas on sputum culture, intravenous antibiotics, usually an aminoglycoside and anti-pseudomonal penicillin (minimum 2 weeks)
- Consider long-term therapy with regular nebulized aminoglycoside to reduce levels of Pseudomonas and reduce subsequent exacerbations and airway inflammation.

Further management

- Self-management plan—patients need an individual plan for exacerbations, which usually involves having a supply of home antibiotics
- Treatment of associated airflow obstruction/wheeze with inhaled steroids and/or bronchodilators
- There is no specific treatment for abnormalities of mucociliary clearance, although β_2 agonists may enhance clearance
- Nebulized DNase (Dornase alpha)—no evidence for the use of this in non-CF bronchiectasis, but it may be useful in severe exacerbations, if the sputum is very tenacious and expectoration is difficult
- N-acetylcysteine
- Annual influenza and pneumococcal vaccinations
- Osteoporosis prophylaxis (if on long-term steroids)
- Reflux treatment if aspiration
- **Immunoglobulin replacement therapy** Patients found to have immunoglobulin deficiency should be referred to an immunologist for further assessment. Intravenous immunoglobulin replacement therapy is usually given one or two monthly, as a day case
- **Surgery** This is the only potential curative treatment, with resection of a single chronically infected lobe occasionally being of benefit. It is less commonly needed these days, as the incidence of single lobe disease related to previous severe childhood pneumonia is falling. Surgery may be indicated for life-threatening haemoptysis
- **Transplant** is most commonly performed for CF bronchiectasis, but referral may be warranted for severe, non-CF related disease.

Complications of bronchiectasis

- Infective exacerbation
- Haemoptysis—small volume haemoptysis (increasing during exacerbations) is common.
- Massive haemoptysis (usually from tortuous bronchial arteries around damaged lung, e.g. bulla) is a life-threatening emergency (see page 25)
- Pneumothorax
- Respiratory failure
- Brain abscess (now very rare)
- Amyloidosis.

Bronchiectasis and aspergillus

- Allergic bronchopulmonary aspergillosis (ABPA)—this excessive immune response to the environmental fungus aspergillus (most commonly *Fumigatus* species) may be the cause of bronchiectasis (suspect particularly if upper lobe disease), as mucus plugs become impacted in distal airways, causing airway damage and subsequent dilatation. See page 262
- Aspergilloma—Aspergillus may colonize damaged airways with formation of a fungus ball (mycetoma) within a previously formed cavity. This is extremely difficult to treat. Most commonly it causes systemic upset and haemoptysis. See page 268.

Adult cystic fibrosis

General principles

Definition and pathophysiology

- Multisystem disease, due to mutations in the gene encoding for the cystic fibrosis transmembrane conductance regulator (CFTR), a complex chloride channel
- CFTR is essential for regulating salt and water movement across membranes
- Faulty regulation causes viscous secretions
- In the lungs, these secretions result in colonization with pathogenic bacteria, causing a massive inflammatory response, including elastase release. This contributes to lung damage and subsequent development of irreversible bronchiectasis
- In the pancreas, the exocrine ducts become blocked by secretions, leading to pancreatic enzyme insufficiency, pancreatic destruction, and diabetes mellitus.

Genetics

- Autosomal recessive
- Gene found on the long arm of chromosome 7
- Carrier frequency of this gene in Caucasians 1 in 25. 1 in 2500 live births have cystic fibrosis
- CF rare in Afro-Caribbeans, but has been seen in patients of Asian origin in the UK and USA
- Heterzygote/carrier advantage in resistance to *E. coli* diarrhoea and cholera has probably led to persistence of CF genotype, despite lethal homozygous form
- More than 1000 different mutations in the CFTR gene are recognized to cause clinical disease
- The most common mutation is $\Delta F508$ and accounts for around 67% of CF alleles in the UK and northern Europe. This is a deletion of 3 nucleotides resulting in the omission of a single amino acid, phenylalanine, at the 508 residue
- 13 other mutations have a frequency of greater than 1%, accounting for 85% of CF alleles altogether. These can be effectively screened for. They include G542X (3.4%), G551D (2.4%), W1282X (2.1%), and 3905insT (2.1%)
- Different mutations may be associated with particular clinical sub-groups. The phenotype–genotype relationship is closest for pancreatic disease
- Non-CFTR 'modifier' genes (such as TNFα, mannose binding lectin, and α_1-antitrypsin), as well as environmental factors, probably further influence the clinical picture and account for phenotypic variation.

Screening In the UK, neonatal heel-prick for immunoreactive trypsin measurement is now offered routinely in some areas. A national screening programme is going to be implemented. Prenatal second trimester fetal ultrasound may identify presence of echogenic bowel, which can occur in CF. These babies can be screened at birth. People with relatives with CF are advised to have pre-conception CF genotyping, as are the partners of a patient with CF.

Diagnosis Patients are usually diagnosed with CF as neonates or children (genetic screening, family history, failure to thrive, meconium ileus, rectal prolapse, cough, recurrent chest infections). Diagnosis is based on compatible clinical findings, with biochemical or genetic confirmation. The sweat chloride test is an important laboratory test, particularly in children. Some patients are diagnosed with CF in adult life. They usually have different alleles leading to a milder phenotype.

Management The ongoing care of CF patients moves to the adult CF centre around the age of 16–18. A multidisciplinary team approach is recommended, consisting of respiratory physician, specialist nurse, physiotherapist, pharmacist, dietician, and psychologist, with regular additional input from gastroenterology and endocrine teams.

This transition can be a difficult time, as the patient begins to take more responsibility for their care and treatment. Some may have periods of rebelling, not taking medications or performing physiotherapy, despite recognizing the need to do so.

Improved treatment and nutrition of CF patients has led to an increase in median survival, to around 30 years. The predicted lifespan for a baby born with CF now is 42 years.

The main management issues for the adult CF patient are:
- **Lung disease**
  - Maintaining lung function
  - Monitoring lung bacteriology, including screening for multi-resistant and transmissible organisms
  - Consideration of referral for heart–lung or liver transplant, if and when appropriate
- **Nutrition**: Nutritional support, weight, enzymes
- **GI**: Annual screening for biliary cirrhosis and portal hypertension
- **Endocrine**
  - Annual screening for CF-related diabetes (CFRD)
  - Annual screening for osteoporosis
- **Fertility advice**
- **Ensuring psychosocial well-being.**

CF pulmonary sepsis: aetiology

Chronic pulmonary sepsis and its complications cause much of the morbidity and mortality of CF patients. The airways of a CF patient are chronically colonized by pathogenic bacteria from an early age. Bronchiectasis is usually established by a young age (around 5 years).

- Patients commonly expectorate variable volumes of purulent sputum, even when well
- When organism levels are high, patients may feel generally unwell or more tired
- They may have symptoms of dyspnoea, increased volume of more purulent sputum, haemoptysis, wheeze, and chest ache
- Examination and CXR can be unchanged from normal
- FEV_1 levels are a valuable marker of infection and tend to decrease
- With effective antibiotic treatment, FEV_1 levels should rise to the pre-infection normal. If they do not, further antibiotics may be necessary, and other diagnoses or unusual organisms should be considered
- In practice: the FEV_1 is the best marker of disease progression and can be used to assess overall decline, as well as to determine an exacerbation and response to treatment (as PEFR would be used in asthma).

Organisms Airway colonization changes over time, as the patient gets older and organisms become more resistant to antibiotics. Goals of management should be initially to prevent infection, then to eradicate it, and finally to control the infection. Material for culture should be collected; most commonly sputum, but BAL if necessary.

Typical progression of organism colonization with time is:

- *Haemophilus influenzae*
- *Staphylococcus aureus*
- *Pseudomonas aeruginosa* worsens lung function and CXR appearance. Most patients with CF are chronically infected with *Pseudomonas* by their early teens. Non-mucoid species colonize initially and these may be asymptomatic or intermittent. These can be eradicated. Mucoid species then follow and permanent eradication is rare. Decreasing this *Pseudomonas* load produces clinical benefit.

Other organisms

- *Stenotrophomonas maltophilia* a Gram-negative bacteria, often with multiple antibiotic resistance
- *Burkholderia cepacia complex* There are at least 10 different strains, or genomovars, of *Burkholderia cepacia*. Some are associated with a worse clinical outcome and some are not. These organisms are resistant to many antibiotics. It is crucial that *Burkholderia cepacia* colonized patients are separated from non-colonized patients, as the organism is highly transmissible. This means separate clinics, separate spirometers, and side rooms on a different ward are necessary. '**Cepacia syndrome**' is the severe worsening of pulmonary infection with septicaemia, which can be rapidly fatal. This is caused by one strain, genomovar III, or

Burkholderia cenocepacia. CF patients infected with this strain are not accepted for transplant, as studies have shown they do less well. However, other *cepacia* strains are accepted
- **MRSA**
- **NTM**.

CF pulmonary sepsis: antibiotics

Antibiotic courses in patients with CF are longer and at higher doses than in non-CF patients. The choice of antibiotics is based on clinical response more than *in vitro* resistance patterns, but recent sputum culture results will also guide therapy. If *Pseudomonas* has previously been isolated, it may need to be covered in the current antibiotic regime.

- In practice, be guided by the last sputum culture result
- It is usually appropriate to give the patient the same regime they had during their last exacerbation, provided there was a good clinical response
- Microbiology advice should be sought if necessary.

Haemophilus influenzae When isolated (usually in young children) should be treated with amoxicillin, co-amoxiclav, second-generation cephalosporin, tetracycline, or chloramphenicol (toxicity risk), even if the patient is asymptomatic.

Staphylococcus aureus A significant pathogen causing exacerbations. Prevention and eradication are important, even if the patient is asymptomatic. In adults, a minimum of 2 weeks of treatment should be given when *Staphylococcus* is cultured, with flucloxacillin, erythromycin if penicillin resistant, tetracycline, fucidin, rifampicin, or clindamycin. There is no published evidence that long-term treatment in adults has any additional benefit.

Pseudomonas aeruginosa

- **Oral antibiotics** The *Pseudomonas* colonized patient who develops a mild exacerbation should receive 2 weeks of an oral quinolone (such as ciprofloxacin), as well as their usual nebulized colomycin. There are problems with resistance, so therefore should not be used more frequently than every 3 months
- **IV antibiotics** should be used when oral and nebulized treatments have failed, or patient is unwell. An aminoglycoside plus a β-lactam are given, which have a synergistic effect when used in combination. Treatment should be for a minimum of 10 days. Once or twice a day aminoglycoside dosing is used in many centres (5–7 mg/kg), rather than 3 times a day, providing high efficacy and fewer toxic effects
  - *Drug levels* should be checked pre and 1 hour post the third dose and adjusted if necessary. Bacterial toxicity is achieved by the high peak and safety is ensured by low trough. Renal function should also be checked during the IV course
  - Some centres, especially in northern Europe, recommend that patients with chronic *Pseudomonas* colonization should receive 2 weeks of IV antibiotic therapy every 3 months routinely. This policy is not widely adopted in the UK, although, as the threshold for starting treatment is low, the number of antibiotic courses is similar using both regimes.

Satisfactory aminoglycoside levels

- od regime: trough < 1 mg/l and repeat in the first week
- tds regimes:
  - Gentamicin/netilmicin/tobramycin: pre 1–2 mg/l, post 9–12 mg/l
  - Amikacin: pre < 10 mg/l, post 28–32 mg/l.

Any reports of dizziness or balance problems may suggest early ototoxicity. This must be taken seriously as there is a cumulative dose effect. The aminoglycoside should be stopped and ENT referral made for middle ear testing.

- **Aerosol anti-pseudomonal antibiotics** Once the patient is chronically *Pseudomonas* colonized, twice daily nebulized colomycin is used long term (1–2 mega units bd in 4 ml saline after physiotherapy), to try and minimize *Pseudomonas* levels. If colomycin causes wheezing, it can either be given in 6 ml saline or salbutamol added. If colomycin is not tolerated or is ineffective, aminoglycosides designed for IV injection can be tried. A new preservative-free form of tobramycin (TOBI) has been developed and has been found in studies to improve pulmonary function and increase weight gain, although it is expensive and its role in long-term management of CF patients in the UK is yet to be established
- **First isolate of non-mucoid *Pseudomonas*** should be treated aggressively with 4–6 weeks of oral ciprofloxacin 750 mg bd and concurrent 6 weeks of nebulized colomycin 1 mega unit bd. 80% of newly infected patients have *Pseudomonas* eradicated by this regime. If this is not successful, they should have IV therapy with 2 drugs and nebulized colomycin.

Burkholderia cepacia is characteristically resistant to antibiotics, including colomycin and aminoglycosides. Conventional IV therapy may be effective. Should be treated with combination of 2 to 3 IV antibiotics, such as ceftazidime and an aminoglycoside. Possible synergistic combinations are chloramphenicol and minocycline, chloramphenicol and ceftazidime, or a quinolone with a β-lactam/carbopenem. Septrin has now also been used.

MRSA is not more pathogenic than *Staphylococcus aureus*. Nebulized vancomycin can be used for persisting sputum colonization, but IV vancomycin or teicoplanin are required for MRSA exacerbations. Oral rifampicin, fucidin, or linezolid have been used.

Macrolides have additional anti-inflammatory effects, as well as being antibiotics. They do not exhibit intrinsic anti-pseudomonal activity, but there is *in vitro* synergy between macrolides and anti-pseudomonal antibiotics. They also seem to improve clinical status compared to placebo or other antibiotics. This is seen with erythromycin, but especially azithromycin, which decreases sputum viscoelasticity. It is administered three times a week and has been found to improve FEV_1 and decrease exacerbations, when used over 5 months, but larger trials are needed to assess its long-term effects.

IV antibiotic administration

- If patients are unwell or if they are commencing a new antibiotic, they should be admitted to hospital. Otherwise the majority of IV antibiotic courses can be administered at home, after an initial assessment and with home support from nursing staff. Many patients are relatively well during courses of IV antibiotics and are able to continue attending work or college, although it can take them considerable extra time to administer the antibiotics
- Courses of IV antibiotics are often administered prophylactically before surgery
- Most antibiotic regimes involve two weeks of IV antibiotics. This may require the siting of an intravenous cannula with a microbiological filter (to make it last longer), or preferably a long-line
- Many patients have an indwelling port-a-cath that can be accessed when required
- Review patients after 1 week of treatment to ensure there is adequate clinical progress. If there is no improvement, review microbiological sensitivities and change treatment as appropriate.

Port-a-caths

- Inserted in patients with difficult IV access, or those needing frequent courses of IV antibiotics
- Usually accessed/needled by a trained nurse, patient, or family member. Should be accessed only with a Gripper needle of the appropriate length; do not use standard needles, which may damage the port
- Should be flushed with 10 ml of 100 u/ml heparin monthly and with 5–10 ml of 10 u/ml heparin at the end of each IV dose
- Avoid taking blood from port-a-cath as this increases the risk of blockage and infection. Other complications include venous obstruction, tip dislocation, and leakage
- If port-a-cath blocks: 20–50 ml heparinized saline gently alternating between irrigation and aspiration may clear small occlusions. Urokinase 25,000 units in 3 ml 0.9% saline instilled into port may help a blockage
- Infected or fractured lines need removal by surgeons.

Antibiotic desensitization Antibiotic sensitivity is a major problem in patients with CF as repeated antibiotic courses are associated with the development of allergic reactions, especially to β-lactams. Rashes are common, but anaphylaxis can occur. Document any drug reactions, provide an Epi-pen, and give first doses of a new antibiotic in hospital. Desensitization regimes can be helpful and are used for specific antibiotics that have previously caused an allergic reaction. Such regimes need to be given at the start of the antibiotic course each time it is used, and during the course if doses are missed for more than one day. Give a dilute antibiotic dose over 20 minutes, followed by slightly stronger concentration, and repeat for 7 concentration strengths until full antibiotic strength is given. Takes 3–4 hours. Stop infusion if any side-effects are noted.

Management of an exacerbation

Diagnosis on 2–4 of the following:
- Increase in productive cough or dyspnoea
- Change in appearance or volume of sputum
- New signs on auscultation
- New CXR signs
- Decreased appetite
- Fall in respiratory function
- Fever
- 10% fall from baseline FEV_1.

Investigations:
- FEV_1
- Oxygen saturation
- Blood gases
- CXR—exclude pneumothorax
- CRP—relatively non-specific, but can be a useful monitoring tool
- Repeat sputum M, C & S, AFBs. Consider Aspergillus precipitins.

Treatment with appropriate antibiotics, O_2, NIV, consider ITU/resuscitation status if necessary—liaise with CF consultant.

Other pulmonary interventions

Physiotherapy Dedicated CF physiotherapists aim to teach effective airway clearance. This improves secretion clearance, decreases airflow obstruction, and improves ventilation. Patients should do this themselves daily on a long-term basis. Several techniques are used: active cycle of breathing control (tidal volume breathing, then deep inspiration and passive expiration, followed by forced expiration to mobilize secretions prior to coughing/huffing), autogenic drainage, with percussion if patients are not clearing their chest well, flutter devices, and positive expiratory pressure mask. More intensive physiotherapy is administered during exacerbations, by family and/or physiotherapist. Physiotherapists also have important role in assessment of functional ability with exercise testing and evaluating treatment and encouraging aerobic exercise.

Recombinant DNase (dornase alfa or Pulmozyme), a nebulized mucolytic that cleaves the DNA from dead neutrophils, decreasing sputum viscosity and aiding its clearance. It is recommended in patients with an FVC > 40% predicted, to improve pulmonary function. It is used once daily 2500 U via a specific nebulizer. It is only continued in patients who gain objective benefit, with improved lung function, for example, 10% improvement in spirometry and shuttle walk test. It is expensive and only effective in 30–40% of people.

Respiratory support Respiratory failure and cor pulmonale can occur with later stage disease. Home oxygen may be required. Nocturnal non-invasive ventilation may be necessary as a bridge to transplant, if the patient has chronic respiratory failure. If support is needed for acute deterioration related to infection with a major reversible component, this may be non-invasive initially, but the patient may need intubation and ventilation. Such decisions should be made with the patient, their family, and their CF consultant. These decisions can be difficult and factors, such as being on the transplant list, may be relevant.

Steroids Short oral courses seem to improve lung function, but side-effects, such as growth impairment, osteoporosis, diabetes, and cataracts, are significant. They are used in ABPA, severe unresponsive exacerbations, and occasionally in terminal care to improve the sense of well-being in a patient.

Immunization Annual influenza, as well as pneumococcal vaccination.

Transplant The role of transplantation in patients with CF is well established. Patients should be considered for transplant when their life expectancy is less than 2 years and their quality of life is severely impaired, despite optimal medical therapy.
- $FEV_1 \leq 30\%$ predicted or $FEV_1 > 30\%$ with rapid progressive deterioration, e.g. increasing number of admissions, rapid fall in FEV_1, massive haemoptysis
- Hypoxia ($PaO_2 < 7.3$ kPa) and hypercapnia ($PaCO_2 > 6.7$ kPa) are associated with a < 50% survival at 2 years without transplantation, and so are useful guidelines, but patients should be referred for assessment on the basis of FEV_1 criteria even in the absence of severe hypoxia/hypercapnia

- Young female patients with rapid deterioration have a poor prognosis and should be considered for early referral.

Some patients do not want a transplant and full psychosocial assessments are necessary. Whilst on the transplant waiting list, the patient should have optimal nutrition and physical care. Average waits are around 1 year and some patients will inevitably die on the waiting list. Heart–lung or bilateral lung transplants are performed. Following transplantation, the main immediate problems are infection and acute rejection. Later, 40% of patients go on to develop bronchiolitis obliterans (see page 388). One-year survival following transplant is around 58%.

Other pulmonary disease

Pneumothorax The risk of spontaneous pneumothorax increases with age. It occurs in around 20% of male CF patients and slightly fewer females. It is associated with a poor prognosis. It should be managed according to the standard pneumothorax guidelines (page 295), with initial aspiration if patient is not breathless and chest tube if this fails. The lung can take some time to reinflate and require prolonged drainage and suction. Continue physiotherapy during this. Lack of resolution may require surgical input, ideally with a limited procedure, such as local abrasion. Pleurodesis should be avoided if possible in those for whom future lung transplant is an option, as it can cause increased bleeding when the pleura is dissected, but this is not an absolute contraindication. Liaise with the transplant centre, as the transplant surgeon may want to perform the pleurodesis.

Allergic bronchopulmonary aspergillosis (see page 262) Difficult to diagnose in CF as nearly 50% of CF patients have Aspergillus hypersensitivity with positive skin prick tests and 25% have positive precipitins. The incidence is around 10%. Should be screened for annually and advice on avoiding compost heaps and hay/stables should be given. ABPA is indicated by:

- Asthma-like symptoms with new CXR changes
- Raised IgE > 500 IU/l or IgE RAST
- Eosinophilia > 500/mm^3 or
- Positive sputum result for hyphae.

Treatment should be with oral steroids for 2 weeks and, if there is a clinical improvement, these should be continued at decreasing doses for 2–3 months. Intensive physiotherapy is also an important part of the treatment regime. There is some trial evidence that antifungal agents, such as itraconazole 200 mg bd for 4 months, should be used in addition and may have a steroid-sparing role. Itraconazole can cause liver dysfunction, so LFTs need monitoring.

Non-tuberculous mycobacteria (see page 256) Significance unclear and treatment may not produce a clinical benefit. Should be screened for annually. If culture positive, repeat twice and consider 12–18 month course of antibiotics.

CF 'asthma' Some CF patients have coexisting asthma and some have asthma-like symptoms of prolonged exhalation, wheeze, and crackles due to underlying lung inflammation. This is difficult to diagnose, as these symptoms and a variable PEFR are found in most CF patients, due to bronchial hyperreactivity. Occurs in 2–37% of patients. Bronchial hyperreactivity found on testing in at least 40% of patients with CF. There may be bronchodilator responsiveness, also bronchodilatation after exercise or nebulized hypertonic saline. Treat with the standard asthma stepwise progression: short-acting bronchodilator, inhaled corticosteroid, long-acting β2 agonist, theophyllines (which may aid mucociliary clearance), leukotriene receptor antagonist (limited evidence in CF, but may decrease eosinophilic inflammation), oral steroids.

Haemoptysis Small volume haemoptysis is common, especially with concurrent infection and advanced disease. Check clotting and platelets; consider group and save. Stop NSAIDs, give IV antibiotics, vitamin K 10 mg od, and tranexamic acid 15–25 mg/kg/day in 4 divided doses.

Massive haemoptysis (>500 ml) usually reflects bronchial artery bleeding and can be fatal. Needs in-patient support and monitoring. Cross-match. Sit upright and give ice-cold drink to cause pulmonary vasoconstriction. Bolus dose of octreotide 50 µg over 15 min, then octreotide infusion 400 µg in 20 ml 5% dextrose at 2.5–5 ml per hour. May require bronchial artery embolization, bronchial artery ligation, or surgical resection, see also page 25.

Non-pulmonary disease

Nutritional management Maintaining good nutrition is directly related to the patient's survival. Nutrition is more problematic as respiratory disease progresses (raised basal metabolic rate, increased work of breathing, ongoing infection, and inflammation). Dietician's input is crucial. High calorie, high protein diets are encouraged. Patients may need dietary supplements or, if necessary, supplemental overnight feeding via nasogastric tube or gastrostomy. Perform weight and body mass index measurements at the annual review. Aim for BMI > 20.

- *Pancreatic enzyme supplementation* to avoid high faecal fat/energy loss. The smallest dose of pancreatin, containing lipase, required to control steatorrhoea should be used. Typical preparations are Creon (contains lipase, protease, and amylase) 10000, 25000, or 40000 and are taken pre-meals. Typically patients will take 10–20 tablets per day. The dietician can educate patients to adjust the dosage according to the fat and protein content of each meal. Constant re-education is often required to optimize enzyme supplementation. High strength pancreatic enzyme preparations have been found to be linked to colonic strictures, or fibrosing colonopathy; hence maximum levels of lipase of 10,000 units/kg/day have been recommended

- *Vitamins* Fat-soluble vitamins are not absorbed well in patients with CF and these need replacement. Vitamins A, D, and E should be started when pancreatic insufficiency is diagnosed and vitamin K if there is evidence of liver disease, with prolonged prothrombin time. Vitamins should be taken at meal times with pancreatin. Vitamin levels should be checked at annual review

- *Salt* tablets in hot weather, due to excessive losses in sweat.

Gastrointestinal disease

- *Distal intestinal obstructive syndrome/abdominal pain* Also known as meconium ileus equivalent. Bloating, abdominal pain, possible palpable caecal mass, and complete or incomplete intestinal obstruction. Abdominal X-ray shows empty colon and ileal distension with air-fluid levels. Occurs secondary to dehydration, or rapidly increased doses of pancreatic enzymes. Rarely needs surgery. Medical treatment with senna and oral acetylcysteine 200 mg tds and gastrograffin 50–100 ml tds for 5 days is usually adequate. If not, perform gastrograffin enema to determine site of obstruction. This can be therapeutic. Oral intestinal lavage with Kleen Prep solution and up to 10 l of fluid over 1–2 days can also be given. The treatment is considered to have worked when fluid is passed from the rectum and symptoms have resolved. If not resolving, may need further imaging to rule out intussusception

- *Reflux* More common in patients with CF than the general population. Symptoms may occur during physiotherapy, which require changes to positioning/tipping. May require treatment with a proton pump inhibitor to prevent development of a Barrett's oesophagus

- *Pancreatitis* Can occur in those patients who are pancreas-sufficient. Seen in up to 15% adults with CF. May present as severe acute attack or chronic recurrent abdominal pain. Not usually as unwell as non-CF patients with pancreatitis. Raised amylase and abnormal USS/CT. Treat with bowel rest, protein pump inhibitor, IV rehydration.

Liver and biliary disease

- *Liver screening—cirrhosis, portal hypertension* Reduced bile production and deranged bile acid composition leads to biliary obstruction, portal tract inflammation and eventual fibrosis and focal biliary cirrhosis. Cirrhosis affects 2–25% of CF patients. Annual screening liver USS is performed, as blood tests can be unhelpful. Established cirrhosis can lead to variceal bleeds, so annual screening endoscopies are performed in those with cirrhosis. Cirrhosis may need treatment with ursodeoxycholic acid, porto-systemic shunts, and sclerotherapy. Liver transplant may be necessary.

Metabolic disease

- *CF-related diabetes (CFRD)* is becoming increasingly common as the median age of survival with CF increases. Pancreatic damage by CF causes decreased insulin secretion. Approximately 50% of 30 year olds will have CFRD. It presents insidiously and non-specifically, with weight loss or fall in lung function and not with ketoacidosis. Screening glucose tolerance test should be performed annually and more frequently in those on overnight enteral feeds or those with clinical symptoms suggestive of diabetes. Once diabetes is diagnosed, patients should not be managed on a hypoglycaemic diet. Lower doses of insulin are usually required than in IDDM. There is no benefit with oral medication. Microvascular complications can occur and annual screening for these should be performed
- *Osteoporosis* Several studies have confirmed an increased incidence of low bone mass in CF and increased fracture risk, particularly ribs. Risk factors include: malabsorption of vitamin D and calcium, low body mass index, decreased physical activity, delayed puberty, steroid use, diabetes. Treatment is with calcium and vitamin D supplements to maintain vitamin D levels, weight-bearing exercises, hormones for delayed puberty, bisphosphonates.

Other organ systems

- *Arthropathy and CF vasculitis* Acute or subacute arthritis occurs in around 5% of patients with CF. It often responds to NSAIDs. Sometimes arthritis is associated with skin lesions, such as purpura or erythema nodosum. Up to 40% may be ANCA positive. Purpuric vasculitis is associated with more severe lung disease
- *Nasal polyps and sinusitis* Nasal polyps occur in 30% and can cause nasal obstruction. Treatment with topical or systemic steroids and decongestants is usually not helpful and polypectomy may be required, often more than once. Asymptomatic sinusitis is common and can cause mucosal swelling. Consider sinus CT if problematic
- *Stress incontinence* occurs in both men and women, caused by coughing. It has been recognized as an increasing problem. Pelvic floor exercises can be taught by physiotherapists.

Other issues

Fertility

Women with CF are usually subfertile. When planning a pregnancy, their physical state should be optimized with antibiotics and nutrition. The outcome of a pregnancy is improved by optimizing and maintaining pulmonary function and weight gain during the pregnancy. Close monitoring throughout is required. Pregnancy does not affect survival when compared to the entire adult female CF population, but impaired pulmonary function with $FEV_1 < 60\%$ predicted is likely to be the main predictor of worse maternal and fetal outcome. Breast-feeding is possible but intensifies the nutritional strain put on the mother. Most CF antibiotics are safe to use in pregnancy, but avoid ciprofloxacin, chloramphenicol, metronidazole, and IV colomycin. Care with aminoglycoside levels.

Men are infertile due to failure of the normal development or blockage of the vas deferens, seminal vesicle, ejaculatory duct, and body and tail of epididymis. Testicular histology is normal and hence one option is surgical sperm retrieval for intracytoplasmic sperm injection (ICSI) into an egg, performed by fertility clinics.

Genetic counselling and screening should be offered to patients with CF and their partners.

Psychosocial support Trained psychologists offer personal and family support regarding education, employment, financial benefits, burden of treatment, and adapting to progressive disease. Pre-transplant psychological assessment is carried out, as well as terminal care and bereavement counselling. Also treat depression, anxiety, and emotional difficulties, with referral to psychiatric services if necessary. Social worker involvement to help with benefit entitlements, travel insurance, disabled car badge, if necessary.

Care of the dying CF patient When all acknowledge that there are no further treatment options, the focus of care should adjust to being palliative, with an emphasis on symptom relief. This can be done at home or in hospital.

Future developments Gene therapy. Replacing CFTR function to prevent progressive airways disease. Work is focusing on finding a suitable vector for delivery, such as nebulizer and airway epithelial implantation. Progress so far has been disappointing, but work is ongoing.

Living-donor lobar transplantation–lobectomy from donor and transplanted into CF patient. Gives improved pulmonary function, which plateaus after 9–12 months.

Further information

Standards for the clinical care of children and adults with cystic fibrosis in the UK 2001. CF Trust.

www.cff.org (USA)

www.cftrust.org.uk, www.cysticfibrosis.co.uk (both UK)

Seeing the patient with CF in clinic

Routine visit

- Fill in paperwork for UK CF database—contains basic data such as height, weight, oxygen saturation, number of hospital admissions, and details of antibiotic use, as well as regular drug details
- Check spirometry, weight, oxygen saturation
- Antibiotics if required.

At the annual review

- Fill in paperwork for UK database for CF—contains basic data such as height, weight, number of days off school/work, number of complications, antibiotic use, organisms cultured, supplemental feeding, fertility, glucose level, transplant status, and treatment compliance
- Weight
- Height (until they stop growing)
- Radiology
  - CXR (calculate the Northern score; see CF annual review documentation)
  - Liver and biliary system USS (Doppler if known cirrhosis)
- Bloods
  - FBC and clotting studies
  - U&E, LFTs
  - Fasting glucose tolerance test
  - HbA1c if established diabetes
  - Aspergillus species RAST and precipitins
  - IgA, IgG, IgM, and IgE
  - Fat-soluble vitamin levels A, D, E, and K, if available
- Sputum
  - M, C&S including *B. cepacia, S. aureus, Aspergillus*, and MRSA
  - NTM
- Urinalysis
  - Dip for glucose, protein and blood
- Physiotherapy review
- Exercise testing (6 minute walk test or shuttle walk test)
- Respiratory function
  - Spirometry
  - Oximetry and, if <92%, a blood gas
  - ± KCO, lung volumes
- Dietician
  - Full assessment and review of dietary intake, enzyme and vitamin use
- CF nurse review
- Psychologist review
- Social worker review
- Doctor review.

Lung transplantation

Patient selection

Lung transplantation was first performed successfully in the early 1980s, and since then the number of candidates for transplantation has increased significantly. However, there is a significant shortage of donor organs, and so an increasing number of patients (up to 10–15%) die on the waiting list. Approximately 100 lung transplants and 50 heart–lung transplants are carried out in the UK annually. Average waiting times in the UK are around 12 months for lung transplantation and 16 months for heart–lung transplantation. Matching is carried out according to size and major blood groups; HLA matching is not carried out.

Underlying conditions Most common diagnoses, in order:
- COPD (including alpha$_1$-antitrypsin deficiency)
- Cystic fibrosis
- Usual interstitial pneumonitis
- Primary pulmonary hypertension
- Pulmonary hypertension secondary to congenital cardiac disease (Eisenmenger's syndrome)
- Others, including sarcoidosis, lymphangioleiomyomatosis, Langerhans' cell histiocytosis, collagen vascular disease related lung disease, bronchoalveolar cell carcinoma (successful transplantation has been carried out, although tumour recurrence in the donor lung is common).

Indications Referral for transplant assessment should be considered in patients with chronic, severe lung disease despite maximal medical therapy, whose life expectancy is 2–3 years or less (so that transplantation would be expected to prolong their survival). Candidates should be functionally disabled but still able to walk, with no significant cardiac, renal, or hepatic impairment. Suggested age limits are 55 years for heart-lung, 60 years for bilateral lung, and 65 years for single lung transplant.

General referral criteria for lung transplantation

- Normal renal function, with creatine clearance > 50 ml/min
- Normal left ventricular function and normal coronary arteries
- Preserved liver synthetic function
- No osteoporosis
- No systemic sepsis
- BMI > 17
- No psychiatric disorder
- No history of malignancy within 5 years (excluding basal cell carcinoma).

Contraindications
Absolute
- Severe extrapulmonary organ dysfunction (including renal, hepatic, and cardiac)
- Acute, critical illness
- Active cancer or recent history of cancer with substantial likelihood of recurrence

- Severe psychiatric illness and non-compliance
- Active or recent (6 months) substance addiction (cigarette smoking, alcohol, narcotics)
- Severe malnutrition (<70% ideal body weight) or obesity (>130% ideal body weight)
- Inability to walk, with poor rehabilitation potential.

Relative
- Chronic medical conditions that are poorly controlled or associated with target-organ damage (osteoporosis, hypertension, diabetes, coronary artery disease)
- Daily requirement for >20 mg prednisolone
- Mechanical ventilation (excluding NIV)—associated with higher mortality
- Extensive pleural thickening (from infection or prior surgery, e.g. pleurodesis)—procedure is technically more difficult
- Active collagen vascular disease
- Pre-operative colonization of the airway with panresistant bacteria in cystic fibrosis: there is no clear data to support exclusion of pan-resistant *Pseudomonas*, although it remains a relative contraindication in some centres. *B. cepacia* colonization, however, is high risk and an absolute contraindication in some centres.

Contentious
- Active extrapulmonary infection (including HIV, hepatitis B and C)
- Non-tuberculous mycobacteria, especially chelonae
- Aspergilloma (ABPA is not generally a contraindication, though patients would not be transplanted during an exacerbation, and would be treated with prophylactic voriconazole)
- Portal hypertension (prophylactic variceal sclerotherapy may be offered).

Further information

International guidelines for the selection of lung transplant candidates *Am J Respir Crit Care Med* 1998; **158**: 335–9

Indications, patient selection and timing of referral for lung transplantation. Glanville AR, Estenne M. *Eur Respir J.* 2003; **22**: 845–52

Specific conditions

Timing of referral This can be difficult; life expectancy should be <2–3 years, but patients must be fit for the procedure during a waiting time of up to 16 months. Disease-specific guidelines are available.

Chronic obstructive pulmonary disease

- FEV_1 < 20% predicted and/or hypercapnia ($PaCO_2 \geq 6.5$ kPa) and/or clinically significant pulmonary hypertension or hypoxaemia, particularly if rapid deterioration in lung function or frequent severe exacerbations, with poor quality of life
- Should be on maximal medical therapy and have completed pulmonary rehabilitation
- Should have stopped smoking for at least 6 months (if in doubt, check with urinary cotinine levels)
- Ideally < 60 years old.

Cystic fibrosis

- $FEV_1 \leq 30\%$ predicted or FEV_1 > 30% with rapid progressive deterioration, e.g. increasing number of admissions, rapid fall in FEV_1
- Hypoxia (PaO_2 < 7.3 kPa) and hypercapnia ($PaCO_2$ > 6.7 kPa) are associated with a <50% survival at 2 years without transplantation, and so are useful guidelines, but patients should be referred for assessment on the basis of FEV_1 criteria even in the absence of severe hypoxia/hypercapnia
- Severe haemoptysis despite embolization
- Increasingly resistant bacteria (including *Burkholderia cepacia*)
- Weight loss, despite enteral feeding
- Young female patients with rapid deterioration have a poor prognosis and should be considered for early referral
- Invasive ventilation is a contraindication in most centres.

Usual interstitial pneumonia

- Symptomatic disease unresponsive to medical therapy (such as 3 months of immunosuppression). An interval assessment (e.g. 3 monthly) is useful in evaluating disease progression
- VC < 60–70% predicted, TLCO < 50%, resting or exercise-induced hypoxaemia, pulmonary hypertension.

Primary pulmonary hypertension

- New York Heart Association (NYHA) functional class III or IV, mean PAP > 55 mmHg, mean right atrial pressure > 15 mmHg, cardiac index <2 l/min/m^2 despite optimal medical therapy.

Eisenmenger's syndrome

- NYHA functional class III or IV despite optimal medical therapy.

Investigations and surgical approaches

Investigations prior to referral Consult transplant referral centre for details and avoid repetition of investigations. Important investigations include full PFTs, tests of exercise performance (e.g. 6-minute walk), sputum microbiology, ECG, Echo, HRCT chest, LFTs, viral serology (e.g. HIV, CMV, hepatitis B and C), 24-hour creatinine clearance, stress Echo, and/or coronary angiography. If on waiting list, inform transplant centre of changes in clinical condition. Remember that the referring physician remains responsible for continuing regular medical care of the patient, to ensure they remain optimally treated during the waiting period, with particular attention to:

- Maintenance of nutrition (may require PEG feeding)
- Avoidance of obesity
- Maintenance of mobility, continuing exercise and rehabilitation
- Monitoring co-morbid disease: heart, kidney, liver, bones
- Early NIV if indicated
- Avoiding intubation, if possible.

Surgical approaches for transplant

Single lung (50% of procedures)
- Technically easier, allows two recipients from one donor
- Used successfully in all patients except CF and bronchiectasis
- Overdistension of the compliant native lung in emphysema is uncommon, but may be problematic.

Bilateral sequential (25%)
- Sequential right and left single lung transplants at one time
- Selective lung ventilation may render cardiopulmonary bypass unnecessary.

Heart–lung (25%)
- Indicated in Eisenmenger's syndrome, or advanced lung disease with concurrent LV dysfunction or coronary disease
- Cor pulmonale is not in itself an indication, as right ventricular hypertrophy resolves rapidly following lung transplantation alone
- Certain patients without cardiac disease (e.g. many patients with cystic fibrosis) may undergo a 'domino' procedure, where they receive a combined heart–lung transplant, because this is technically easier, and their healthy heart is then used for a patient needing a heart transplant.

Living lobar transplantation
- Bilateral grafting of lower lobes from two living adult donors to replace lungs of child or small adult
- Appears to be safe for the donor, with lung volume reductions of about 15%, but potential for 300% overall mortality (2 donors and one recipient)
- Not widely performed in the UK.

Follow-up

Patients are usually discharged about one month after transplant, following post-transplant bronchoscopy, with BAL and biopsy. They will be followed up closely by their transplant centre, but may also attend general respiratory clinics intermittently between transplant centre visits. Be alert to possible complications (pages 386–9). Spirometric values are generally very stable from 3 months after transplantation, and sustained falls ≥10–15% warrant further investigation. Remember drug interactions (particularly cyclosporin and tacrolimus) if new medications are added. Check immunosuppressant drug blood levels and perform routine blood tests according to the local transplant centre policy.

Outcomes

Survival

- Survival rates: 75% 1-year, 58% 3-year, 44% 5-year. Median survival is 3.7 years
- Compared with patients on the waiting list, lung transplant conveys a survival benefit to patients with CF and UIP, but not emphysema
- Rate of death is highest in first year (infection, primary graft failure)
- Risk factors for early death are pre-existing pulmonary hypertension, ventilator-dependence, recipient age >50, donor age >50
- No survival difference between single, and double-lung transplant.

Functional

- Lung function usually normalizes after bilateral transplant and markedly improves following single-lung transplant. In COPD, FEV_1 increases to 50–60% of predicted value after single lung transplant
- Arterial oxygenation rapidly normalizes
- Six-minute walk distance typically doubles; most patients resume active lifestyle although fewer than 40% of patients return to work
- Limited data on quality of life: initial improvement suggested, but effects after one year are unclear.

Future developments are likely to address both the shortage of donor organs (e.g. living lobar transplantation, the 'non-heart beating donor', xenotransplantation, and further research in lung preservation) and the development of more effective treatments for chronic rejection (new immunosuppressive drugs, induction of immune tolerance).

Routine surgery after lung transplant

Routine surgery >3 months after transplant can be carried out locally, but inform the transplant centre. Routine antibiotic prophylaxis is adequate; there is no increased risk of SBE. The morning dose of *calcineurin inhibitor* (cyclosporin, tacrolimus) should be omitted, as there is a risk of nephrotoxicity with hypovolaemia.

Further information

Lung transplantation. Trulock EP *Am J Respir Crit Care Med* 1997; **155**: 789–818

Lung transplantation. Arcasoy SM, Kotloff RM *NEJM* 1999; **340**(14): 1081–91

Complications 1

Early graft dysfunction

- Characterized by pulmonary infiltrates, hypoxaemia, and diffuse alveolar damage or organizing pneumonia on biopsy; not uncommon during first few days after transplant. Clinical severity ranges from very mild acute lung injury to acute respiratory distress syndrome
- Presumably related to preservation and ischaemia–reperfusion injury
- Exclude other causes e.g. volume overload, pneumonia, rejection, occlusion of venous anastomosis, aspiration
- Treatment is supportive (mechanical ventilation)
- High mortality (up to 60%).

Airway complications

- Anastomotic stenosis most common and typically occurs weeks–months after transplant; suggested clinically by localized wheeze, recurrent pneumonia, or suboptimal lung function. Treat with stent placement via bronchoscopy
- Complete dehiscence of bronchial anastomosis now rare, and requires immediate surgery or retransplantation
- Partial dehiscence is managed conservatively: drain pneumothorax, reduce steroid dose.

Infection

Bacterial

- May occur early, soon after transplant, or late; associated with bronchiolitis obliterans
- Most commonly due to Gram-negative organisms, particularly *Pseudomonas aeruginosa*
- Recipients with cystic fibrosis are not at greater risk than other patients.

CMV

- CMV-seronegative recipients from seropositive donors are at particular risk of severe infection, including pneumonitis; this is usually treated successfully with ganciclovir
- Ganciclovir prophylaxis probably results in later, less severe infection.

Aspergillus

- *Aspergillus* frequently colonizes the airways after lung transplant, but clinically apparent infection develops in only a small proportion of patients
- Peak disease incidence at two months after transplant
- Sites of disease include airways (may lead to mucosal oedema, ulceration, and pseudomembranes; usually responds to itraconazole, voriconazole, or amphotericin B), lung parenchyma, fresh bronchial anastomosis, and disseminated aspergillosis (associated with high mortality).

Drug-related Immunosuppressive drugs must be taken lifelong following transplantation. Agents used include cyclosporin or tacrolimus, azathioprine, mycophenolate mofetil, and prednisolone. They are associated with many side-effects and drug interactions. Cyclosporin and tacrolimus blood levels need to be closely monitored.

Complications 2

Acute rejection

- Very common, particularly within 3 months of transplant. Rare after 12 months
- Asymptomatic, or may be associated with malaise, fever, dyspnoea, cough, hypoxia. May present similarly to pneumonia or COP
- CXR may be normal or show non-specific infiltrates
- Most reliable sign is fall in spirometry >10%, although this does not distinguish from other complications, particularly infection
- Refer back to the transplant centre if these problems develop within 3 months of the transplant
- Ideally confirm histologically: transbronchial biopsies are safe, and typically show perivascular lymphocytic infiltrates
- Treatment: IV methylprednisolone pulses. The majority of patients respond quickly
- Acute rejection is the main risk factor for the development of chronic rejection
- Acute rejection is an uncommon cause of breathlessness after 3 months, and other common causes of SOB should be considered.

Chronic rejection

- A significant problem, accounting for poor long-term prognosis following lung transplant
- Uncommon in first 6 months but prevalence subsequently increases steadily, affecting 60–70% of patients at 5 years
- Clinically: insidious onset with breathlessness and cough, and progressive airflow obstruction on spirometry
- Manifest histologically as **bronchiolitis obliterans**, a fibroproliferative process affecting small airways. Histological confirmation is difficult: transbronchial biopsies have a low sensitivity, so a clinical diagnosis of 'bronchiolitis obliterans syndrome' is defined as an unexplained and sustained fall in FEV_1 to <80% of peak value post-transplant
- CXR unhelpful; HRCT may show expiratory air trapping and peripheral bronchiectasis
- *P. aeruginosa* colonization is common, with recurrent purulent tracheobronchitis
- Treatment involves increased immunosuppression, and if effective this acts only to reduce the rate of disease progression. Infection is treated aggressively
- Prognosis is poor: mortality is 40% within 2 years of diagnosis; the rate of decline variable
- Retransplantation is the only definitive treatment and is controversial.

Recurrence of primary disease Documented in sarcoidosis, lymphangioleiomyomatosis, giant cell interstitial pneumonitis, diffuse panbronchiolitis, and bronchoalveolar cell carcinoma.

Malignancy Increased risk of certain malignancies, e.g. non-Hodgkin's lymphoma (and other post-transplant lymphoproliferative diseases), skin, lip, vulval, and perineal carcinomas, *in situ* cervical cancer, and Kaposi's sarcoma. Most lymphomas appear within the first year, and the lung allograft is the most common site of involvement. Post-transplant lymphoproliferative disease may present with CXR nodules, tonsillar enargement, peripheral lymphadenopathy, skin nodules, and bowel complications, such as intussusception. These patients should be referred back to the transplant centre for treatment, rather than the local haematologist. The usual treatment is a reduction in immunosuppression or rituximab.

Differential diagnosis of CXR nodules following transplant

- Nocardia
- Aspergilloma
- TB
- Pseudomonas
- Post-transplant lymphoproliferative disease
- Disease recurrence
- Primary malignancy.

Chapter 32

Pulmonary hypertension

Classification

Definition Pulmonary hypertension is a mean pulmonary artery pressure (PAP) > 25 mmHg with a pulmonary capillary or left atrial pressure < 15 mmHg.

A rise in pulmonary artery pressure can be due to:
- Increased pulmonary blood flow, e.g. atrial septal defect
- Increased resistance in the pulmonary vascular bed, e.g. hypoxia, pulmonary embolism
- Elevated pulmonary venous pressure, e.g. left ventricular failure.

WHO classification of pulmonary hypertension, 2003

1 Pulmonary arterial hypertension
- Idiopathic pulmonary arterial hypertension (IPAH, previously known as primary pulmonary hypertension)
- Familial pulmonary arterial hypertension (FPAH)
- Related to:
  - Collagen vascular disease
  - Congenital systemic to pulmonary shunts
  - Portal hypertension
  - HIV infection
  - Drugs/toxins: anorectic agents (fenfluramine, dexfenfluramine), rape seed oil, others
  - Very likely: amphetamine, L-tryptophan
  - Possible: meta-amphetamines, cocaine, chemotherapy agents
  - Other (glycogen storage diseases, haemoglobinopathies, myeloproliferative disorders, hereditary haemorrhagic telangiectasia, splenectomy)
- Associated with significant venous or capillary involvement
  - Pulmonary veno-occlusive disease
  - Pulmonary capillary haemangiomatosis.

2 Pulmonary venous hypertension
- Left-sided atrial or ventricular heart disease
- Left-sided valvular heart disease.

3 Pulmonary hypertension associated with hypoxaemia
- Chronic obstructive pulmonary disease
- Interstitial lung disease
- Sleep disordered breathing
- Alveolar hypoventilation disorders
- Chronic high altitude exposure.

4 Pulmonary hypertension due to chronic thrombotic and/or embolic disease

- Thromboembolic obstruction of proximal pulmonary arteries
- Obstruction of distal pulmonary arteries
  - Pulmonary embolism (thrombus, tumour, ova, parasites, foreign material)
  - *In situ* thrombosis
  - Sickle cell disease.

5 Pulmonary hypertension associated with miscellaneous disorders

- Inflammatory
  - Langerhans' cell histiocytosis
  - Sarcoidosis
  - Other.
- Extrinsic compression of the central pulmonary veins
  - Fibrosing mediastinitis
  - Lymphadenopathy/tumours.

Primary pulmonary hypertension (PPH)

Definition Primary pulmonary hypertension (PPH) or idiopathic pulmonary arterial hypertension (IPAH) is a rare disease of uncertain aetiology. The mean pulmonary artery pressure is > 25 mmHg with a pulmonary capillary or left atrial pressure < 15 mmHg. By definition there is no demonstrable cause. The presence of resting pulmonary hypertension is significant, as more than 70% of the vascular bed must be lost for the pulmonary arterial pressure to rise.

Epidemiology The incidence of PPH in Europe and the USA is 1–2 cases per million population per year. The mean age at diagnosis is 36, with a female preponderance of about 2.1:1. Although rare, it is important to diagnose, as it affects a young age group and has an extremely poor outcome without treatment.

Pathophysiology Vasoconstriction and secondary thickening of peripheral 'resistance' blood vessels in association with thrombosis lead to raised pulmonary vascular resistance. This leads to further structural vessel changes, due to proliferation of vascular smooth muscle cells. The mechanism for this is poorly understood, but the identification of the gene for familial PPH (which codes for BMPR2—bone morphogenetic protein receptor type II, a receptor in the transforming growth factor beta (TGFβ) family) has implicated TGFβ in the pathogenesis. The BMPR2 family of proteins is related to TGFβ, and is involved in cell apoptosis. It is hypothesized that defective signalling via this pathway may result in abnormal endothelial proliferation and cell growth in response to various insults, with an inability to terminate the proliferative response to injury. Endothelin-1, a potent vasoconstrictor, has also been implicated in the disease. The genetic abnormality may have to be accompanied by some additional environmental factor to cause PPH.

Aetiology

Sporadic PPH—a number of risk factors have been identified for sporadic PPH, and BMPR2 mutations may be present in up to 25%. The identified risk factors for PPH have in common an ability to damage the pulmonary endothelium, which may provoke an excessive proliferative response, progressing to PPH. In a proportion of patients no risk factors are found.

Familial PPH—a familial predisposition is seen in 6–10% of cases, where the disease is transmitted in an autosomal dominant fashion. Incomplete penetrance and anticipation are seen, with presentation at a younger age in successive generations. The responsible gene has been localized to chromosome 2 (locus 2q 31–32). Abnormal cardiovascular responses to exercise have been demonstrated in asymptomatic carriers of BMPR2.

Prognosis is variable, depending on haemodynamic compromise, and response to vasodilator therapy, with cardiac index, right atrial pressure, and mean pulmonary artery pressure at presentation being linked to prognosis. The median survival from diagnosis is 3–4 years. There is no cure and mean survival without treatment is 2 years.

Patients in New York Heart Association (NYHA) classes III and IV have a poorer prognosis than those in classes I and II. All patients are at risk of progressive right heart failure and sudden death.

PPH: clinical features

The symptoms of primary pulmonary hypertension are non-specific, leading to a delay in diagnosis (on average of around 3 years from first symptoms). The mean age at diagnosis is 36.

Presenting features

- Exertional breathlessness, due to the inability to increase cardiac output with exercise
- Chest pain (right heart angina)
- Syncope, due to a fall in blood pressure on exercise
- Palpitations
- Oedema, or other signs of right-sided fluid overload.

Examination Signs consistent with right heart fluid overload and right ventricular hypertrophy, including:

- Raised JVP, with giant V waves
- Right ventricular heave and tapping apex beat
- Wide splitting of S2 with loud P2
- Murmur of tricuspid regurgitation
- Hepatomegaly
- Ascites
- Peripheral oedema
- Hypoxia and exercise desaturation.

Investigations These are aimed at making a diagnosis of primary pulmonary hypertension by excluding possible underlying causes for the pulmonary hypertension. In 85% of patients presenting with symptoms caused by established pulmonary hypertension, a CXR and ECG will be abnormal.

- **CXR** may show enlarged pulmonary arteries and an enlarged cardiac silhouette, with pruning of peripheral vessels
- **ECG** Right axis deviation and RVH
- **Arterial blood gas** Hypoxia and hypocapnia, with a fall in oxygen saturation on exercise
- **Pulmonary function tests** The lung volumes may be normal, or show a mild restrictive or obstructive defect with a reduced TLCO
- **HRCT chest** to exclude underlying lung disease
- **Ventilation-perfusion scanning/CTPA** to exclude chronic thromboembolic disease as a cause
- **Echocardiography** The most useful diagnostic test in pulmonary hypertension. Typically shows right heart enlargement with paradoxical interventricular septum movement, and tricuspid regurgitation. Pericardial effusions may be present. The pulmonary artery pressure can be estimated from the tricuspid regurgitation jet, using Doppler techniques
- **Right heart catheterization** to confirm the exact pulmonary artery pressure and cardiac output (with a Swann–Ganz catheter, by thermodilution). This is usually performed in parallel with vasodilator

testing in a specialist centre. Also needed to exclude a left to right intracardiac shunt
- *Selective pulmonary angiography* if the CTPA is inconclusive
- *Blood tests* Routine tests, including autoantibodies (anti-centromere antibody, anti SCL-70, and RNP if connective tissue disease suspected as a cause), HIV, TSH, thrombophilia screen, serum ACE.

PPH: general management

The diagnosis of primary pulmonary hypertension (or IPAH) is made when all other causes have been excluded. The management in this section applies to primary pulmonary hypertension.

General management

- **Anticoagulation** All patients with pulmonary hypertension are at risk of venous thromboembolism and intrapulmonary thrombus, because of sluggish pulmonary blood flow, dilated heart chambers, venous stasis, and an enforced sedentary lifestyle, and therefore should be on life-long warfarin. A small thrombus can have catastrophic effects in a patient who is already severely compromised. Studies show an increased survival with warfarin in PPH, which may reflect reversal of an underlying pro-thrombotic state, as well as the prevention of *in situ* thrombus formation. Additional beneficial effects are seen when combined with a vasodilator. There is no published data on the use of warfarin in secondary pulmonary hypertension
- **Long-term oxygen** Hypoxaemia is due to a combination of reduced cardiac output, ventilation/perfusion mismatching, and right–left shunting through a patent foramen ovale
- **Diuretics and digoxin** Diuretics may be useful for the treatment of oedema, but excess preload reduction may limit their usefulness. Digoxin has been shown to improve cardiac output acutely in PPH, though its longer-term effects are not known
- **Immunization** Annual influenza and one-off pneumococcal vaccination
- **Contraception** Pregnancy is poorly tolerated in PPH. Tubal ligation is recommended, as combined oral contraceptives increase the risk of venous thromboembolism.

A **national pulmonary hypertension service** was set up in the UK in 2002, to coordinate diagnosis and treatment in 5 regional centres, recognizing the need to provide best care (with complex interventions) and optimize funding for expensive treatments. The five centres at the time of publication are

- London—Hammersmith Hospital
  - Royal Brompton Hospital (adult congenital heart disease)
  - Royal Free Hospital (connective tissue disease)
  - Great Ormond Street Hospital for Children (children)
- Cambridge—Papworth Hospital
- Sheffield—Royal Hallamshire Hospital
- Newcastle—Freeman Hospital
- Glasgow—Western Infirmary.

Recent guidelines suggest referral to a specialist centre after CXR, ECG, simple spirometry, and echocardiogram (but not cardiac catheterization, as this should be done in parallel with a vasodilator study in a specialist centre).

Recommendations on the management of pulmonary hypertension in clinical practice. *Heart* 2001; **86**: S1

PPH: vasodilator therapy

The rationale for the use of vasodilators in PPH is based on impaired production of the vasodilators nitric oxide and prostacyclin and over-production of the vasoconstrictor endothelin by the pulmonary endothelium. *Vasodilator responsiveness* is measured at right heart catheterization with incremental doses of a short-acting vasodilator administered, such as prostacyclin, epoprostenol, or adenosine. Patients are defined as responders or non-responders. A responder has a significant (usually >20%) reduction in mean pulmonary artery pressure (PAP) and pulmonary vascular resistance, with an unchanged or increased cardiac output and minimally changed systemic blood pressure. Only about 25% of patients are responders.

Calcium channel blockers

- High-dose nifedipine (30–240 mg daily) and diltiazem (120–900 mg daily) are recommended in patients with a positive acute vasodilator response (and normal right heart function). They reduce PAP and mortality. Their acute vasodilator response is maintained long term. They are unlikely to be beneficial in acute vasodilator challenge non-responders
- Side-effects include hypotension and oedema, which may limit use
- Amlodipine has more selective vasodilating properties, and at doses of 2.5–5 mg daily may be useful in those intolerant of the other agents, or if right ventricular function is impaired
- Calcium antagonists should be started in hospital, and titrated with careful monitoring
- Verapamil is not used, because of its negative inotropic effects.

Prostaglandin analogues Prostaglandins are potent vasodilators. They inhibit platelet aggregation and have antiproliferative and cytoprotective properties. Benefits with prostaglandin therapy are also seen in pulmonary hypertension due to anorectic agents, intracardiac shunts, chronic thromboembolic disease, sarcoidosis, and connective tissue disease. Side-effects include jaw pain, diarrhoea, and arthralgias; also infection, thrombosis, and pump failure, resulting from the continuous and complex delivery system needed for the drug. Prostaglandin therapy is expensive, costing between £40,000 and £60,000 per year.

- *Epoprostenol (Flolan)* This potent vasodilator acts on receptors related to cAMP. It is a prostacyclin analogue (PGI_2). It probably has its effects as a selective pulmonary vasodilator and potentially through vascular remodelling and platelet adhesion. It has been shown to improve exercise capacity and improve haemodynamics. Long-term treatment improves survival. It is inactive within the circulation after 5 minutes, and therefore needs to be given by continuous intravenous infusion via a portable pump and Hickman line
- *Treprostinil* is a prostacyclin analogue that can be given sub-cutaneously as it has greater *in vivo* stability than epoprostenol
- *Iloprost* is a prostacyclin analogue (working via epoprostenol vascular endothelial receptors) and is more potent than epoprostenol. It also needs to be given by continuous intravenous infusion. A benefical effect is also seen with nebulized iloprost and studies are ongoing

- Prostacyclin analogues have been shown in placebo-controlled trials to improve 6-minute walk and improve haemodynamics
- A beneficial haemodynamic response is seen chronically in acute vasodilator response non-responders. Despite this negative acute response, these patients have the greatest survival benefit from prostaglandin therapy
- Prostaglandin treatment doubles the time on the lung transplantation waiting list, and improves transplantation outcomes. Improved haemodynamics may lead to some patients coming off transplant waiting lists
- Failure to show improved exercise capacity following one month's treatment with prostaglandin therapy is an indication for lung transplantation
- Tolerance develops to intravenous prostaglandin therapy, with increasing dose requirements over time. The mechanism for this is unclear.

Endothelin receptor antagonists Endothelin has effects on pulmonary endothelium, causing smooth muscle cell proliferation. Plasma levels are raised in patients with various forms of pulmonary hypertension.

- *Bosentan* A novel oral endothelin receptor A and B antagonist that improves 6-minute walk, increases cardiac output, and decreases pulmonary artery pressure and pulmonary vascular resistance compared to placebo. Side-effects include liver enzyme abnormalities.

Nitric oxide/L-arginine Endothelial production of nitric oxide is reduced in PPH. Treatment with continuous inhaled nitric oxide has been successful. The acute pulmonary vascular response to nitric oxide predicts response to oral calcium antagonists. Chronic use is limited by expensive and complicated delivery systems. Trials are underway to assess the effect of replacement of the substrate for nitric oxide, L-arginine.

Phosphodiesterase inhibitors e.g. sildenafil (Viagra) prolong the vasodilatory effects of nitric oxide, and are currently licensed for erectile dysfunction. A small placebo-controlled trial has demonstrated the drug's ability to attenuate the PAP rises seen with hypoxia in 10 normal controls. It appears to be as effective as inhaled nitric oxide in PPH. A small trial has demonstrated favourable effects of sildenafil in combination with iloprost in a group of patients with PPH or chronic thromboembolic PHT. It also has anti-platelet activity. Larger trials are ongoing.

PPH: surgical treatments, end of life care, and future developments

Surgical treatments

Atrial septostomy Creation of a right–left shunt by balloon atrial septostomy aims to increase systemic blood flow, by bypassing the pulmonary circulation, particularly in patients with syncope or severe right heart failure. It is a palliative procedure, and can be used for symptom control prior to transplantation, with the defect being closed at the time of transplant. Arterial desaturation occurs following the procedure, but is normally offset by the increased cardiac output seen, with increased oxygen delivery. It is not indicated in severe left heart failure or in patients with impaired left ventricular function.

Transplantation Improves survival and quality of life in patients with pulmonary hypertension. In those with preserved left ventricular function, lung transplant is the procedure of choice. Return of normal right ventricular function is found after transplantation.

- As for all diseases needing transplantation, timing of referral and operation is crucial, as response to medical therapy is poor and the organ availability is limited
- The incidence of obliterative bronchiolitis appears to be higher post-transplantation for PPH, though the reason for this is uncertain.

End of life care Palliative care may be warranted to improve symptoms such as fatigue, breathlessness, abdominal bloating, nausea, and pain (see page 650).

Future developments Combination therapies are likely to be used more commonly in the future. A number of agents are currently being investigated, including L-arginine, vasoactive intestinal peptide (VIP), and drugs with anti-proliferative effects such as simvastatin and rapamycin. Also being investigated are newer endothelin antagonists, such as ambisentan.

Secondary pulmonary hypertension: causes

The majority of patients with pulmonary hypertension seen by a respiratory specialist will have secondary pulmonary hypertension due to chronic hypoxic lung disease, such as COPD. In this case, the pulmonary hypertension is often an incidental finding in a patient with a chronic respiratory disease.

Chronic hypoxia causes pulmonary vasoconstriction due to changes in the pulmonary endothelium, including down regulation of endothelial nitric oxide synthetase.

COPD with pulmonary hypertension has a much poorer prognosis than COPD without pulmonary hypertension. In patients with a PAP < 25 mmHg, the 5 year survival is >90%. In those with a PAP > 45 mmHg, the 5 year survival is <10%. Whether this is due to the pulmonary hypertension itself, or whether the pulmonary hypertension is a marker of hypoxia and disease severity is unclear.

Chronic thromboembolic pulmonary hypertension is a rare cause of secondary pulmonary hypertension, due to incomplete clot resolution following treatment for an acute pulmonary embolic event. It occurs in no more than 0.1% of pulmonary embolic event survivors. The pathogenesis is uncertain, with no consistent defect in fibrinolytic activity demonstrated. Antiphospholipid antibodies are present in 10–20% of patients. The diagnosis is not usually made until advanced pulmonary hypertension is present. Progressive pulmonary hypertension seems to result from changes in the small peripheral resistance vessels in the vascular bed, as opposed to being due to progressive pulmonary events. Secondary hypertensive changes, probably induced by high pulmonary artery pressures, lead to incremental increases in right ventricular afterload, with increasing pulmonary hypertension, ultimately leading to right ventricular failure.

Collagen vascular disease Secondary pulmonary hypertension develops in up to one-third of patients with scleroderma, and is most frequently seen as an isolated phenomenon in patients with limited cutaneous disease. It can also occur secondary to interstitial lung disease, and has a very poor prognosis. Life expectancy is <1 year in patients with collagen vascular disease and isolated pulmonary hypertension, with a gas transfer of <25% of normal. Obliteration of the alveolar capillaries and arteriolar narrowing is induced by both the primary vascular disease and by interstitial fibrosis (if it is present).

Other connective tissue diseases, including rheumatoid arthritis and SLE, can also lead to secondary pulmonary hypertension. There is an association with Raynaud's phenomenon and a female predominance is seen.

Drugs and toxins Damage to the pulmonary artery endothelium can be caused by drugs, e.g. anorectic agents such as fenfluramine, dexfenfluramine, cocaine, and amphetamines. The clinical syndrome can be indistinguishable from PPH. A careful history must therefore be taken.

The absolute risk for pulmonary hypertension with anorectic agents is 28 cases per million person-years of exposure. Pulmonary hypertension can develop within days of starting the drug.

HIV infection Pulmonary hypertension is seen in up to 1 in 200 people who are HIV positive, in the absence of AIDS. It is hypothesized that HIV-infected macrophages release vasoactive cytokines that lead to endothelial damage and proliferation. Antiretroviral drugs may have a beneficial effect on pulmonary haemodynamics.

Congenital heart disease and shunts Volume and pressure overload caused by left heart abnormalities (including mitral valve disease), constrictive pericarditis, and left to right intracardiac shunts, e.g. atrial and ventricular septal defects, lead to secondary pulmonary hypertension.

Portal hypertension Porto-pulmonary hypertension, seen in patients with portal hypertension (of whatever cause), is probably due to the failure of the liver to remove vasoactive substances from the portal circulation, with their resultant accumulation and presentation to the pulmonary arterial endothelium.

Alveolar hypoventilation e.g. due to neuromuscular disease. Respiratory acidosis increases hypoxic vasoconstriction, thereby increasing secondary pulmonary hypertension.

Hypothyroidism is also recognized as a cause.

Secondary pulmonary hypertension: management

In this group of patients the diagnosis is usually made from echocardiography, and the treatment is optimal management of the underlying lung disease, with the addition of oxygen and diuretics. Recent guidelines on the management of pulmonary hypertension suggest that the management protocol for patients with primary pulmonary hypertension (see page 398) may also be suitable for patients with secondary hypertension, but there is limited evidence for most of it in this context. In particular the evidence for treating pulmonary hypertension in hypoxic COPD, other than with long-term oxygen therapy, does not yet exist. Current studies will establish if agents such as calcium channel blockers, sildenafil, or warfarin are of benefit in patients with secondary pulmonary hypertension.

Disease specific management

- *Chronic thromboembolic pulmonary hypertension* Patients with chronic thromboembolic pulmonary hypertension have a five year survival of < 10%, if the PAP > 50 mmHg. Pulmonary thromboendarterectomy is the treatment of choice. This is the surgical removal of organized thrombotic material. This aims to strip away the pulmonary arterial endothelium, starting proximally and extending out to remove all clot in the subsegmental levels. It is done on cardiopulmonary bypass with circulatory arrest. The PAP usually falls within 48 hours of surgery. Operative mortality is <10% in experienced hands

- *Scleroderma* Up to 70% of patients with systemic sclerosis have a positive acute vasodilator response, but treatment with vasodilators may not confer a survival advantage. Oral calcium antagonists are poorly tolerated (due to worsening of oesophageal dysmotility). Patients with systemic sclerosis (particularly if anti-centromere antibody positive) should be screened for pulmonary hypertension, even if no symptoms are present.

Further information

Recommendations on the management of pulmonary hypertension in clinical practice. *Heart* 2001; **86** (S1): i1–i13

Primary pulmonary hypertension. Peacock A. *Thorax* 1999; **54**: 1107

Diagnosis and management of pulmonary arterial hypertension: ACCP evidence-based clinical practice guidelines. *Chest* 2004; **126**: suppl.

Patient group, www.pha-uk.com

Pulmonary thromboembolic disease

Epidemiology and pathophysiology

Definition A pulmonary embolism (PE) is a clinically significant obstruction of part or all of the pulmonary vascular tree, usually caused by thrombus from a distant site.

Epidemiology

- The overall annual incidence is 60–70/100,000, with a UK annual death rate of 100/million
- PE may account for up to 15% of all post-operative deaths. It is the commonest cause of death following elective surgery, and the commonest cause of maternal death
- Post mortem studies have consistently shown a frequency of 7–9%, and large in-patient studies have shown a frequency of around 1%, with a mortality of 0.2%. The mortality is much higher in patients with serious underlying co-morbid disease
- The incidence is likely to be stable, but improved diagnostic methods mean that it is probably reported more frequently.

Pathophysiology

- 75% of thrombi are generated in the deep venous system of the lower limbs and pelvis, probably initiated by platelet aggregation around venous valve sinuses. Activation of the clotting cascade leads to thrombus formation, with Virchow's triad (venous stasis, injury to the vessel wall, and increased blood coaguability) predisposing to thrombus formation. Venous stasis is increased by immobility and dehydration, and leads to local accumulation of platelets and clotting factors. In addition, coagulation factors may be altered in various disease states, e.g. in the acute phase response, malignancy, and autoimmune disease
- 20% of leg thrombi embolize, with a higher incidence in above knee clots than below knee clots. Large clots may lodge at the bifurcation of the main pulmonary arteries causing haemodynamic compromise. Smaller clots will travel more distally, infarcting the lung and causing pleuritic pain. These are more commonly multiple and bilateral and are found most often in the lower lobes, where blood flow is greatest
- Thrombi can also develop in the right heart following myocardial infarction
- Septic emboli are found in endocarditis, in association with intraventricular septal defects (paradoxical emboli), AV shunts, or with central venous access.

Haemodynamic effects of PE depend on the size of the clot and which area of the pulmonary vascular tree it subsequently obstructs, as well as the pre-existing state of the myocardium and pulmonary parenchyma.

- As the pulmonary vasculature in a healthy lung has a large capacitance, the mean pulmonary artery pressure (PAP) does not rise until at least 50% of the vascular bed has been occluded
- As the PAP rises, right ventricular afterload increases, with a resulting increase in right ventricular end diastolic pressure

- The right ventricle will start to fail acutely as the PAP reaches over 40 mmHg
- This causes a reduction in pulmonary blood flow, leading to reduced left ventricular filling and a reduction in systemic blood pressure
- The secondary effects are much worse if right-sided filling cannot be maintained, if for example, the patient is dehydrated, hypovolaemic, or erect
- Hypoxia results from reduced cardiac output, low mixed venous PaO_2 and higher perfusion to the remaining alveoli leading to ventilation/perfusion mismatching in the unaffected lung
- Hypoxia will be worse if there is a larger premorbid V/Q spread, e.g. in the elderly and those with pre-existing lung disease. It is therefore possible for a young healthy person to have a normal PaO_2 and A–a gradient following a PE
- A patient with a PAP of ≥ 40 mmHg cannot have *acute* PE as this pressure cannot be achieved acutely. In this setting, the raised PAP raises the possibility of *chronic* thromboembolic disease, pulmonary hypertension, or another cause of raised PAP.

Aetiology

Risk factors can be divided into major and minor factors. This division is important for an assessment of clinical probability.

Risk factors for venous thromboembolism (VTE)

Major risk factors (relative risk x 5–20)

Surgery	Major abdominal/pelvic surgery
	Orthopaedic surgery (especially lower limb)
	Post-operative intensive care
Obstetrics	Late pregnancy (higher incidence with multiple births)
	Caesarean section
	Pre-eclampsia
Malignancy	Pelvic/abdominal
	Metastatic/advanced
Lower limb problems	Fracture, varicose veins
Reduced mobility	Hospitalization
	Institutional care
Previous proven VTE	

Minor risk factors (relative risk x 2–4)

Cardiovascular	Congenital heart disease
	Congestive cardiac failure
	Hypertension
	Central venous access
	Superficial venous thrombosis
Oestrogens	Oral contraceptive pill
	(especially third-generation higher oestrogen containing)
	Hormone replacement therapy
Miscellaneous	Occult malignancy
	Neurological disability
	Thrombotic disorders
	Obesity
	Inflammatory bowel disease
	Nephrotic syndrome
	Dialysis
	Myeloprofilerative disorders
	Behçet's disease

Risk of malignancy Occult cancer will be present in 7–12% of patients presenting with idiopathic venous thromboembolism (VTE). Malignancy may be detected by careful clinical assessment, routine blood tests, and chest radiography. Screening for malignancy in these patients is not recommended, unless suspected clinically. These patients are more likely to have a poor prognosis, because of regional spread or distant metastases at diagnosis.

Inherited thrombophilias

- 25–50% of patients with VTE have an identifiable inherited thrombophilia, e.g. antiphospholipid syndrome, deficiency of antithrombin III, a prothrombin gene defect, protein C or protein S deficiency
- These usually need to interact with an additional acquired risk factor to cause VTE
- Factor V Leiden deficiency is present in 5% of the population, and 20% of patients presenting with thrombosis
- Current recommendations do not advocate routine screening for inheritable thrombophilias, unless in specific circumstances (see below), as the number needed to test to prevent an episode of VTE would be very high. In addition, detecting a heritable thrombophilia does not predict a significantly higher rate, or earlier occurrence of VTE, in the absence of a secondary risk factor.

Those in whom thrombophilia testing is recommended:

- Patients with recurrent venous thrombosis
- Patients < 40 with venous thrombosis with no obvious risk factors
- First venous thromboembolism with a clear family history in first degree relatives
- Thrombosis secondary to pregnancy, oral contraceptive pill, hormone replacement therapy
- Thrombosis at an unusual site—cerebral, mesenteric, portal, or hepatic veins.

All but factor V Leiden deficiency and the prothrombin gene mutation need to be tested for when the patient is off anticoagulants.

'Economy class syndrome' Thromboembolic disease associated with long distance sedentary travel, with increasing incidence of disease with increasing distance travelled. A 2001 study of 135.29 million passengers showed an incidence of PE of 1.5 cases/million for travel over 5000 km, compared with 0.01 cases/million for travel under 5000 km. For travel over 10,000 km, the incidence increased to 4.8 cases/million.

Clinical features

Acute PE typically presents in four main ways:
- *Circulatory collapse in a previously well patient*
  Hypotension ± loss of consciousness in 1%. Usually due to extensive pulmonary artery occlusion from massive PE causing marked hypoxia and hypocapnia (due to hyperventilation) and acute right heart failure, with raised JVP and fainting on sitting up. ECG may be normal, show sinus tachycardia or right heart strain. Echocardiogram shows pulmonary hypertension and right ventricular failure
- *Pulmonary infarction and haemoptysis* (in 60%)
  ± pleuritic pain. Arterial blood gases may be normal, and ECG changes uncommon. Localizing signs may be present, e.g. pleural rub
- *Isolated dyspnoea* (in 25%)
  Defined as acute breathlessness in the absence of haemorrhage or circulatory collapse. The thrombus is more likely to be central, with hypoxia on blood gases. The patient may have sudden onset and unexplained breathlessness, in the presence of risk factors for VTE
- *Collapse, poor reserve* (in 10%)
  May be due to a small PE, often in an elderly patient with limited cardiorespiratory reserve. These patients can rapidly decompensate with even a relatively small PE. The clinical findings may be non-specific and reflect the underlying disease process, rather than the PE itself.

Chronic thromboembolic disease This typically presents with more insidious onset breathlessness over the course of weeks to months, due to increasing load of recurrent small volume clot.

Dyspnoea and tachypnoea (defined as a respiratory rate > 20) are the commonest presenting features and are absent in only 10% of patients.

Consider PE in the differential diagnosis of:
- Unexplained shortness of breath
- Collapse
- New onset atrial fibrillation
- Signs consistent with right heart failure
- Pleural effusion.

Examination of patient with PE
- May be normal
- Tachycardia and tachypnoea are common
- Atrial fibrillation
- Reduced chest movement (due to pain)
- Pleural rub
- Classically loud P2 and splitting of the second heart sound, with a gallop rhythm (acute right heart strain)
- Hypoxia (with hypocapnia due to hyperventilation, and an increased alveolar–arterial gradient) BUT PaO_2 may be in the normal range in young, healthy individuals
- Low grade fever
- Signs of DVT (common, in around 25%)
- Right heart failure—low cardiac output and raised JVP with reduced BP and perfusion pressure.

Diagnosis of acute PE

The diagnosis of a pulmonary embolism can be difficult and involves a clinical assessment of probability. This takes risk factors, clinical presentation, and clinical signs into account. Tests are then performed, tests that may add weight to the clinical decision, rather than being stand alone diagnostic tests. Therefore the estimation of the pre-test clinical probability of PE is of vital importance in interpreting the tests performed.

Pre-test clinical probability scoring systems One example is the BTS pre-test clinical probability scoring system, shown in the box below.

A standard assessment of **pre-test clinical probability** might include:
a) Patient has clinical features compatible with PE:
  • raised respiratory rate
  • ± haemoptysis
  • ± pleuritic chest pain.
Plus 2 other factors:
   1. Absence of another reasonable clinical explanation
   2. Presence of a major risk factor (see box, page 410)

• a) plus 1 and 2: HIGH pre-test clinical probability
• a) plus 1 or 2: INTERMEDIATE pre-test clinical probability
• a) alone: LOW pre-test clinical probability.

The Wells and Geneva pre-test probability scores are similar to the above, but include separate scores for clinical features such as heart rate, haemoptysis, and blood gas estimates (Geneva). Local scoring systems may be in place. These scoring systems should always be used with D-dimer testing.

D-dimer testing has an important role in diagnosing and excluding PE, and should only be used with a pre-test clinical probability assessment. D-dimers are sensitive for thromboembolism, but not specific. They are rarely in the normal range in cases of acute thromboembolism, but they are not a valid screening test for PE on its own. D-dimers are generated as a result of fibrinolysis, which occurs in many clinical situations, including sepsis, pneumonia, neoplasia, inflammatory disease, and pregnancy.
• The sensitivity ranges from 87 to 99%, depending on the assay used (ELISA (Vidas) or red cell agglutination (SimpliRED)). Specificity is poorer, around 60–70% (so a large number of false positives)
• The different assays have different performance characteristics and these should be known before incorporating them into diagnostic algorithms
• D-dimer testing for PE has been validated as an out-patient test, but not in in-patient groups
• A low or intermediate pre-test clinical probability score, combined with a negative D-dimer has a 92% sensitivity at excluding PE.

D-Dimer test interpretation

- A negative D-dimer test reliably excludes PE in patients with a low (SimpliRED) or intermediate pre-test clinical probability (Vidas). These patients do not need further imaging
- A negative test is unhelpful in those with a high clinical probability (and therefore should not be done in this situation)
- A positive result needs further investigation
- The D-dimer becomes less useful the longer the period spent in hospital (i.e. increasing false positives), due to clot formation at venepuncture sites, venous stasis due to bed rest, etc.

Assessment and documentation of pre-test clinical probability in PE is paramount. This enables accurate clinical assessment, and may obviate the need for imaging.

An alternative explanation should be sought when PE is excluded.

Investigations

- *ECG* Non-specific changes are frequent. Most commonly sinus tachycardia. Atrial fibrillation, right bundle branch block, anterior T wave inversion (indicating R ventricular strain) are common. The S1Q3T3 pattern is uncommon
- *CXR* No specific features are characteristic in PE, but it may reveal another pathology. Small effusions are present in 40% (80% are exudates, 20% transudates). Focal infiltrates, segmental collapse, and raised diaphragm can also occur
- *Arterial blood gas* may be normal, especially in the young and healthy. Hypoxia and hypocapnia, due to hyperventilation, with an increased A–a gradient are more common
- *D-dimer* (see page 415)
- *CTPA* is the gold standard investigation, and is now recommended as the initial imaging technique in suspected non-massive PE. It has a sensitivity of >95%, and may enable an alternative diagnosis to be made if PE is excluded. It should be performed within 1 hour in suspected massive PE, and within 24 hours of suspected non-massive PE. It needs specialist reporting
- In those with a high clinical probability, but negative CTPA the options are:
  - PE has been excluded, stop anticoagulation, or
  - Perform further imaging (leg ultrasound, conventional pulmonary angiogram).

In one large prospective multicentre study, with all patients investigated with CTPA and leg ultrasound, those with negative tests and low or intermediate clinical probability were not anticoagulated. Only 0.2% had a definite PE after 3 months of follow-up. Those with negative tests, but high clinical probability were investigated further, and PE was identified in 5% (Lancet 2002; 360: 1914).

- *Isotope lung scanning* (ventilation/perfusion or V/Q scan)—mostly now superseded by CTPA. May be useful as a first-line imaging investigation in patients with a normal CXR and with no concurrent cardio-pulmonary disease, in whom a negative scan would reliably exclude a PE. Scans are reported as low, intermediate, or high probability and the report's meaning must be interpreted in light of the pre-test clinical probability score. Further imaging is necessary for those in whom:
  - The scan is indeterminate
  - There is discordant lung scan and clinical probability.

The clinical significance of the V/Q scan report is:

- Normal = no PE
- Low or intermediate pre-test clinical probability *plus* low probability scan = PE excluded
- High pre-test clinical probability *plus* high probability scan = PE diagnosed
- Any other = need further imaging.

Other imaging techniques

- **Leg ultrasound**—around 70% of patients with a proven PE have a proximal DVT; hence leg imaging can be used as an alternative to lung imaging in those with clinical DVT. A single examination is not adequate to exclude subclinical DVT (venography is more sensitive). It is safe to withhold anticoagulation in patients with suspected DVT and a single negative leg ultrasound, but these data cannot yet be extrapolated to those presenting with suspected PE. If positive, they exclude the need for further imaging. Up to 50% of patients with a clinically obvious DVT will have a high-probability V/Q scan
- **Conventional pulmonary angiogram** is available in a few specialist centres only, where catheter fragmentation of large clots may be of therapeutic benefit. Now mostly superseded by CTPA
- **CT venography** is an emerging area. It can be combined with CTPA to image the pelvic leg veins simultaneously
- **Echocardiogram** is diagnostic only in massive PE. The transoesophageal route is more sensitive, enabling visualization of intrapulmonary and intracardiac clot. May give prognostic information
- **Transthoracic ultrasound** is used uncommonly. May show peripheral infarcts with peripheral pulmonary emboli
- **Cardiac troponin** A rise indicates acute right heart strain. For prognostic information only; has no role in decision making.

Management

Management of acute massive PE

Acute massive PE has a mortality of 20%.
1. Oxygen—100%
2. IV access. Send baseline bloods, including clotting. Perform ECG.
3. Analgesia if required; consider opiates.
4. Management of cardiogenic shock—fluids and inotropes may be required in sub-massive or massive PE to maintain right ventricular filling.
5. Start IV heparin unless active GI bleeding or intracerebral haemorrhage:
   • Bolus dose 5000–10,000 units or 80 IU/kg
   • Maintenance infusion of 1300 IU/hr or 18 units/kg/hr
   • Adjust infusion rate until APTT is 1.5–2.5 × control. Check APTT 4–6 hours after initial bolus and 6–10 hours after any dose change. When APTT is in the therapeutic range, check it daily.
6. Investigation to confirm PE depends on clinical state of patient. Ideally perform urgent echocardiogram and, if this is non-diagnostic, perform a CT scan, but not delaying for more than one hour. It may however be unwise to move the sick patient to the radiology department for a CT and, if they have circulatory collapse and are peri-arrest, with PE being the most likely cause, confirmation of the diagnosis should not be sought, but treatment prioritized. Remember aortic dissection, cardiac tamponade, and acute MI can mimic PE.
7. Thrombolysis if collapsed or hypotensive, if no active GI bleeding or intracerebral haemorrhage:
   • Alteplase 100 mg over 2 hours given peripherally
   • Or streptokinase 250 000 units in 20 minutes with 100 000 units/h for 24 hours (plus hydrocortisone to prevent further circulatory instability)
   • Or urokinase 4400 IU/kg in 10 minutes and 4400 IU/kg/h for 12 hours.
Stop the heparin during thrombolysis and restart afterwards.
In cardiac arrest due to suspected massive PE, 50 mg IV alteplase immediately may be life-saving.
8. Consider liaising with cardiothoracic centre to consider embolectomy, particularly if thrombolysis is contraindicated.

Low molecular weight heparin (LMWH) is as effective as standard unfractionated intravenous heparin, and should be given to patients with intermediate or a high pre-test clinical probability prior to imaging.
Unfractionated heparin should be considered in massive PE (faster onset of action) as a first dose bolus prior to commencement of LMWH.
Oral anticoagulation should only be commenced once PE is proven. Target INR 2.0–3.0 (when achieved, heparin can be stopped). Some centres now advocate out-patient anticoagulation for PE, as well as DVT. Data suggest that is as safe as in-patient anticoagulation, in centres with a well-established out-patient DVT service.

Length of warfarin anticoagulation
• Temporary risk factor: 4–6 weeks. This is an area of some debate

- First episode of idiopathic PE: 3 months is currently recommended (though ongoing BTS study is comparing 3 and 6 months anticoagulation)
- Recurrent idiopathic PE: no guidelines exist; length of treatment depends on individual circumstances, with risk of bleeding balanced with risk of recurrent event, and often long-term anticoagulation
- Persisting risk factors: lifelong anticoagulation may be recommended.

Side-effects
- The risk of bleeding increases with age and concurrent illness
- Higher bleeding rate with concomitant aspirin use, and previous gastrointestinal bleed
- Risk of bleeding relates to duration and intensity of anticoagulation.

Thrombolysis There is emerging evidence to support the use of thrombolysis in certain subgroups of patients with PE; however this is a controversial area, and the risk/benefit analysis of this treatment must always be carefully considered.

Massive PE causing circulatory collapse. Current BTS guidelines (2003) support the use of early thrombolysis. In practice, thrombolysis is usually given to the acutely unwell/peri-arrest patient, when the history and physical findings are suggestive of massive PE, in the absence of another reasonable explanation. There is rarely time for imaging or investigations in this situation.

Non-massive PE More controversial. Some evidence now supports the use of intravenous alteplase in addition to intravenous heparin in the treatment of haemodynamically stable submassive PE, in association with pulmonary hypertension or right ventricular dysfunction. Current BTS guidelines recommend thrombolysis only for patients with clinically massive PE.

Contraindications None absolute; rarely a consideration in the life-threatening situation. Risk of major haemorrhage is 3–4 times that of heparin, with a higher incidence of bleeding in the elderly. Active bleeding or recent intracerebral bleed are contraindications.

Embolectomy Rarely done, and only in life-threatening massive PE. Options include surgical embolectomy (few regional centres only) and mechanical clot fragmentation via right heart catheterization.

IVC filter placement There is little evidence to show improved survival, or reduction in recurrent PE rate with IVC filters, and changing to low molecular weight heparin may be as effective. IVC filters may however be indicated in:
- Acute VTE in patients with an absolute contraindication to anticoagulation
- Patients with massive PE who survive (in whom a second PE may be fatal)
- Recurrent VTE despite adequate anticoagulation
- Post-pulmonary thromboendarterectomy in pulmonary hypertension.

Further information

Heparin plus Alteplase compared to heparin alone in patients with submassisve pulmonary embolism. Konstantinides S et al. NEJM 2002; **347**: 1143–50

Special circumstances

Pregnancy and thromboembolic disease

- The incidence of DVT ± PE in pregnancy is 1 in 1000, rising to 2 in 1000 in puerperium. The risk of PE in pregnancy is greater with increasing maternal age and with increasing gestational age, and more PEs occur during pregnancy than after delivery. 20–30 times increased risk with Caesarean section, compared to normal vaginal delivery. Fatal PE is one of commonest causes of maternal death in pregnancy (1/100,000 pregnancies)
- D-dimers are raised in the normal pregnancy and so are unhelpful in the investigation of thromboembolic disease
- There are no published data regarding the risk to the fetus of CTPA, but the average fetal radiation dose of CTPA is less than that of a ventilation perfusion scan
- Warfarin is teratogenic and is contraindicated in pregnancy, although it is safe in breast-feeding
- In those with antenatal thromboembolic disease, low molecular weight heparin (LMWH) is used. Close to delivery, this is changed to unfractionated heparin, as it is easier to monitor and to reverse its effects. It is unclear whether heparin should be stopped or the dose reduced at the time of delivery
- Anticoagulation should be continued for 6 weeks after delivery, or 3 months following initial episode, whichever is longer.

Thromboembolic disease and the oral contraceptive pill/HRT

- The OCP, pregnancy, and hormone replacement therapy (HRT) increase the risk of PE, but the incidence of fatal PE is low (estimated at 1/100,000 OCP users, with a median age of 29)
- Risk of fatal PE is twice as high amongst those taking third-generation pills
- Previous history of DVT or PE is a contraindication to the OCP
- Meta-analyses show a relative risk of VTE of 2.1 in HRT users (highest in the first year of use).

Flight prophylaxis for thromboembolic disease

- For patients with high risk of a PE, that is, previous VTE, within 6 weeks of surgery, or current malignancy, the 1997 BTS Guidelines recommend: low dose aspirin, low molecular weight–heparin, or formal anticoagulation (INR 2–3) prior to flying
- For those of moderate or low risk, graduated or compression stockings with or without pre-flight aspirin is suggested.

Future developments

Thrombolysis Further research is ongoing regarding the use of thrombolysis in non-massive PE and more data is likely in the next few years.

Low-intensity warfarin therapy A reduced target INR of 1.5 to 2.0, may be used. A study of a cohort of patients treated for up to 4.3 years, following 6 months of standard warfarin therapy for idiopathic venous thromboembolism led to a 48% reduction in recurrent VTE, major haemorrhage, or death compared to placebo (Ridker et al, NEJM 2003; 348: 1425).

Ximelagatran is a novel oral direct thrombin inhibitor with a wide therapeutic range that does not need anticoagulation monitoring. It can cause liver function derangement in up to 6% of patients, and therefore needs LFT monitoring. It is now licensed in some European countries but there are concerns over toxicity.

Further information

BTS guidelines for the management of suspected acute pulmonary embolism. *Thorax* 2003; **58**: 470–84

Seminar: pulmonary embolism. Goldhaber SZ. *Lancet* 2004; **363**: 1295–305

Rare causes

Air embolism Air is found within the arterial or venous circulation. Small amounts of air can be tolerated, but large amounts can lodge in the pulmonary vasculature and cause mechanical obstruction and death. Rare.
Causes Neck vein cannulation, intrauterine manipulations (such as criminal abortion, where a frothy liquid is passed under pressure into the uterus), bronchial trauma, or barotrauma causing air to enter the pulmonary vein and left heart. Air in the left ventricle causes impairment to venous filling and subsequent poor coronary perfusion as air enters the coronary arteries.
Diagnosis Arterial air emboli may cause dizziness, loss of consciousness, and convulsions. Air may be seen in the retinal arteries or from transected vessels. *Venous* air emboli may cause raised venous pressure, cyanosis, hypotension, tachycardia, syncope, and a 'mill-wheel' murmur over the praecordium.
Treatment Patients should lie on their right side, with head down and feet up, to allow air to collect and stay at the cardiac apex. From here it can be aspirated via thoracotomy.

Amniotic fluid embolism is estimated 1 in 25,000–80,000 live births. It is the third commonest cause of maternal death, and the most common cause of death in the immediate post-partum period. Usually catastrophic, 80% of women die, 20–50% of these in first hour. Anaphylactic-type response to amniotic fluid entering the circulation is seen. Amniotic fluid enters circulation because of torn fetal membranes, which can occur in Caesarean section, uterine or cervical trauma, or uterine rupture. It has a thromboplastic effect, causing disseminated intravascular coagulation and thrombi to form in pulmonary vessels. Not all women react in this way to amniotic fluid. It is more common in older, multiparous mothers, who have had short tumultuous labour, often involving uterine stimulants.
Clinically presents with sudden onset respiratory distress, hypoxia, bronchospasm, cyanosis, cardiovascular collapse, pulmonary oedema, convulsions, coma, and cardiac arrest. Coagulopathy with intractable uterine bleeding and uterine atony is seen.
Diagnosis is clinical. Fetal debris/cells can be identified in blood sampled from the maternal pulmonary artery, but this is not pathognomonic.
Treatment is supportive whilst the thrombi clear from the maternal lungs. Maintain the circulation with fluids and ionotropes. Respiratory support with oxygen and ventilation may be needed. Correct coagulopathy with fresh frozen plasma and packed cells. Control placental bleeding.

Fat embolism Common pathological finding following long bone fractures. Occurs especially with lower limb fractures—pelvis and femur. Commoner in fractures that have not been immobilized. Can also occur after prosthetic joint replacement, cardiac massage, liver trauma, burns, bone marrow transplant, rapid high altitude decompression, and liposuction. Generally occurs in the young and previously healthy. Presents 24–72 hours post-fracture. Marrow fat enters the circulation and lodges in the lungs, causing mechanical obstruction.

Classically presents with hypoxia, coagulopathy, with transient petechial rash on neck, axillae, and skin folds and neurological disturbance, such as confusion, disorientation, or sometimes coma. Stable patients may deteriorate with low-grade fever, petechial rash, hypoxia, and confusion. Jaundice and renal dysfunction are possible.

Diagnosis is usually made clinically in a patient with a lower limb fracture presenting with tachypnoea and hypoxia. Fat globules can be identified in the urine. CXR shows bilateral alveolar infiltrates. ARDS can develop.

Treatment is with early immobilization of fracture, fluid replacement, oxygen, and supportive care.

Septic and tumour emboli are also causes.

Sarcoidosis

Aetiology and pathology

Definition
- A multisystem inflammatory disorder, of unknown cause
- Characterized by non-caseating granulomata and CD4 Th1-biased T cell response in affected organs
- Commonly involves the respiratory system, but can affect nearly all organs
- 50–60% of people have spontaneous remissions; others may develop chronic progressive disease.

Aetiology Incidence varies with population studies, from 5 to 100/100,000, according to geographic distribution. UK incidence is about 5–10/100,000. Commoner in African-Americans, West Indians, and the Irish. Commonly presents between ages of 20 and 40. Unusual in children and the elderly. Typically more aggressive disease in Black populations than in Caucasians—especially with skin disease, peripheral lymphadenopathy, bone marrow, and liver involvement.

Genetics Familial and ethnic clustering of cases suggest a genetic predisposition. Best evidence of HLA association comes from recent 'ACCESS' study, showing HLA-DRB1*0301 is associated with susceptibility of disease in Blacks and Whites. Also a genome-wide scan for susceptibility genes in familial sarcoidosis has been performed, pointing to a locus on chromosome 6.

Pathology Sarcoidosis is caused by an immunological response:
- Unknown antigenic stimulus triggers CD4 (helper) T cell activation and expansion. This response is exaggerated and Th1-biased, with resultant interferon gamma and IL-2 production from these T cells
- There is concomitant macrophage activation and immune granuloma formation, which is enhanced by interferon gamma
- Granulomata themselves cause increased local fibroblast stimulation and hence fibrosis
- Metabolic activity of macrophages causes raised ACE (angiotensin converting enzyme) levels in serum, lung tissue, and bronchoalveolar fluid. Increase in T cell activity causes B lymphocyte stimulation, which can cause raised serum immunoglobulins and immune complexes
- In most patients, response resolves over 2–5 years.

Delayed-type hypersensitivity reactions are depressed in sarcoidosis. This is thought to be due to the migration of lymphocytes to the active compartment (lungs), with resultant peripheral blood lymphopenia. Seen as a decreased response to tuberculin, mumps virus, and *Candida albicans* antigens. This is not thought to be clinically significant.

Sarcoid-like reactions are reported in association with malignancy and also in HIV patients starting on antiretroviral therapy (very rare). Non-caseating pulmonary granulomas are found, but there are no other symptoms or signs of sarcoidosis.

Differential diagnosis of granuloma on lung biopsy

- Sarcoidosis
- Tuberculosis
- Extrinsic allergic alveolitis
- Wegner's granulomatosis
- Primary biliary cirrhosis
- Granulomatous orchitis
- Langerhans' cell histiocytosis
- Leprosy
- Tertiary syphilis
- Brucellosis
- Berylliosis
- Silicosis
- Hypogammaglobulinaemia
- Fungal infections—coccidioidomycosis
- Schistosomiasis
- Cat scratch fever
- Lymphoma
- Giant cell arteritis
- Polyarteritis nodosa
- Takyasu's arteritis
- Crohn's disease
- De Quervain's thyroiditis.

Further information

Familial sarcoidosis is linked to the major histocompatability complex region. Schurmann M, Lympany PA et al. Am J Respir Crit Care Med 2000; **162**: 8 61–4

HLA-DQB1 and HLA-DPB1 genotypes in familial sarcoidosis. Schurmann M, Bein G et al. Respir Med 1998; **92**: 649–52

Chest disease: clinical features

More than 90% of patients with sarcoidosis have thoracic involvement, with an abnormal CXR. Pulmonary sarcoidosis can be an incidental CXR finding.

Clinical features There are probably at least 2 distinct clinical courses:

- **Löfgren's syndrome** Mild acute disease, which is usually non-progressive. Presents with fever, bilateral hilar lymphadenopathy, erythema nodosum, and arthralgia. Occurs particularly in Caucasians. Has a good prognosis and resolves completely and spontaneously in 80% within 1–2 years. A minority may develop lung disease
- **Persistent progressive infiltrative lung disease**
  - *Hilar/mediastinal lymphadenopathy* May be asymptomatic or cause cough or chest pain. Often bilateral and symmetrical, but can be unilateral and asymmetrical. Can be associated with systemic symptoms of malaise and arthralgia, which are helped by nonsteroidal anti-inflammatory drugs. Benign course.

    Important to exclude other causes of lymphadenopathy, such as TB and lymphoma. May need HRCT and lymph node aspirate or biopsy.

    Does not require systemic steroid treatment.

    Stage I: 85% resolve spontaneously over 2 years, 15% develop lung infiltrates. The average time for bilateral hilar lymphadenopathy resolution is 8 months
  - *Interstitial lung involvement* May be asymptomatic or cause morbidity and mortality, with dyspnoea, cough, chest ache, or frank pain and malaise. Pulmonary infiltrates on CXR. Can return to normal over time, or can progress to fibrosis and respiratory failure. Lung function tests may be normal, or may show a restrictive defect with reduced transfer factor.

    Differential diagnosis: other interstitial lung disease, malignancy, infection.

Radiological classification of thoracic sarcoidosis

Stage 0	Normal
Stage I	Hilar lymphadenopathy
Stage II	Hilar lymphadenopathy and parenchymal infiltrate
Stage III	Parenchymal infiltrate
Stage IV	Fibrosis

Seeing a patient with possible sarcoidosis in clinic:

- Make diagnosis—clinically, HRCT ± histology
- Assess extent/severity/presence of extrapulmonary involvement—CXR, PFT, ECG, eyes, rash, renal function, serum calcium, liver function, immunoglobulins, and ACE (latter two can be raised in active sarcoidosis)
- Stable or progressive?—CXR, PFT (VC ± KCO), oximetry, ACE, urea (if renal involvement)
- Treatment?

Differential diagnosis of bilateral hilar lymphadenopathy on CXR

- Sarcoidosis
- Tuberculosis
- Lymphoma
- Coccidioidomycosis and histoplasmosis
- Leukaemia
- Berylliosis
- Hypogammaglobulinaemia and recurrent infections.

Further information

Two year prognosis of sarcoidosis: the ACCESS experience. Judson MA, Baughman RP *et al. Sarcoidosis Vasc Diffuse Lung Dis* 2003; **20**: 204–11

Chest disease: management

Diagnosis is based on a characteristic clinical picture, plus:
- Histological evidence of non-caseating granuloma in any tissue
- Characteristic picture on imaging (thoracic HRCT scan or gallium scan)
- Lymphocytosis on bronchoalveolar lavage (BAL).

Other diseases capable of producing similar clinical and histological picture, particularly tuberculosis and lymphoma, should be excluded.

Investigations

- *HRCT* Micronodules in a subpleural and bronchovascular distribution. Fissural nodularity and bronchial distortion. Irregular linear opacities, ground-glass shadowing related to bronchovascular bundles, and nodular or ill-defined shadows. Air-trapping due to small airway granulomata common. Endobronchial disease in 55%. Possible honeycomb lung. Hilar and mediastinal lymphadenopathy
- *Bronchoscopy (transbronchial biopsy, bronchial biopsy, or broncho-alveolar lavage)* may not be necessary if there is no diagnostic doubt clinically and radiologically. Positive yield of bronchial biopsy is 41–57%. Higher if visible abnormal mucosa. Positive yield of transbronchial biopsy is 40–90%. BAL in sarcoidosis shows a CD4:CD8 ratio of >3.5. If this test is not available, a lymphocytosis of >2 × 10^5 cells/ml supports the diagnosis, but is not diagnostic. (Lymphocytosis is also seen in UIP, COP, hypersensitivity pneumonitis, and smokers)
- *Mediastinoscopy* for central or paratracheal nodes or open lung biopsy: 90% positive yield. May be necessary to exclude lymphoma
- *Biopsy other affected areas* such as skin, liver, etc. if indicated, as these may be easier to biopsy in order to make a diagnosis
- *Mantoux/Heaf test* may show minimal reaction/grade 0 in sarcoid (peripheral cutaneous anergy to tuberculin due to migration of T cells to active sites of disease). A positive Mantoux or Heaf test therefore make sarcoidosis less likely as a diagnosis, although does not necessarily make tuberculosis more likely as the diagnosis
- *Kveim test* No longer performed clinically, due to risks of transmissible diseases. It involved injecting homogenized splenic tissue from a patient with sarcoidosis to see if a granulomatous reaction occurred.

Monitoring disease There is no single measurement to assess all the aspects of patients with sarcoidosis. Clinical examination and serial measurements are key.

- **PFT** TLCO provides most sensitive measurement of change, although a properly performed VC is probably adequate for clinical purposes. Likely to improve with steroids
- **CXR** may improve with time or treatment
- **ACE** (angiotensin converting enzyme) levels increased in up to 80% of patients with acute sarcoidosis. Levels become normal as disease resolves. Can be useful to monitor the clinical course. Levels suppressed by steroids and when steroids are stopped levels usually increase, unrelated to sarcoidosis activity. This is not a specific test. False positives include TB
- **Calcium** may rise with active sarcoidosis or in the summer months. This may cause renal impairment, so urea should also be checked
- **BAL** not performed routinely to assess progress of sarcoidosis, but changes in proportions of cells seen in lavage would indicate improvement
- **PET** scan may be positive in areas of disease activity. Not reliable for studying brain or heart. Limited studies of serial data
- **Gallium scan** rarely used now, as non-specific and expensive. Areas of active inflammation are positive, with a classic 'panda pattern'. Positive areas soon become negative with steroid use. Bowel and liver positive anyway, so disease cannot be charted in these areas.

General management

Most patients with pulmonary sarcoidosis do not require treatment. Asymptomatic CXR infiltrates are usually monitored.

Indications for immunosuppressive treatment

- Increasing symptoms, deteriorating PFTs, and worsening CXR infiltrates
- Cardiac sarcoidosis
- Neurosarcoidosis
- Sight-threatening ocular sarcoidosis
- Hypercalcaemia
- Lupus pernio
- Splenic, hepatic, or renal sarcoidosis.

Starting drug treatment

- When required, treatment is usually with steroids initially
- Give high doses, such as 40 mg prednisolone/day, to control active disease. Rarely need more than 40 mg/day. Usually give this high dose for 4 weeks and then reduce if there has been a response
- **Maintenance dose** of around 5–15 mg, to control symptoms. Leave on this dose for a few months and then slowly reduce steroid dose further. Maintain on low dose of prednisolone (5–7.5 mg/day or alternate days) for prolonged period of 6–12 months, to consolidate resolution, before considering complete withdrawal
- Some patients, especially those with progressive pulmonary sarcoidosis, may require longer treatment
- **Relapses** often occur when treatment is stopped and may require the reintroduction of steroids, or the increase of steroid dose. Duration and dose of steroids is dictated by site and response to treatment
- Avoid futile steroid treatment for end-stage disease, such as honeycomb lung
- If steroid treatment fails, or sarcoidosis is life-threatening, other immunosuppressive regimes may be indicated. Pulsed high-dose intravenous methylprednisolone is an option, which can be particularly useful for neurosarcoidosis
- In cases where prolonged immunosuppression is required, or if steroid side-effects cannot be tolerated, other immunosuppressive drugs should be considered. Possibilities include azathioprine and methotrexate. There is limited data for their use in sarcoidosis
- Patients who have troublesome symptoms related to sarcoidosis, such as arthralgia, skin disease, fever, sweats, ocular symptoms, systemic symptoms such as fatigue, may require symptomatic steroid treatment. Lower initial doses such as 20 mg/day are likely to be sufficient to gain symptomatic control and doses can then be reduced
- Prescribe gastric and bone protection with steroids when necessary.

Other drugs used in sarcoidosis

(See page 625 for more information regarding immunosuppressive drugs)

- **Methotrexate** Given once/week 10–25 mg po for 6-month trial. Avoid if hepatic or renal failure. Side-effects: GI upset, stomatitis, pneumonitis, myelosuppression. Teratogenic. Low oncogenic potential. Monitor FBC incl. MCV, AST, ALT every 2 weeks for 3 months, then monthly. Do not use for >2 years. Useful for chronic sarcoidosis and cutaneous disease
- **Azathioprine** Used in neurosarcoidosis and stage II/III pulmonary sarcoidosis with partial/no steroid response. Use with low-dose prednisolone. Side-effects: myelosuppression, GI upset, stomatitis, idiosyncratic reaction–fever, rash. Low oncogenic potential. No gonadal toxicity. Check FBC every 2 weeks for 3 months, then monthly
- **Cyclophosphamide** IV pulsed, for neurosarcoidosis unresponsive to steroids. Toxicity profile limits use. (See page 628)
- **Anti-malarials** Chloroquine and hydroxychloroquine 200 mg od/bd. For skin and hypercalcaemia. Steroid sparing. Can be given with steroids and other immunosuppressant in severe sarcoidosis Side-effects: rarely, ocular toxicity
- **Others** new, unproven efficacy: cyclosporin, thalidomide, TNFα inhibitors.

Prognosis There are no prognostic markers in sarcoidosis, apart from:

- *Good prognosis* Löfgren's syndrome has complete resolution in 80% of people
- *Poorer prognosis with chronic disease* Lupus pernio, nasal mucosa involvement, chronic uveitis, chronic hypercalcaemia, nephrocalcinosis, neural involvement, age greater than 40 and Black race
- Prognosis according to CXR appearance

  Stage II: 50% cases recover spontaneously in 2 years, 30–40% require systemic steroids, 10–15% require long-term steroids

  Stage III: Worse prognosis. Only 30% show significant improvement with steroids.

Transplant Consider if patient has end-stage lung disease, rapidly progressive disease despite treatment, or if they are oxygen dependent. Sarcoidosis is a rare indication for lung transplant. Granulomata recur in transplanted lung, but do not cause higher rates of graft failure.

Extra-thoracic disease 1

Varies according to ethnic origin and sex of patient.

Systemic symptoms are common, such as fever, sweats, loss of appetite, weight loss, fatigue, malaise, chest pain, dyspnoea, and cough. Polyarthralgia often affects the knees, ankles, wrists, and elbows and can be improved by NSAIDs.

Hypercalcaemia Granulomata convert vitamin D_3 to active 1,25 dihydroxycholecalciferol. This causes enhanced calcium absorption from intestine. Sunlight also increases levels of vitamin D and calcium. High calcium may cause systemic effects and is often associated with renal damage and hypercalciuria. Commoner in Caucasians and in men.

Treatment Steroids, often low dose once calcium level controlled. Decrease dose when calcium level satisfactory. Some patients may only need steroids during the summer months. Hydroxychloroquine can also be used.

Skin 25% of patients have skin involvement. More common in women.

Erythema nodosum Raised papules, nodules, or plaques, usually on shins. Also tender, indurated, or bruised appearance. Firm and often have shiny appearance. Nodular change involving different tattoo colours recognized and is characteristic of sarcoidosis. Sarcoid tissue may arise in old scars, or cause scar hypertrophy.

Lupus pernio is a bluish tinge that occurs on nose, cheeks, and ears. It is associated with chronic disease.

Diagnosis Usually easily biopsied.

Treatment Initially with topical preparations. Lupus pernio should be treated with systemic steroids. Hydroxychloroquine or methotrexate may be necessary. Role of long-term tetracyclines for cutaneous sarcoidosis under investigation.

Eye Common, occurring in 25+ % of cases, especially women and Afro-Caribbeans.

Uveitis (acute or chronic), episcleritis, scleritis, glaucoma, conjunctivitis, and retinal involvement can occur. May be asymptomatic, or cause painful red eye, with photophobia, lacrimation, and blurred vision. Pupil irregular or constricted. Untreated, can cause visual impairment.

Lacrimal involvement in sarcoidosis gives keratoconjunctivitis sicca—dry eye with diminished tear secretion. Painful red eyes. Treat with artificial tears.

Diagnosis Assessment by an ophthalmologist with slit lamp examination if any ocular symptoms. Some recommend that all newly diagnosed patients with sarcoidosis have slit lamp examination. Mild asymptomatic eye involvement is common. May need conjunctival biopsy, if no evidence of sarcoid elsewhere.

Treatment Local steroids are commonly used, if there is no other indication for systemic steroids. However, if it does not respond, systemic steroids should be used.

Heart Cardiac sarcoidosis occurs in 5% of patients with pulmonary disease. Post mortem studies show cardiac sarcoidosis is present in 25%, so is often undiagnosed. Patients may present with chest pain or, more commonly, are found to have conduction defects on the ECG. These may be benign and asymptomatic, like first-degree heart block, but more significant arrhythmias can occur, the first indication of which may be sudden death. Myocardial granulomata can occur in any part of the heart. Commonly they occur in the interventricular septum, where they can affect nodal and conducting tissue. The left ventricular wall can be affected, with fibrosis causing reduced compliance and contractile difficulties, leading to cardiac failure. Aneurysms can form, and pericarditis can occur. Valvular dysfunction due to infiltration of the papillary muscles is rare. The clinical course can be uncertain.

Diagnosis Echocardiogram may show signs of cardiomyopathy—usually restrictive. MRI, technetium scan, or gallium scan show nonsegmental fixed defects. Biopsy is diagnostic but can be difficult as sarcoidosis is patchy. Not recommended in general. ECG and 24-hour tape may be helpful in investigation.

Treatment Must be treated with systemic steroids 20–40 mg prednisolone/day, which improve symptoms and ECG and Echo features. These should be slowly reduced, but intractable arrhythmias may need continued high dosage. May need other immunosuppressants. Investigate with 24-hour tape if uncertain. Amiodarone, pacemaker, implantable defibrillator, or heart transplant may be necessary.

In clinic Perform a screening ECG on all patients with sarcoidosis perhaps every 6 months.

Extra-thoracic disease 2

Kidney Degree of renal involvement in 35% of patients with sarcoidosis. Rarely can present with renal failure, obstructive uropathy, nephrolithiasis, or urinary tract disorder. Nephrocalcinosis is a common cause of chronic renal failure. Often associated hypercalcaemia or other manifestation of sarcoidosis.

Diagnosis Renal biopsy with granulomata found in interstitium, but this is rarely needed in this context. Search for pulmonary sarcoidosis.

Treatment Steroids ± hydroxychloroquine for hypercalcaemia.

CNS Involved in 4–18% of patients. Can affect any part of the peripheral or central nervous system. Can present as a peripheral nerve or cranial nerve lesion. Most common is lower motor neuron facial nerve palsy, with optic nerve involvement being next commonest. Mononeuritis multiplex recognized. May be less specific, with psychiatric features. Hypothalamic granulomata may cause diabetes insipidus, appetite disturbance, or hypersomnolence.

Diagnosis Difficult, but may be made easier if there is another sign of systemic sarcoidosis, for example bilateral hilar lymphadenopathy. Lumbar puncture may show a raised CSF ACE and an increased lymphocyte count. Confirm with biopsy if possible—cerebral or meningeal tissue if no pulmonary involvement.

Treatment Must be treated with steroids, but often quite resistant to treatment. May need to try further immunosuppressants.

Musculoskeletal Arthralgia is common in sarcoidosis, but arthritis is unusual. Arthralgia commonly affects the ankles and feet, but also hands, wrists and elbows. Subacute, proximal myopathy can occur, as well as bone cysts, especially of terminal phalanges. The latter show little response to systemic steroids.

Diagnosis Granuloma seen on muscle biopsy.

Treatment NSAIDs; steroids may be necessary.

GI 60% of liver biopsies on patients with sarcoidosis show granuloma. Frequently asymptomatic. Hepatomegaly unusual, but can get portal fibrosis and cirrhosis. LFTs suggestive if 3 × normal, especially ALP and γGT.

Diagnosis Biopsy

Treatment Steroids—may reduce size of liver and improve LFTs.

Haematological Splenomegaly can occur and may be massive, causing abdominal discomfort. Massive spleen may require splenectomy to avoid rupture. Associated anaemia, neutropenia, and thrombocytopenia. Lymphopenia often seen.

ENT Nasal or laryngeal granuloma. Sinus invasion. Parotid and other salivary gland enlargement, dry mouth.

Rarely: breast disease, ovarian or testicular masses.

Further information

American Thoracic Society/European Respiratory Society/World Association of Sarcoidosis and other Granulomatous Disorders statement on sarcoidosis. *Eur Respir J* 1999; **14**: 735–7

Guidelines for the diagnosis and assessment of diffuse parenchymal lung disease. *Thorax* 1999; **54** (suppl. 1): S1

Two year prognosis of sarcoidosis: the ACCESS experience. Judson MA, Baughman RP *et al*. *Sarcoidosis Vasc Diffuse Lung Dis* 2003; **20**: 204–11

World Association of Sarcoidosis and other Granulomatous Disorders website, *www.pinali.unipd.it/sarcoid*

Chapter 35

Idiopathic interstitial pneumonias

Overview

Definition The IIPs comprise a group of diffuse lung diseases of unknown aetiology that primarily involve the pulmonary interstitium—the area between the alveolar epithelium and capillary endothelium as well as the septal and bronchovascular tissues that make up the fibrous framework of the lung. These primarily interstitial processes, however, also frequently involve the airways, vasculature, and alveolar airspaces. The underlying pathological process is one of varying degrees of inflammation and fibrosis.

The terminology used to describe the IIPs may be confusing; these conditions have been subject to much re-classification, reflecting the lack of understanding of their underlying aetiology and pathogenesis. Usual interstitial pneumonia (UIP) is the commonest IIP, and is the histological pattern of cryptogenic fibrosing alveolitis (CFA). The other IIPs are distinct disease entities and are all rare. They all represent a subgroup of interstitial (or diffuse parenchymal) lung diseases.

Diagnosis Made from a combination of clinical, HRCT, and histological features—distinguish from other causes of diffuse lung disease (see Chapter 7). Histological patterns are the most specific and form the basis for the current classification of IIPs. Surgical lung biopsy is recommended for most cases of suspected IIP with the exception of patients exhibiting typical clinical and HRCT features of UIP. Transbronchial biopsies have a very limited role due to the generally patchy distribution of the IIPs, although they may be useful in the diagnosis of acute interstitial pneumonitis (AIP) and cryptogenic organizing pneumonia (COP), as well as the exclusion of other causes of diffuse lung disease (e.g. sarcoidosis).

Treatment The optimal treatment of many of the IIPs is poorly understood, and there is a lack of supportive data from randomized controlled trials. Steroids and immunosuppression are the mainstay of treatment, but these are often ineffective and have significant side-effects. Treatment may alter both the HRCT and histological pictures, and if possible should be delayed until a diagnosis has been made.

The conditions currently included within the classification of idiopathic interstitial pneumonias, together with their key clinical, imaging, and histological features and prognosis, are presented in the table opposite and discussed in detail in the remainder of this chapter. They are listed in order of frequency.

Further information

ATS/ERS. International Multidisciplinary Consensus Classification of the Idiopathic Interstitial Pneumonias. *Am J Respir Crit Care Med* 2002; **165**: 277–304

Idiopathic interstitial pneumonias: summary of key features

Usual interstitial pneumonia (UIP) [idiopathic pulmonary fibrosis (IPF), or cryptogenic fibrosing alveolitis (CFA)]	*Idiopathic* *Onset* over years *HRCT* fibrosis, honeycombing, minimal ground-glass, subpleural and basal distribution *Histology* areas of interstitial fibrosis (made up of foci of proliferating fibroblasts) interspersed with normal lung (temporal and spatial heterogeneity), minimal inflammation *Prognosis* poor
Non-specific interstitial pneumonia (NSIP)	*Idiopathic or disease-associated* *Onset* over months–years *HRCT* diffuse ground-glass, fine reticulation, minimal honey-combing *Histology* varying degrees of inflammation and fibrosis, more uniform appearance than UIP *Prognosis* variable, can be good
Cryptogenic organizing pneumonia (COP) [idiopathic bronchiolitis obliterans organizing pneumonia, BOOP]	*Idiopathic or disease-associated* *Onset* over months *HRCT* areas of consolidation, basal, subpleural, and peribronchial predominance *Histology* alveolar spaces 'plugged' with granulation tissue, ± extension into bronchioles *Prognosis* generally good
Acute interstitial pneumonia (AIP)	*Idiopathic* Many similarities to ARDS *Onset* over days *HRCT* diffuse ground-glass and patchy consolidation *Histology* diffuse alveolar damage: interstitial oedema, intra-alveolar hyaline membranes, followed by fibroblast proliferation and interstitial fibrosis *Prognosis* poor
Respiratory bronchiolitis-associated interstitial lung disease (RB-ILD)	*Idiopathic*, occurs in smokers *Onset* over years Symptoms usually mild *HRCT* centrilobular nodules, ground-glass, thick-walled airways *Histology* pigmented macrophages in bronchioles *Prognosis* good
Desquamative interstitial pneumonia (DIP)	*Idiopathic*, occurs in smokers *Onset* over weeks–months *HRCT* ground-glass *Histology* pigmented macrophages in alveolar air spaces (perhaps a more extensive form of RB-ILD), temporally uniform appearance *Prognosis* good
Lymphoid interstitial pneumonia (LIP)	*Idiopathic or disease-associated* *Onset* over years *HRCT* ground-glass, often reticulation *Histology* diffuse interstitial lymphoid infiltrates *Prognosis* variable

Usual interstitial pneumonia (UIP): diagnosis

Definition Chronic interstitial pneumonia of unknown cause characterized histologically by temporal and spatial heterogeneity, with areas of fibrosis and architectural distortion interspersed with areas of normal lung. This occurs as different areas of lung are in varying stages of evolution of the pathological process. UIP is the histological appearance of cryptogenic fibrosing alveolitis (also known as idiopathic pulmonary fibrosis).

Epidemiology Prevalence figures vary from 6 to 14/100,000, although prevalence may be 175/100,000 in patients >75 years old. Slightly more common in males. Mean age at presentation 67. Familial form well-described but very rare.

Causes and pathophysiology The development of fibrosis was previously thought to reflect a response to chronic inflammation resulting from an unknown initial injury. This key role of inflammation in the pathogenesis of UIP has been questioned, however, based partly on the observations that inflammation is not a major feature on pathological specimens, and that responses to 'anti-inflammatory' treatment with steroids are often poor. An alternative theory is that repeated lung injury leads to wound healing and fibrosis, and this concept of 'fibrosis without inflammation' has been demonstrated both in animal models and other human diseases. The nature of the lung injury remains obscure: postulated triggers include inhalation of metal dust and wood dust, smoking, or exposure to the Epstein–Barr virus. Cytokine production (e.g. plasminogen activator inhibitors, matrix metalloproteinases, transforming growth factor-β) by alveolar epithelial cells may play an important role in the development of fibrosis. Host genetic factors are also likely to be important in modifying the wound-healing response.

Clinical features

- Typically presents with gradual onset exertional breathlessness and cough; average of 9 months of symptoms prior to presentation
- 5% of patients are said to be asymptomatic, although this is likely to be an underestimate
- Arthralgia occurs in about 20%
- Fine basal late inspiratory crackles
- Clubbing in up to 50%
- Cyanosis and cor pulmonale in severe disease.

Investigations

- **Blood tests** Raised ESR and CRP and mild anaemia may occur; positive rheumatoid factor and/or ANA may occur at low titres in the absence of associated connective tissue disease

- *PFTs* Typically restrictive pattern with reduced vital capacity and transfer factor; smokers may exhibit coexisting obstructive defect. Oxygen saturations are frequently reduced, particularly on exertion; ABGs may demonstrate type I respiratory failure
- *CXR* Peripheral and basal reticular shadowing, may extend to other zones, sometimes with honeycombing; rarely may be normal
- *HRCT* features include bilateral, peripheral, and subpleural reticulation, with honeycombing, traction bronchiectasis, architectural distortion, and minimal or no ground-glass change. Predominantly basal initially, more extensive later in disease course. Extent of disease on CT correlates with physiological impairment. Predominant ground-glass appearance suggests an IIP other than UIP—consider lung biopsy
- *BAL* is not routinely required and is rarely helpful. Typically shows neutrophilia, sometimes mild eosinophilia. Marked eosinophilia (>20%) or lymphocytosis (>50%) should raise possibility of alternative diagnosis
- *Lung biopsy* (via VATS or thoracotomy) if there is diagnostic doubt
- *Gallium and DTPA* scanning are seldom of use in clinical practice.

Histology Fibrosing pattern characterized by temporal and spatial heterogeneity: patches of active fibroblastic foci (reflecting acute injury) are interspersed with honeycombing/architectural distortion (reflecting chronic scarring) and areas of normal lung, reflecting varying stages of evolution of the disease process in different areas of lung. Interstitial inflammation is minimal.

Diagnosis can be confidently made in most cases on the basis of clinical and HRCT findings. Lung biopsy is not generally required in patients with typical clinical and HRCT features of UIP, but should be considered in the presence of unusual features (e.g. predominant ground-glass/nodules/consolidation/upper lobe involvement on HRCT, or young patient). When required, biopsies should be obtained at VATS or thoracotomy; transbronchial biopsies provide smaller samples, which rarely give diagnostic information due to the patchy distribution of disease.

Differential diagnosis
- Left ventricular failure (a common clinical misdiagnosis in UIP, and patients are often prescribed inappropriate diuretics)
- Asbestosis (may mimic clinically and radiologically; occupational history and presence of pleural plaques may suggest this diagnosis)
- Connective tissue disease (may mimic clinically and radiologically, and precede extrapulmonary manifestations of disease)
- Chronic hypersensitivity pneumonitis (suggested by typically upper/mid zone predominance, micronodules, ground-glass, areas of reduced attenuation)
- Drug-induced lung disease.

UIP: management 1

Treatment choices are hindered by a lack of well-conducted, placebo-controlled trials. There is currently no evidence that any drug treatment improves survival or quality of life. Drugs should not be used routinely, but may be considered in a closely observed trial of therapy. They may be of benefit in patients with other IIPs misdiagnosed as UIP. Drug treatments include:

- **Oral corticosteroids** Prior to the recent reclassification of IIPs, studies suggested that oral corticosteroids may improve lung function (in around 20–30% of patients) and symptoms (in around 50%). However, these studies probably included patients with conditions other than UIP that are associated with a better treatment response and prognosis (e.g. NSIP). Significant side-effects may affect at least a quarter of patients (e.g. hyperglycaemia necessitating insulin, osteoporosis, myopathy, peptic ulcer disease, cataracts, raised intraocular pressure, psychosis). Consider septrin prophylaxis (960 mg 3 x/week) against PCP
- **Azathioprine** in combination with prednisolone may improve survival compared with prednisolone alone, although again this may reflect studies undertaken on individuals with IIPs other than UIP. Side-effects appear to be uncommon. Use of azathioprine alone has not been investigated
- **Cyclophosphamide** does not appear to improve survival and side-effects are common
- **Colchicine** appears to have a comparable effect to prednisolone and may be better tolerated
- Penicillamine and cyclosporin have not been studied in detail.

Management protocol The following recommendations are adapted from the BTS Guidelines. In all cases they should be considered in the context of the individual patient's clinical condition, co-morbidity, and wishes, particularly in view of the often unpredictable disease course, unknown efficacy of treatment, and high frequency of serious side-effects.

Initial assessment and decision to treat On presentation all patients should have full clinical assessment, pulmonary function tests, and HRCT chest. In general, decisions regarding treatment are based on severity and rate of progression of symptoms, changes in pulmonary function, and HRCT appearance. Predominant ground-glass appearance on HRCT suggests an IIP other than UIP, and may be associated with steroid responsiveness—consider lung biopsy prior to starting treatment. Predominantly reticular patterns are usually less steroid-responsive.

Indications for trial of treatment

Severe or rapidly progressive symptoms
Predominantly ground-glass appearance on HRCT (consider lung biopsy) Consider in the context of a reticular pattern on HRCT if lung function significantly impaired or patient requests treatment.

If mild/moderate symptoms or a long history, and without predominant ground-glass on HRCT (i.e. a reticular/mixed pattern), consider with-holding treatment and follow-up within 3 months. If stable on follow-up, review 3-monthly for at least 1 year and regularly thereafter; consider trial of treatment if lung function deteriorates or symptoms worsen.

Monitoring Disease progression and response to treatment are best assessed by serial measurements of VC and TLCO; document them at each clinic attendance. Changes in VC or TLCO of 10–15% or more are considered significant in terms of assessing treatment response or disease progression. Changes in symptoms such as exercise tolerance and cough frequency/severity may also be useful.

Recommended treatment Oral prednisolone (0.5 mg/kg) is the mainstay of treatment. Consider IV methylprednisolone in very ill patients. Re-assess lung function after 1 month (some recommend treating for a longer period before response to therapy is formerly assessed, e.g. 3–6 months):

- Improvement (increase in VC or TLCO by 10–15% or more) or stable: slowly reduce prednisolone dose (e.g. reduce by 5 mg weekly to 20 mg and review—if no worse, reduce by 5 mg a month to maintenance dose of 10 mg and continue at 10 mg for one year, and consider further reduction after this). Consider combination treatment with azathioprine (regimens vary, an example is initial daily dose of 50 mg for 4 weeks, then increase by 50 mg each week to maximum of 2–3 mg/kg although do not exceed 150 mg daily; check WCC weekly until established on maximum dose for two weeks, then check WCC and LFTs every 6–8 weeks). Azathioprine is used less frequently in patients with a predominantly ground-glass HRCT appearance, who may be treated with prednisolone alone
- Deterioration (decrease in VC or TLCO by 10–15% or more): quickly reduce prednisolone dose (e.g. reduce by 10 mg weekly to 10 mg daily, and more slowly after this). Supportive treatment (see below). Consider lung transplant referral.

Patients who are unable to tolerate treatment

- Consider trial of azathioprine alone if prednisolone is not tolerated
- Consider trial of cyclophosphamide if azathioprine is not tolerated
- Colchicine may be tried as an alternative to prednisolone alone.

Further information

BTS guidelines on the diagnosis, assessment and treatment of diffuse parenchymal lung disease in adults. British Thoracic Society. *Thorax* 1999; **54** (suppl. 1): S1–30

UIP: management 2

Supportive treatment Consider use of home oxygen if very limited by breathlessness and in respiratory failure. Use of oxygen during exercise may improve exercise tolerance. Encourage pulmonary rehabilitation program, if no contraindications. Cough may be troublesome—consider oral codeine. Opioids (e.g. oramorph) are frequently required for palliation of severe breathlessness.

Lung transplantation Patients with UIP are often referred for consideration of transplantation too late, and most die whilst on the waiting list (which is around 12 months in the UK). Single lung transplant in UIP leads to an 80% survival at 1 year and 55% at three years. Consider referral following failure of first-line treatment in symptomatic patients aged < 65 years, with TLCO and/or VC <60% predicted, resting hypoxaemia, and/or pulmonary hypertension.

Causes of acute deterioration in patients with previously stable UIP

- Accelerated decline of UIP—mechanism poorly understood; biopsy often shows diffuse alveolar damage
- Pneumothorax—collapsed lung is often relatively resistant to re-expansion, making treatment difficult
- Infection (especially if immunocompromised), e.g. PCP
- Pulmonary embolism
- Acute deterioration may also occur post-operatively following major surgery, e.g. cardiac or orthopaedic—the reasons behind this are unclear.

Prognosis is variable: some decline rapidly, others remain stable or decline slowly over years. Several studies have demonstrated a median survival of 2.5–3.5 years. Improved survival may be associated with young age, less advanced disease, female sex, and absence of advanced fibrosis and honeycombing on biopsy. Predominantly ground-glass appearance on HRCT independently predicts treatment response and survival. Death is commonly due to respiratory failure and/or infection. Risk of developing lung cancer is increased.

Future developments Therapeutic agents currently under evaluation include the antifibrotic pirfenidone, interferon γ-1b (inhibits fibroblast proliferation and downregulates transforming growth factor β), and oral septrin (as a disease-modifying agent; pilot studies have been promising).

Non-specific interstitial pneumonia (NSIP)

Definition The term NSIP is a description of a histological pattern rather than a specific clinical entity. This form of IIP is poorly understood, and may be subject to further re-classification in the near future. Patients with NSIP on lung biopsy have a generally better prognosis and greater response to steroids when compared to patients with UIP. NSIP may be idiopathic or occur in association with other systemic conditions, most notably connective tissue diseases.

Epidemiology Typically affects younger patients than UIP, with age of onset 40–50 years. May rarely affect children.

Causes/associations
- Idiopathic
- Connective tissue disease (NSIP may be the first manifestation of disease)
- Hypersensitivity pneumonitis
- Drugs
- Infection
- Immunodeficiency (including HIV, post-bone marrow transplant, chemotherapy).

Clinical features There are few specific clinical features that help distinguish NSIP from other IIPs. Described features include:
- Breathlessness, cough
- Weight loss is common
- Onset gradual or subacute, typical symptom duration before diagnosis varies 0.5–3 years
- Crackles at lung bases, later more extensive
- Clubbing in a small proportion of patients.

Investigations
- *HRCT* frequently shows diffuse, symmetrical ground-glass change, with or without reticulation and traction bronchiectasis. The confluent and homogeneous appearance contrasts with the patchy, heterogeneous distribution seen in UIP. Honeycombing is rare
- *PFTs* typically restrictive pattern, but impaired gas transfer in only 50%. Desaturation on exertion is common
- *BAL* lymphocytosis common
- *Lung biopsy*
- Investigations to exclude underlying disease (see above).

Histology Variable, ranging from a predominantly 'cellular' pattern (mild–moderate interstitial inflammation, no fibrosis) to a 'fibrotic' pattern (interstitial fibrosis, more homogeneous appearance than in UIP and lack of fibroblastic foci or honeycombing, lung architecture may be relatively preserved). NSIP may be subclassified based on the relative proportions of inflammation and fibrosis: NSIP 1 (primarily inflammation), NSIP 2 (inflammation and fibrosis), and NSIP 3 (primarily fibrosis). Features of both NSIP and UIP are sometimes seen on biopsies from the same individual—in such cases, the diagnosis is considered to be UIP.

Diagnosis Clinical and HRCT features are non-specific and surgical lung biopsy is required for diagnosis. Consider the presence of associated diseases (see list above).

Management Treatment is with corticosteroids (see page 445 for example of protocol). Additional immunosuppressive treatments may be considered in patients who fail to respond to corticosteroids alone (see page 445).

Prognosis Variable. Most patients improve or remain stable on treatment. 'Cellular' pattern on biopsy is associated with a good prognosis. Disease progression to death occurs, but is unusual.

Cryptogenic organizing pneumonia (COP)

(formerly bronchiolitis obliterans organizing pneumonia, BOOP)

Definition Cryptogenic organizing pneumonia (COP) is a disease of unknown cause characterized by 'plugging' of alveolar spaces with granulation tissue that may also extend up into the bronchioles. In addition to the 'cryptogenic' form, organizing pneumonia may also occur in the context of other diseases (see below). Use of the name 'BOOP' is no longer recommended, as it erroneously suggests a previous primarily airways disease and is easily confused with bronchiolitis obliterans, a distinct disease entity.

Epidemiology More common in non-smokers. Mean age of onset 55 years, although can affect any age. Males = females.

Causes of organizing pneumonia
- Cryptogenic (COP)
- Organizing pneumonia secondary to:
  - Infection (including pneumonia, lung abscess, bronchiectasis)
  - Drug reaction or radiotherapy
  - Connective tissue disease (particularly myositis, rheumatoid arthritis, Sjögren's)
  - Diffuse alveolar damage
  - Hypersensitivity pneumonitis
  - Eosinophilic pneumonia
  - Inflammatory bowel disease
  - Post-bone marrow transplant
  - Lung malignancy or airways obstruction
  - Pulmonary infarction.

Clinical features
- Typically short (<3 month) history of breathlessness and dry cough, often with malaise, fevers, weight loss, and myalgia. Often presents as a 'slow to resolve chest infection', frequently after several courses of antibiotics
- Breathlessness is usually mild, although a minority of patients experience severe breathlessness and rapid onset of respiratory failure and sometimes death
- Examination may be normal or reveal crackles. Clubbing is absent.

Investigations
- **Blood tests** Raised CRP and ESR, neutrophilia
- **PFTs** Mild-moderate restrictive pattern is typical, although mild airways obstruction may also be seen in smokers. Mild hypoxaemia is common
- **CXR** classically shows patchy consolidation, sometimes with nodular shadowing. May present as a solitary mass on CXR
- **HRCT** Areas of consolidation with air bronchograms, sometimes with associated ground-glass or small nodules. Often basal, subpleural, and peribronchial. May migrate spontaneously. Reticulation may suggest poor response to treatment. Less common appearance is as a solitary

mass that may cavitate and that is often mistaken radiologically for a lung cancer. Septal thickening may occur
- *TBB* often confirms diagnosis, but there is concern that the relatively small samples may not effectively exclude associated diseases. Usually adequate in patients with typical clinical and HRCT features who are subsequently followed up closely. Surgical lung biopsy (at VATS) is otherwise required
- *BAL* if performed, shows lymphocytosis, neutrophilia, and eosinophilia.

Histology Alveolar spaces 'plugged' with granulation tissue (fibrin, collagen-containing fibroblasts, often with inflammatory cells), sometimes with extension up into the bronchiolar lumen. Patchy. Lack of architectural distortion. Examine for evidence of underlying cause, e.g. infection, vasculitis.

Diagnosis Usually made on the basis of clinical and HRCT features and transbronchial biopsy. Surgical lung biopsy may be required in atypical cases or if an underlying disease is suspected. Remember that the histological finding of 'organizing pneumonia' is non-specific, and search for secondary causes (see list above). Lung cancers may be surrounded by patches of organizing pneumonia, and biopsy of these areas in patients with a solitary lung mass may give misleading results.

Differential diagnosis
- Infective consolidation
- Connective tissue disease, vasculitis
- Lymphoma, alveolar cell carcinoma
- Lung cancer (when COP presents as lung mass).

Management Steroids are the mainstay of treatment. Optimal dose and duration unknown. Typical initial dose of oral prednisolone is 0.75 mg/kg daily. Slowly taper the dose over a period of several months (see page 445 for example). Additional treatment with azathioprine or cyclophosphamide may be considered in patients with minimal response to steroids; intravenous pulses of cyclophosphamide may be tried in addition to steroid treatment in critically ill patients.

Prognosis Generally good. Most patients respond to steroids, and improve within a week of starting treatment. Consider alternative diagnosis (e.g. lymphoma) if no improvement on steroid doses >25 mg/day. Relapse is common on reduction of steroid dose, and treatment courses of 6–12 months are usually required. A minority improve spontaneously. Lack of steroid response and progressive respiratory failure and death are rare but well-documented.

Further information
Organising pneumonia. Cordier J-F *Thorax* 2000; **55**: 318–28

Acute interstitial pneumonia (AIP)

Definition Rapidly progressive form of interstitial pneumonia characterized histological by diffuse alveolar damage. May be considered as an idiopathic form of ARDS. Formerly known as Hamman–Rich syndrome.

Epidemiology Poorly described. Mean age of onset is 50, but may occur at any age. Patients often previously healthy.

Clinical features

- Often preceded by 'viral'-type illness, with systemic symptoms, e.g. fevers, tiredness, myalgia, arthralgia
- Rapid onset (over days) of breathlessness; usually presents <3 weeks after symptom onset
- Widespread crackles on examination.

Investigations

- *CXR* Bilateral diffuse airspace shadowing with air bronchograms, progressing to widespread reticulation and ground-glass; often spares costophrenic angles, heart borders, and hila
- *HRCT* Bilateral diffuse ground-glass and patchy airspace consolidation in early stages; later traction bronchiectasis, cystic change, reticulation
- *PFTs* Restrictive, reduced gas transfer. Often profound hypoxia and respiratory failure
- *BAL* Increased total cells, red blood cells, and haemosiderin. Non-diagnostic, but may be useful in excluding infection
- *Lung biopsy* required for diagnosis. Transbronchial biopsy may be diagnostic; the risk of pneumothorax is higher in mechanically ventilated patients (about 10%), although serious complications are rare. Surgical lung biopsy is otherwise required.

Histology Diffuse alveolar damage: hyaline membranes, oedema, interstitial inflammation, and alveolar septal thickening, progressing to organizing fibrosis and sometimes honeycombing.

Diagnosis based on lung biopsy and exclusion of causes of ARDS.

Differential diagnosis

- ARDS (ARDS is of known cause, whereas AIP is idiopathic; often otherwise indistinguishable on clinical and histological grounds)
- Accelerated decline of UIP (with diffuse alveolar damage on biopsy)
- Connective tissue disease (causing diffuse alveolar damage)
- Diffuse infection (community-acquired pneumonia, PCP, CMV)
- Drug-induced pneumonitis
- Acute hypersensitivity pneumonitis
- Acute eosinophilic pneumonia
- Cardiogenic pulmonary oedema
- Pulmonary haemorrhage/vasculitis.

Management No treatment demonstrated to be of benefit. In practice, treat infection (including consideration of unusual organisms) and consider steroids (often given at high dose, e.g. intravenous methyl-prednisolone). High flow oxygen. ITU admission, and mechanical ventilatory support usually required.

Prognosis Overall mortality at least 50%, although difficult to predict in individuals. Survivors may stabilize, develop chronic, progressive interstitial lung disease, or experience recurrent exacerbations.

Respiratory bronchiolitis-associated interstitial lung disease (RB-ILD)

Definition 'Respiratory bronchiolitis' is a pathological term referring to the accumulation of bronchiolar pigmented macrophages in cigarette smokers, and is asymptomatic in nearly all cases. A minority of smokers with respiratory bronchiolitis, however, develop a form of interstitial lung disease known as respiratory bronchiolitis-associated interstitial lung disease (RB-ILD). The exact relationship between RB-ILD and DIP is unclear—they may be considered as different forms of the same underlying disease, with DIP associated with a more extensive accumulation of macrophages throughout alveolar spaces.

Epidemiology Invariably occurs in current or previous smokers, typically >30 pack years. Male:female 2:1. Usual age of onset 30–40 years.

Clinical features
- Usually mild breathlessness and cough
- Small proportion have severe dyspnoea and respiratory failure
- Often crackles on examination.

Investigations
- **PFTs** often show restrictive or combined obstructive and restrictive picture, with mildly impaired gas transfer
- **CXR** Thick-walled bronchi, reticular or ground-glass change, may be normal
- **HRCT** Centrilobular nodules, ground-glass change, thick-walled airways, often with associated centrilobular emphysema
- **BAL** typically reveals pigmented alveolar macrophages.

Histology Accumulation of pigmented brown macrophages in terminal bronchioles. Patchy, bronchiolocentric distribution. These findings are frequently incidental in smokers, and so the diagnosis of RB-ILD requires consideration of clinical and imaging features in conjunction with histology.

Management Smoking cessation is the mainstay of treatment. Corticosteroids are occasionally used, with uncertain benefit.

Prognosis Generally good, although limited available data. Patients who refrain from smoking tend to improve. Progression to severe fibrosis is not documented. It is not known whether RB-ILD progresses to DIP.

Desquamative interstitial pneumonia (DIP)

Definition Interstitial lung disease that occurs in smokers and is associated with the pathological finding of abundant pigmented macrophages located diffusely throughout alveolar air spaces. It may represent a more extensive form of RB-ILD, in which macrophages are restricted to peribronchiolar regions. The term DIP is misleading, as desquamation of epithelial cells is not responsible for the histological findings as previously thought; a more accurate term is 'alveolar macrophage pneumonia', although this is not in widespread use.

Epidemiology Very rare. Majority of patients are smokers, although may also occur following inhalation of inorganic dusts, including passive inhalation of cigarette smoke. Typically occurs aged 30–50.

Clinical features Onset of breathlessness and cough over weeks–months is typical. Clubbing is common.

Investigations
- **PFTs** Mild restrictive pattern common, sometimes with reduced gas transfer
- **CXR** may be normal, or may demonstrate reticular or ground-glass pattern particularly affecting lower zones
- **HRCT** Ground glass seen in all cases, typically lower zone or peripheral predominance. Reticulation and honeycombing may be present, although tend to be mild
- **BAL** Increase in pigmented macrophages.

Histology Diffuse accumulation of pigmented macrophages in alveolar air spaces. Changes are uniform.

Diagnosis Clinical and HRCT features are non-specific and surgical lung biopsy is required for diagnosis.

Management Smoking cessation. Corticosteroids are often used, although their efficacy has not been studied.

Prognosis Usually good prognosis. Improvement in ground-glass on HRCT may correlate with response to treatment. Survival 70% after 10 years. Fluctuating course with remissions and relapses may occur.

Lymphoid interstitial pneumonia (LIP)

Definition Interstitial pneumonia characterized by diffuse lymphoid infiltrates and often lymphoid hyperplasia. Previously considered to be a precursor to pulmonary lymphoma, and difficult to distinguish from lymphoma histologically, it is now considered a distinct entity and is thought to only rarely undergo neoplastic transformation.

Epidemiology Very rare. Commoner in women. May occur at any age.

Causes/associations
- Idiopathic
- Connective tissue disease—particularly Sjögren's syndrome, also rheumatoid arthritis, SLE
- Immunodeficiency, e.g. HIV
- Infection, e.g. PCP, hepatitis B
- Autoimmune disease, e.g. haemolytic anaemia, Hashimoto's thyroiditis, pernicious anaemia, chronic active hepatitis, primary biliary cirrhosis, myasthenia gravis
- Drugs.

Clinical features Gradual onset breathlessness and cough over several years. Fever, weight loss may occur. Crackles may be heard on examination.

Investigations
- **Blood tests** Mild anaemia may occur; poly- or mono-clonal increase in serum immunoglobulins is common
- **CXR** Lower zone alveolar shadowing or diffuse honeycombing
- **HRCT** Predominant ground-glass change, often with reticulation and sometimes honeycombing and nodules
- **BAL** Non-clonal lymphocytosis
- Investigations to identify underlying cause (see above).

Histology Diffuse interstitial lymphoid infiltrates, predominantly involving alveolar septa, sometimes with lymphoid hyperplasia or honeycombing. Cellular NSIP, follicular bronchiolitis, and lymphoma may give similar appearances.

Management Steroids are frequently used and often appear to improve symptoms.

Prognosis Progression to extensive fibrosis occurs in around one-third of patients.

Hypersensitivity pneumonitis

Causes

Definition Group of lung diseases caused by inhalation of organic antigen to which the individual has been previously sensitized. Hypersensitivity pneumonitis (HP; previously termed extrinsic allergic alveolitis) is often divided into 'acute' and 'chronic' forms based on the time-course of presentation. Acute HP often follows a short period of exposure to a high concentration of antigen, and is usually reversible. Chronic HP typically follows a period of chronic exposure to a low antigen dose and is less reversible. These two presentations may overlap and 'subacute' forms of the disease are recognized.

Epidemiology Exact prevalence unknown. At least 8% of budgerigar and pigeon keepers and up to 5% of farmers may develop HP. Hypersensitivity pneumonitis is thought to be more common in non-smokers (mechanism unclear, may reflect inhibition of alveolar macrophage function by smoke).

Causes Many different antigens have been reported to cause HP, ranging from the relatively common (bird-fancier's lung and farmer's lung in the UK; summer-house HP in Japan) to the more unusual and exotic (shell lung—proteins on mollusc shells; pituitary snuff–taker's disease; sericulturist's lung—silk worm larvae proteins; sax lung—yeast on saxophone mouthpieces). Important examples are listed in the table below.

Causes of hypersensitivity pneumonitis—examples

Antigen	Sources	Diseases
Organisms		
Thermophilic actinomycetes (*Micropolyspora faeni*, *Thermoactinomyces vulgaris*), *Aspergillus* spp	Mouldy hay; sugarcane; compost; mushrooms; contaminated water in humidifiers and air conditioners	Farmers' lung; bagassosis; compost lung; mushroom workers' lung; humidifier lung
Aspergillus clavatus	Mouldy barley	Malt workers' lung
Trichosporon cutaneum	House dust	Summer-house HP (Japan)
Cladosporium spp	Ceiling mould	Hot tub lung
Animal protein		
Bird proteins	Bloom on bird feathers and droppings	Bird fancier's lung
Rat proteins	Rat droppings	Rat lung
Chemical		
Toluene diisocyanate	Paints	Isocyanate HP

Pathophysiology Pathogenesis of HP is not fully understood, and may involve T-cell mediated immunity and granuloma formation (type IV hypersensitivity) and/or antibody–antigen immune complex formation (type III hypersensitivity). It is not an atopic disease, and is not characterized by a rise in tissue eosinophils or IgE (type I hypersensitivity); this may in part be due to the small particle size of offending antigens, which tend to be deposited more distally in the air-spaces than the larger particles associated with asthma. Lung histology specimens typically reveal an interstitial inflammatory infiltrate, often with accompanying bronchiolitis and organizing pneumonia. Non-caseating granulomata are often present, and typically are ill-defined and single (cf. sarcoidosis, where granulomata are well-defined and are grouped subpleurally or near bronchi). Chronic HP is characterized by fibrosis, and often the absence of granulomata and airways involvement, particularly if antigen exposure has ceased.

Diagnosis

Clinical features

Acute HP

- Breathlessness, dry cough, and systemic symptoms (fever, chills, arthralgia, myalgia, headache) occur 4–8 hours after exposure to antigen
- Examination: crackles and squeaks on auscultation, fever
- In the absence of ongoing exposure, symptoms settle spontaneously within 1–3 days. Episodes may be recurrent.

Chronic HP

- Progressive exertional breathlessness, dry cough, sometimes systemic symptoms (weight loss) over course of months–years. May be history of acute episodes
- Examination: crackles and squeaks on auscultation, clubbing rare, may be features of cor pulmonale.

Investigations

- **Imaging: acute HP**
  - **CXR** Diffuse small (1–3 mm) nodules or infiltrates, sometimes ground-glass change, apical sparing. Normal in up to 20% of cases
  - **HRCT** Patchy ground-glass change and poorly defined nodules. Areas of increased lucency (enhanced on expiratory HRCT) occur due to air trapping from bronchiolar involvement
  - Both CXR and HRCT appearances may quickly normalize following removal from antigen exposure
- **Imaging: chronic HP**
  - **CXR** Typically upper- and mid-zone reticulation
  - **HRCT** Diffuse well-defined centrilobular nodules, ground-glass change, increased lucency from air trapping. May mimic UIP
- **PFTs** Typically restrictive pattern with reduced gas transfer and lung volumes; mild obstruction is also sometimes observed. Hypoxia may occur
- **Bloods** Acute hypersensitivity pneumonitis associated with neutrophilia but not eosinophilia. Inflammatory markers often increased
- **Serum antibody (IgG) precipitin** results are presented either as an ELISA or as a number of precipitin lines, referring to the number of different epitopes an individual responds to. Precipitins to organic antigens are found in 90% of patients, but are also present in up to 10% of asymptomatic farmers and 50% of pigeon breeders. Precipitin levels often fall in the absence of ongoing antigen exposure
- **BAL** lymphocytosis (>40% of cells) is a typical finding, but not in itself diagnostic
- **Transbronchial or surgical lung biopsy** may be required in cases of diagnostic uncertainty. TBB may provide insufficient tissue for adequate histological analysis
- **Inhalation antigen challenge** may be unpleasant, and is not recommended routinely.

Diagnosis is based on the combination of history of antigen exposure and typical clinical and HRCT features. The most diagnostically useful clinical features are an onset of symptoms 4–8 hours after exposure, a history of recurrent episodes of symptoms, the presence of weight loss, and the finding of crackles on examination. An absence of serum precipitins is very unusual but described. Atypical presentations require further investigation to support the diagnosis, such as BAL lymphocytosis or characteristic histological features on lung biopsy.

Differential diagnosis
- Atypical pneumonia
- Idiopathic interstitial pneumonias (particularly UIP and COP)
- Sarcoidosis
- Vasculitis
- Occupational asthma (e.g. from isocyanates)
- Drug-induced lung disease (including pesticides)
- Organic dust toxic syndrome (follows very high levels of exposure to agricultural dusts, symptoms transient, benign course)
- Silo-filler's disease (variable respiratory manifestations following exposure to nitrogen dioxide in silos; ranges from mild bronchitis to fatal bronchospasm).

Management

Management centres on antigen avoidance, which is frequently difficult. If complete removal from antigen is unrealistic (e.g. farmers), measures to reduce exposure may be of benefit (such as respiratory protection with high performance, positive pressure masks; avoidance of particularly heavy exposure; improved ventilation and use of air filters; drying of hay prior to storage).

In acute HP, symptoms typically resolve following cessation of antigen exposure, and treatment usually not required. Removal from exposure may also result in symptomatic and physiological improvement in chronic HP, although this is less certain and established pulmonary fibrosis is often irreversible.

When treatment is required, corticosteroids are frequently used although there is a lack of randomized controlled evidence to support this. Steroids may hasten the resolution of impaired pulmonary function in acute HP, although their effect on long-term outcome is unclear. A typical regimen is prednisolone 40–60 mg daily for up to a month, and then slowly reduce dose over several months. Inhaled steroids have not been studied in detail, although may be of some benefit.

Prognosis Highly variable. Prognosis is usually excellent following removal from antigen exposure in acute HP, although progression to respiratory failure and death may very rarely occur after short-term exposures of very high intensity. Recurrent episodes of acute HP do not necessarily progress to chronic HP and fibrosis, and chronic HP may develop in the absence of previous acute HP episodes. Development of chronic HP with ongoing exposure may eventually lead to cor pulmonale and death, although again this is variable and many patients do not exhibit disease progression despite chronic exposure. Persistent, low-dose exposure (e.g. budgerigar in the house) may be more likely to progress to the chronic, fibrotic form of HP than intermittent high-dose exposure (e.g. pigeon fanciers), which predisposes more to episodes of acute HP.

Further information

Hypersensitivity pneumonitis Schuyler M. Lesson 6, Volume 14 in PCCU Education Series online at *www.chestnet*

Bronchiolitis

Pathophysiology and causes

Definition and epidemiology Bronchioles are small airways of diameter <2 mm, lined by bronchial epithelium and with no cartilage in their walls. Terminal bronchioles lead to alveoli. Considerable numbers of bronchioles need to be affected by disease before a patient becomes symptomatic. When they are affected, they cause increased airway resistance. Bronchiolitis is poorly understood.

Disease seems to affect bronchioles in two main ways:
- As a process affecting the bronchioles in isolation, with non-specific injury causing subsequent epithelial damage and inflammation
- As a bronchiolitis associated with other airway disease, where the bronchiolitis may be more of an incidental finding along with other pathologies, e.g. COP, hypersensitivity pneumonitis, RB-ILD, Langerhans' cell histiocytosis.

Pathophysiology is unclear. There is probably an initial injury to the epithelium of the bronchioles with subsequent inflammation. Adjacent alveoli are often also involved. There are two main pathological patterns of bronchiolitis. Both can exist in the same patient:
- *Proliferative bronchiolitis* More common of the two patterns. Non-specific reaction to bronchiolar injury, with organizing exudate within the bronchiolar lumen. Proliferation of intraluminal fibrotic buds, called Masson bodies, seen in bronchioles, alveoli, and alveolar ducts. Often associated alveolar wall inflammation and foamy macrophages in alveolar spaces. May completely or partially resolve. Tends to be more responsive to steroid treatment. The pathology merges with that of COP (see page 450)
- *Constrictive bronchiolitis* Rare. Concentric narrowing of the bronchiolar wall due to cellular infiltrates ± smooth muscle hyperplasia, which may cause extrinsic compression, obliteration, distortion, mucus collection, peribronchiolar fibrosis, and scarring. Patchy in distribution. Typically progressive and unresponsive to steroid therapy. Usually leads to respiratory failure and death.

In practice, these are the commonest situations in which a diagnosis of bronchiolitis is useful:
- Viral bronchiolitis (RSV)
- Post-lung transplant (obliterative bronchiolitis)
- Post-bone marrow transplant
- Connective tissue disease (usually rheumatoid arthritis)
- In association with interstitial lung disease and airways disease
- *Rare but important:* Japanese panbronchiolitis.

Causes of bronchiolitis

Proliferative bronchiolitis (associated with organizing pneumonia)

Commoner causes
- COP (see page 450)
- Hypersensitivity pneumonitis (see page 457)
- Chronic pulmonary eosinophilia (see page 474)
- Connective tissue disease—rheumatoid arthritis, polymyositis, dermatomyositis (see page 487)
- Post bone marrow, heart and lung transplant
- Organizing acute infection—mycoplasma, legionella, influenza, CMV, HIV, PCP.

Rarer causes
- ARDS (see page 519)
- Vasculitides, including Wegener's granulomatosis (see page 501)
- Drug-induced reactions, such as L-tryptophan, busulfan, cocaine
- Chronic thyroiditis
- Ulcerative colitis
- Radiation or aspiration pneumonitis
- Distal to bronchial obstruction
- Common variable immunodeficiency syndrome.

Constrictive bronchiolitis

Commoner causes
- Connective tissue disease, particularly rheumatoid arthritis, especially women in their 50s and 60s, with longstanding rheumatoid arthritis. May be related to penicillamine therapy
- Infection—viral (adenovirus, RSV, influenza, parainfluenza), mycoplasma.

Rarer causes
- 'Chronic rejection phenomenon' in heart, lung, bone marrow transplants—affects up to 65% of lung transplant patients after 5 years post-transplant and is the primary cause of late death, bronchiolitis obliterans syndrome (see page 388). Patients taking statins post-transplant have a lower incidence of this; reasons unclear
- Japanese panbronchiolitis
- Following inhalation injury: mineral dusts, such as asbestos, silica, iron oxide, aluminium oxide, talc, mica, coal, sulphur dioxide, nitrogen oxide, ammonia, chlorine, phosgene—may develop cough days to weeks after exposure
- Drug reaction
- Hypersensitivity reactions
- Ulcerative colitis
- Cryptogenic. Rare, mostly women > 40. Cough and dyspnoea. PFT: progressive airflow obstruction and air trapping. KCO decreased, no bronchodilator response.

Management

Clinical features Insidious onset of cough and dyspnoea, over weeks to months. There may be an associated medical history, such as a transplant, connective tissue disease, or vasculitis, or a history of mineral dust or drug exposure. Possible history of recent viral illness.

Investigations

- **PFTs** Obstructive defect may be found, with no bronchodilator reversibility, particularly in constrictive bronchiolitis. Proliferative bronchiolitis can cause a restrictive or mixed defect
- **CXR** can be normal, or may show hyperinflation, especially with constrictive bronchiolitis, diffuse infiltrates with proliferative bronchiolitis, which may be migratory
- **HRCT** can be very helpful and may be performed prone in full expiration. (Prone CT is used to minimize any gravity-dependent changes.) Normal bronchioles are too small to be seen, although indirect signs of disease may be hyperinflation, air trapping, causing a mosaic pattern and subsegmental atelectasis. Bronchioles with thickened walls due to inflammation and dilatation may be seen, the 'tree in bud' appearance. CT is also useful to assess for signs of associated interstitial lung disease
- **Open or thoracoscopic lung biopsy** may be required to make the diagnosis, as transbronchial biopsies are usually inadequate. The small airways must be carefully examined.

Management

- Treat any underlying disorder
- Cough suppressants
- Long-term macrolide antibiotics, such as erythromycin 200–600 mg/day may improve symptoms, lung function, and mortality, especially in those with *diffuse panbronchiolitis* and *cryptogenic bronchiolitis*. Erythromycin lowers the neutrophil count by an unknown mechanism and reduces the number of lymphocytes
- Steroids are effective in cases of proliferative bronchiolitis and can treat the associated organizing pneumonia. They may also be beneficial in bronchiolitis due to inhalation injury, both in early and later stages. Relapses of the bronchiolitis may occur on stopping the steroids.

Bronchiolitis: specific conditions

Diffuse panbronchiolitis/Japanese panbronchiolitis This is a distinct condition involving both the upper and lower respiratory tracts, with bronchiolar inflammation and chronic sinusitis. It occurs particularly amongst the Japanese and is rarely found outside the Far East, although this may be due to a lack of disease recognition. An infectious aetiology has been postulated as the cause of this disease, but no organism has been consistently identified. It can be familial and is associated with HLA-Bw54 in Japan. It is more prevalent in men, with a mean age at presentation of 50. It occurs particularly in non-smokers and there is a history of chronic sinusitis that precedes the chest symptoms often by years. Patients have a productive cough with purulent sputum, exertional dyspnoea, wheeze, and weight loss. There may be signs of progressive respiratory failure and cor pulmonale. Chest examination may reveal crackles and wheezes.

- **PFTs** are obstructive, although may show a mixed pattern, with minimal airway hyperresponsiveness. kCO is reduced
- **CXR and CT** may show diffuse ill-defined nodules, bronchiectasis, and air trapping
- **Cold agglutinins** may be positive, although mycoplasma tests are negative
- **BAL** shows marked neutrophilia
- **Sputum cultures** may show growth of *Haemophilus influenzae, Streptococcus pneumoniae, Klebsiella pneumoniae,* or *Staphylococcus aureus,* which should be treated
- **Open or thoracoscopic lung biopsy** may provide the definitive diagnosis, although this may not be considered necessary in areas where panbronchiolitis is prevalent. Bronchiolar histology is characteristic although not pathognomonic, with transmural infiltrate of lymphocytes, plasma cells, and foamy macrophages. The intraluminal exudates may be organized to form a polypoid plug.

Treatment is with low-dose erythromycin 400–600 mg/day for 2–6 months, which confers a significant survival benefit, most likely related to its anti-inflammatory effects, rather than its antibacterial effects. Untreated, 50% 5-year mortality.

Acute bronchiolitis This is an infective illness, common in infants, who present with wheezing, tachypnoea, respiratory distress, and tachycardia. It is most commonly caused by respiratory syncytial virus (RSV), but also adenovirus, influenza, parainfluenza, mycoplasma, and chlamydia. In adults, acute bronchiolitis is caused by the same organisms, but is less severe.

- **CXR** may be normal, or show hyperinflation, occasionally with patchy opacities, consolidation, and collapse
- **Histologically** there is acute and chronic inflammation of bronchioles, with necrosis, sloughing, oedema, and inflammatory exudates in the bronchiolar lumen.

Treatment is supportive, with oxygen, fluids, steroids, and bronchodilators if severe.

Further information

Bronchiolar disorders. Ryu JH et al. Am J Respir Crit Care Med 2003; **168**: 1277–92

Eosinophilic lung disease

Eosinophilic lung disease

Definition Pulmonary eosinophilias are disorders classically associated with CXR infiltrates and a raised blood eosinophil count, although eosinophilic infiltration of the lung can occur *without* blood eosinophilia.

- Eosinophils are phagocytes that are produced in bone marrow and circulate for up to 10 hours before localizing in tissues
- Their blood levels are usually tightly regulated
- In health they accumulate in the GI tract mucosa, but they may be attracted to other tissues by chemoattractant mechanisms, including mast cell activation and complement activation
- Eosinophils can survive in the tissues for weeks if appropriate cytokines are present
- Persisting high eosinophil levels cause tissue damage, due to their pro-inflammatory effects
- Eosinophils accumulate in allergic or hypersensitivity disease, parasitic infections, and cancer
- Steroids and severe sepsis both decrease eosinophil levels
- Asthma can cause a raised eosinophil count, especially if there is associated eczema, but an absolute eosinophil count of $> 1 \times 10^9$/l is very unusual and raises the possibility of an alternative diagnosis, such as Churg–Strauss syndrome
- Normal eosinophil counts are below 0.4×10^9/l (1–3% of peripheral WCC)
- Counts of 0.4×10^9/l upwards can be seen in pulmonary eosinophilia.

Causes of CXR infiltrates ± blood eosinophilia

Condition	Characteristic points
Asthma with allergic broncho pulmonary aspergillosis (ABPA)	Known asthma, with worsening symptoms, over weeks to months. Associated systemic symptoms. Raised blood eosinophil count, positive aspergillus skin test, raised IgE, raised aspergillus precipitins
Simple pulmonary eosinophilia (Löffler's syndrome)	Foreign travel. Symptoms for days to weeks. Cough, malaise, anorexia, rhinitis, night sweats, fever, dyspnoea, wheeze. Sputum contains eosinophils and larvae. Low-level blood eosinophilia
Tropical pulmonary eosinophilia	Foreign travel. Symptoms for weeks to months, with remissions and relapses. Cough, wheeze, sputum, dyspnoea, chest pain, fever, weight loss, fatigue. Sputum contains eosinophils. Raised blood eosinophil count, high IgE
Chronic pulmonary eosinophilia	Symptoms for weeks–months, with associated systemic symptoms. Cough, sputum, haemoptysis, dyspnoea, recent onset asthma, fever, weight loss, night sweats. Sputum eosinophilia, but blood levels can be normal
Acute eosinophilic pneumonia,	Short duration of symptoms, < 5 days. Fever, cough, dyspnoea, and myalgia. Unwell, hypoxic. High BAL eosinophil count, no blood eosinophilia
Hypereosinophilic syndrome	Symptoms for weeks–months. Associated systemic symptoms and other organ involvement. Fever, weight loss, cough, night sweats, pruritus. High blood eosinophil count
Churg–Strauss syndrome	Rhinitis, past history of asthma. Other organ involvement. Associated systemic symptoms. Longer duration of symptoms, weeks–months. Blood eosinophilia and eosinophilic tissue infiltration
Drug-induced pulmonary eosinophilia	Recent new drug. Possible associated skin reaction. Symptoms within hours–days. Spectrum of illness, from mild to severely unwell, with cough, dyspnoea, fever, and hypoxia. Eosinophilic tissue infiltration, but blood eosinophilia not universal

Causes of eosinophilic lung disease 1

Asthma and ABPA (see page 262)

- Fever or worsening asthma symptoms may be caused by type 1 and 2 hypersensitivity reactions to *Aspergillus fumigatus*
- Untreated can cause central bronchiectasis
- *CXR* shows fleeting shadows
- *Blood* eosinophilia
- *Aspergillus skin prick test* is positive and serum aspergillus IgG precipitins are positive. IgE levels are raised
- **Treatment** is with steroids, and antifungal agents may be necessary.

Simple pulmonary eosinophilia (Löffler's syndrome)

- Caused by parasitic infection, usually *Ascaris lumbricoides*, but also *strongyloides* and *ankylostoma*
- Occurs worldwide, especially in SE Asia, Africa, Central and South America
- The eggs of the parasite are found in the soil and are ingested. After 10–14 days, larvae migrate from the intestine via lymph and blood to the liver and lung. From the lung, they pass up the bronchial tree to be swallowed, to develop into roundworms in the gut
- The passage of larvae through the lung causes an allergic reaction. This may be asymptomatic, but may cause cough, malaise, anorexia, rhinitis, night sweats, low-grade fever, occasional wheezing, and dyspnoea. The illness lasts around 2 weeks
- *CXR* shows transient bilateral shadows that are discrete and perihilar. They disappear usually between 6–12 days, but can take up to 1 month
- *Sputum* also contains eosinophils and larvae
- *Blood eosinophilia* at a low level
- *Stool examination* reveals parasites, but only 2–3 months later when the adult worms are passed
- **Treatment** is with an antihelminth agent, such as mebendazole for 3 days or levamisole as a single dose. Steroids may be necessary if the pulmonary manifestations are severe.

Tropical pulmonary eosinophilia

- Hypersensitivity to migrating larvae of filarial worms, *Wucheria bancrofti* and *Brugia malayi*, similar to Löffler's syndrome
- Occurs in the Indian subcontinent, SE Asia, and the South Pacific islands
- Insidious onset of cough, wheeze, sputum, dyspnoea, and chest pain, with associated fever, weight loss, and fatigue. Symptoms last for weeks to months, with remissions and relapses
- **Examination** reveals crepitations
- *CXR* shows bilateral uniform mottling of the lung fields, especially in the middle and lower zones. There may be cavitation and pleural effusion
- *Sputum and BAL* contain eosinophils

- *PFTs* may be obstructive initially, but can become restrictive in long-standing untreated cases
- *Histology* shows eosinophilic bronchopneumonia and eosinophilic abscesses
- *Blood eosinophil count* is raised. IgE is raised
- *Filarial complement test* is positive
- **Treatment** is with a filaricide, diethylcarbamazine, for 3 weeks. This rapidly improves symptoms.

Drug-induced pulmonary eosinophilia

- Pulmonary shadowing develops within hours to days of starting the drug and resolves usually within one week of stopping it
- It is due to an allergic reaction in the pulmonary vessel wall caused by the drug and occurs again on drug rechallenge
- There may be an associated skin reaction
- The drug should be avoided in the future and steroids given if necessary
- Severity of illness varies, from mild to severely unwell, with cough, dyspnoea, fever, hypoxia. May occur in those with concomitant asthma
- Tissue eosinophilia, but may not have blood eosinophilia
- Possible drugs include: ampicillin, carbemazepine, chlorpropamide, cocaine (inhaled), diclofenac, inorganic chemicals, such as nickel, methotrexate, nitrofurantoin, penicillin, phenytoin, sodium aminosalicylate, sulphonamides, tetracycline.

Causes of eosinophilic lung disease 2

Chronic pulmonary eosinophilia
- Unknown cause
- Women:men = 2:1. Occurs in middle age
- Insidious onset over weeks to months, with cough, sputum, possibly haemoptysis, dyspnoea, recent onset asthma, weight loss, night sweats, and high fever. Differential diagnosis includes TB
- **Diagnosis** is usually clinical and radiological, but may need BAL or open lung biopsy
- **CXR** shows peripheral dense opacities with ill-defined margins (photographic negative of pulmonary oedema)
- **CT** shows peripheral air space infiltrates
- **Sputum** eosinophilia
- **BAL** eosinophil count high
- **Blood** eosinophilia may not occur. ESR is raised
- **Treatment** is with steroids, such as prednisolone 30–40 mg/day, and improvement is usually rapid, with the CXR clearing within 2–3 days and normal in 2 weeks. Decrease steroid dose once stable, but continue for 6 months
- Relapses common when steroids stopped and they may need further courses.

Acute eosinophilic pneumonia
Unknown cause, occurs in any age or sex. Presents with fever, cough, dyspnoea, and myalgia.
Diagnostic criteria:
- Acute febrile illness of <5 days duration
- Hypoxic respiratory failure
- Interstitial or alveolar CXR infiltrates
- BAL eosinophils >25%
- No parasitic, fungal, or other infection
- Prompt and complete response to steroids
- Failure to relapse after stopping steroids.

May be unwell and hypoxic, requiring ventilatory support. No peripheral blood eosinophilia. High-dose steroids should be given until the respiratory failure resolves and then the dose can be tapered over 2–4 weeks.

Hypereosinophilic syndrome
- Unknown cause. Rare
- Most common in men aged 30 to 40
- Present with fever, weight loss, night sweats, cough, and pruritus
- **Diagnosis** based on:
  - Marked blood eosinophilia of $>1.5 \times 10^9$/l for 6 months or more
  - Signs and symptoms of eosinophilic tissue infiltration on histology
  - No evidence of another cause of eosinophilia
- **Pulmonary involvement** with interstitial infiltrates and pleural effusions on CXR. **Cardiovascular involvement** also occurs, with myocarditis, endocardial fibrosis, restrictive cardiomyopathy, valvular damage, and mural thrombus formation. These may cause considerable morbidity and mortality. Skin may be involved with urticaria and

angioedema; CNS involved with encephalopathy, arterial and venous embolism, peripheral neuropathy or mononeuritis multiplex; GI tract with gastritis, nausea, diarrhoea, alcohol intolerance and hepato- or splenomegaly; joints with effusions and Raynaud's. Kidney and muscles can also be infiltrated by eosinophils. Can be fatal

- **Blood** eosinophil levels may be as high as 70%. IgE levels are high
- **Treatment** is with high-dose steroids (e.g. 60 mg prednisolone), which improves about 50% of cases. May need to use other immunosuppressants, such as cyclophosphamide, hydroxyurea, azathioprine, or interferon alpha. Treatment should be tapered according to falling eosinophil counts and end-organ improvement.

Churg–Strauss syndrome (see page 510)

- Severe asthma, blood eosinophilia, and pulmonary infiltrates occur as part of a small and medium vessel vasculitis
- There may be eosinophilic tissue infiltration
- ANCA usually, but not always positive
- Treatment with steroids and immunosuppression.

Pneumoconioses

Overview and causative mineral dusts

- Pneumoconioses are non-neoplastic pulmonary diseases caused by the reaction of the lung to the inhalation of mainly mineral, but also organic dusts
- Inhaled particles of dust size < 5 µm reach the terminal airways and alveoli and settle on the epithelial lining. From here they are slowly cleared by macrophages or alveolar cells. They may pass into the lymphatic system, be cleared via the airway, or remain in the alveolus
- The dust particles can lead to an inflammatory reaction within the lung, depending on their physical and chemical properties
- The inflammation causes characteristic alterations in pulmonary structure and radiological abnormalities
- Of the diseases caused by inhalation of mineral dusts, many are becoming less common in the UK, due to improved protection of workers from dusts and decreasing levels of mining. Newer industrial nations may see increasing numbers of cases of pneumoconiosis
- Organic dusts causing hypersensitivity pneumonitis and extrinsic asthma are discussed on pages 458 and 105. Asbestos-related diseases are discussed separately on page 318.

Causative mineral dusts

Mineral dust	Disease	Examples of exposure
Coal dust	Simple pneumoconiosis Progressive massive fibrosis Caplan's syndrome	Coal mining, especially hard coal
Silica	Silicosis Caplan's syndrome	Foundry work, sandblasting, stone cutting, hard rock mining
Asbestos	Asbestosis Benign asbestos-related pleural disease Mesothelioma Lung cancer	Mining, milling, and fabrication. Installation and removal of insulation
Beryllium	Acute berylliosis Beryllium granulomatosis	Mining, fabrication of electrical and electronic equipment, workers in nuclear and aerospace industry
Iron oxide	Siderosis	Welding
Barium sulphate	Baritosis	Mining
Tin oxide	Stannosis	Mining
Aluminium	Like silicosis (bauxite worker's lung, Shaver's disease)	Mining, firework, painting, and armament manufacture

Types of mineral dust exposure

Non-fibrous mineral dusts
- Silicosis
- Coal workers' pneumoconiosis
- Mixed mineral dusts containing quartz: slate, kaolin, talc, non-fibrous clays

Fibrous mineral dusts
- Asbestos
- Other mineral fibres

Metal dusts and fumes
- Iron, aluminium, beryllium, cobalt.

Chest disease in coal miners It was recognized many years ago that coal miners had higher levels of respiratory disease than the general population. Coal miners can get any or all of:
- Chronic bronchitis
- COPD
- Pneumoconiosis.

They may be eligible for compensation for all of these.

It has been difficult to establish the independent effects of coal dust due to high smoking rates amongst miners. However, it is now thought that coal dust contributes to the COPD and bronchitis caused by smoking, because:
- Miners have an increased prevalence of cough, sputum, and decreased FEV_1 when compared to non-miners. The risk of cough increases with increasing dust exposure
- FEV_1 declines in proportion to the amount of dust exposure
- In smokers the response to dust is probably different to that of non-smokers, with worse disease at a given level of exposure.

In the past, tuberculosis has been a major problem amongst miners and their families, relating to their socio-economic conditions.

SWORD is the Surveillance of Work-related and Occupational Respiratory Disease scheme run in the UK to monitor the numbers of patients with occupational lung diseases. Patients with a clinical diagnosis of an occupational lung disease are confidentially reported by respiratory or occupational health physicians.

Further information
www.dti.gov.uk/coalhealth

Coal-workers' pneumoconiosis

This is the condition caused by the deposition of coal dust within the lung and its associated inflammatory reaction.

There are two types:
- Simple pneumoconiosis, which can progress to
- Complicated pneumoconiosis, also known as progressive massive fibrosis (PMF).

These are common diseases amongst coal miners who work in poorly ventilated conditions. The risk of pneumoconiosis varies with different compositions of coal from different geographical areas but, the larger the amount of dust to which the miner is exposed, the greater the risk of developing pneumoconiosis. It is now rare for miners under the age of 50 to be diagnosed with pneumoconiosis in the UK.

Pathology

Simple pneumoconiosis Coal dust is inhaled into the alveolus and is engulfed by macrophages, to form a black stellate lesion, the coal macule. This causes cytokine release and subsequent inflammatory cell recruitment, leading to fibroblast activation. These coal macules are found throughout the lung, especially in the upper zones of the upper and lower lobes, and often associated with surrounding bronchiolar dilatation. They are not palpable. Regional lymph nodes also become blackened. In time, larger nodules develop, containing reticulin and collagen between the macrophages, and associated bronchiolar dilatation leading to focal emphysema is seen.

PMF occurs on this background, but with aggregation of the fibrotic nodules to form larger lesions, 2–10 cm diameter. Macroscopically, these look like large black scars, extending from the lung parenchyma to the chest wall. The central area of these nodules may be necrotic and the outer rim is firm and collagenous. It is not understood what causes the progression of small nodules to PMF, although continued exposure to coal dust in the presence of simple pneumoconiosis makes this development more likely.

Clinical features

Simple pneumoconiosis is usually asymptomatic with no associated clinical signs. This is a relatively benign disease.

Progressive massive fibrosis is usually associated with cough, productive of mucoid or blackened sputum, and breathlessness, particularly on exertion, and may in time lead to the development of cor pulmonale. Examination is unremarkable, with no clubbing and no crepitations audible (the presence of crepitations suggests a different diagnosis).

Investigations

- **CXR** In *simple pneumoconiosis* there is nodular shadowing, with nodules of varying size, up to 10 mm, particularly in the upper and middle zones. Pneumoconiosis can be graded according to the number of different sized nodules, p = < 1.5 mm, q = 1.5–3 mm and r = 3–10 mm. Nodule numbers increase with increasing dust inhalation and usually stop forming when the miner has left the work environment. *PMF is diagnosed* when one or more opacities of > 1 cm diameter are present, on the background of simple pneumoconiosis. These lesions are often located in the upper lobes and enlarge, becoming increasingly radiodense and clearly demarcated with time. They may distort the adjacent lung and cause emphysema. The lesions continue to progress out of the work environment
- **HRCT** of *simple pneumoconiosis* shows parenchymal nodules 1–10 mm in size, with upper zone predominance. *In PMF*, nodules of > 1 cm are seen, with irregular borders and associated parenchymal distortion and emphysema. Larger lesions may have cavitation and necrosis. They may also have areas of calcification
- **PFTs** Simple pneumoconiosis: FEV_1 and FVC are normal, although TLCO may be slightly decreased. *PMF*: signs of airway obstruction due to emphysema, and restriction due to loss of lung volumes. TLCO is reduced.

Management Minimization of dust exposure with improved mine ventilation, respirator provision, and monitoring of dust levels. Miners have CXR every 4 years and are moved to less dusty work if they show signs of pneumoconiosis, to prevent the development of PMF. Miners with signs of coal workers' pneumoconiosis are entitled to industrial injury benefits from British Coal. No increased risk of lung cancer with pneumoconiosis or PMF.

Caplan's syndrome Miners with seropositive rheumatoid arthritis or positive serum rheumatoid factor can develop large well-defined nodules. These occur on a background of simple pneumoconiosis and in those with a relatively low coal dust exposure. They may be multiple and may cavitate. They cause no significant functional impairment and have no malignant potential.

Silicosis

This is a chronic nodular densely fibrosing pneumoconiosis, caused by the prolonged inhalation of silica particles.

- Long lag time of decades between exposure and clinical disease
- Insidious onset, progressive
- Larger radiological opacities than those seen in coal-workers' pneumoconiosis, and more rapid progression
- The pattern of disease depends on the level and duration of the silicone dust exposure.

Silica is present mostly as crystalline quartz, which is mined and quarried and used in industries, such as ceramics, brick-making, and stone masonry. It is becoming less prevalent in Western societies, due to changes in silica working conditions.

Pathology Quartz and cristobalite forms of crystalline silica cause silicosis. When they accumulate within the airways, lymphocytes and alveolar macrophages engulf the particles and are removed into the lymphatic system. Any remaining silica dust causes focal aggregations of macrophages, which are in time converted into fibrosing nodules. Silica dust can cause surfactant secretion from the alveolus due to local irritation. This leads to further macrophage recruitment. Large nodules are formed by the aggregation of smaller nodules.

Different types of silicosis There are four types, and the distinction is often not clear:

- *Acute silicosis* is caused by intense exposure to fine dusts, such as those produced by sand blasting. It may become apparent in workers within a few months to a year of starting work. Rapid deterioration over 1–2 years, with treatment being ineffective. Rare now, due to regulation of silica levels in the work place
  - *Clinically* dry cough, shortness of breath, and a feeling of tightness on breathing deeply. Rapid deterioration over a few weeks. Fine crepitations are heard over the lower zones bilaterally. Respiratory failure
  - *CXR* Patchy bilateral lower air space consolidation, which may look like pulmonary oedema
  - *Pathology* Irregular fibrosis adjacent to alveolar spaces filled with a lipoproteinaceous exudate, similar to that found in alveolar proteinosis
- *Subacute silicosis* This is the classic picture of silicosis, which is now quite rare. Dry cough, gradual onset of shortness of breath
  - *CXR* Upper and mid-zone nodules are present, measuring between 3 and 5 mm diameter. Initially indistinct, but become clearer with time. Nodules coalesce and calcify and can progress to progressive massive fibrosis (PMF). Associated calcified hilar lymphadenopathy (egg shell calcification) and possible pleural thickening. Nodules continue to develop with continued exposure, but due to long lag time will also develop when patient stops being exposed. In some cases with heavy exposure to silica, patients may develop progressive upper zone fibrosis with sparse nodularity

- *PFTs* Slow decline, including TLCO, with mild restrictive pattern, unless the silicosis has caused emphysema, when obstructive or mixed picture is seen
- *Pathology* Dust particles within the alveoli are phagocytosed by macrophages. They are removed to the lymphatics, where they lodge and cause diffuse inflammatory change. Layers of collagen are deposited around the dust particle. Nodules are found within the secondary pulmonary lobule, where they cause fibrosis
- *Chronic silicosis* occurs with lower dust concentrations than those seen in active silicosis
  - *CXR* A few upper and mid-zone nodules occur, which become calcified after 10 years or so. There is no associated parenchymal distortion. There may be associated hilar lymphadenopathy

  If there is further silica exposure, this disease may progress, with coalescence of nodules.
- *Silicotuberculosis* Increased likelihood of active TB infection in people with silicosis, most likely due to the reactivation of quiescent lesions. Silica within the lung is thought to affect the efficacy of the macrophage at clearing *Mycobacterium tuberculosis*. TB can be difficult to diagnose, due to multiple pre-existing CXR nodules. Cavitation may occur, which does not occur with silicosis alone. Haemoptysis, fever, and new soft CXR opacities should prompt sputum examination and BAL.

  Confirmed TB should be treated with the usual 3 or 4 drug regime. Non-tuberculous mycobacterial infection is also more common.

Management Prevention of silicosis by monitoring and minimizing dust levels with adequate ventilation. Masks can be useful for short-term use, if the high levels of dust are transiently unavoidable. Disability benefits available from the Department of Social Security. Small increased risk of lung cancer with silicosis and associated PMF.

Berylliosis

Beryllium is a light, strong industrial metal. It is mined and often used as an alloy in the manufacture of fluorescent tubes for lighting and televisions, radiological equipment, in atomic reactors, and in heat-resistant ceramics. Cases of berylliosis are now rare, as beryllium levels have been tightly regulated to avoid sensitization. However, due to the long latent period between exposure and granuloma formation, as well as accidental beryllium exposure, cases are still occurring. There are two types of disease:

- **Acute beryllium disease** is an acute alveolitis due to the direct effects of high-dose inhaled beryllium fumes. There is subsequent widespread airway oedema and pulmonary oedema, which causes dyspnoea, cyanosis, and widespread inspiratory crepitations. CXR shows pulmonary oedema. It may be self-limiting if mild, but if severe is usually fatal. Corticosteroids may prevent progression, but the patient is often left with residual pulmonary impairment
- **Subacute and chronic berylliosis** is a hypersensitivity-type skin or pulmonary disease that occurs a long time after beryllium exposure in a minority of individuals. It can be clinically indistinguishable from sarcoidosis. It has also been seen in the wives of beryllium workers and those who live near beryllium refineries. Inhalation of beryllium or the exposure of beryllium to a skin abrasion causes initial sensitization in 2–19% of exposed individuals. Only low levels of exposure are required for this. There is a cell-mediated immune response, with the production of numerous inflammatory cytokines, which cause granulomatous inflammation. Following a long latent period, which may be months to 10 years plus after exposure, non-caseating granulomatous tissue reactions occur in the lungs or on the skin. Similar to sarcoidosis. There is a genetic predisposition to the response to beryllium exposure and it is HLA-mediated (HLA-DPB1(Glu69)). HLA status could be used to identify workers at high risk of berylliosis (but is not routinely at present).

Clinical features of chronic berylliosis

- **Symptoms** Cough, dyspnoea. Macular skin lesions, which do not spontaneously resolve
- **Signs** No clubbing or crepitations in early disease, but both occur with established fibrosis. Hepato/splenomegaly and macular skin lesions. Do not get uveitis or erythema nodosum.

Investigations

- **CXR** Fine reticulonodular appearance throughout both lungs. Finer nodules than those seen in sarcoidosis. Progression to irregular interstitial fibrosis, with irregular linear opacities seen in the lung bases. Hilar lymphadenopathy can occur, but always in association with interstitial lung disease
- **HRCT** Subpleural micronodular change, thickened interlobular septae, traction bronchiectasis, and honeycombing. There may be ground-glass shadowing
- **BAL** High levels of T-lymphocytes

- *PFTs* Restrictive defect, with decreased KCO
- *Pathology* Non-caseating granuloma. May be indistinguishable from sarcoidosis. May develop irregular fibrosis with bulla and cyst formation
- **No single test to distinguish berylliosis from sarcoidosis.**

Management Corticosteroids to try and prevent disease progression. Continue indefinitely as few patients gain complete resolution of symptoms, CXR or PFTs. Annual screening of beryllium-exposed workers with CXR. If they develop breathlessness or skin rashes, this may be an indication to start oral steroids to delay progression to interstitial fibrosis.

Prognosis Progressive disease, although those with very low exposure who develop CXR changes may find they resolve. Associated delayed skin sensitivity (anergy) to tuberculin. Granulomata do not spontaneously resolve, although can be excised if causing problems, such as troublesome lesions on the skin. Interstitial fibrosis occurs in the lungs, which is progressive and leads to cyanosis and death. Other complications include pneumothorax, hypercalcaemia, hypercalciuria, and nephrocalcinosis.

Differential diagnosis

- Sarcoidosis
- Tuberculosis.

In clinic:

- Ask patients with suspected sarcoidosis about possible exposure to beryllium
- Monitor PFTs and CXR to assess disease response or progression.

Connective tissue disease and the lung

Differential diagnosis and standard tests to consider

Patients with connective tissue diseases can develop pulmonary complications, for which they might be referred to a chest physician. Patients typically present with symptoms of dyspnoea, cough, fever, or chest pain. They may often be on immunosuppressive drugs.

Differential diagnosis

In practice, the main differential diagnosis lies between:

Opportunistic pulmonary infection

- May be in those on immunosuppressive drugs, or functionally immunosuppressed from underlying disease
- Any usual organism, also TB, NTM, PCP, fungi, CMV
- Often acute onset with non-specific features of low-grade fever, productive cough, raised inflammatory markers
- Can be very unwell and need full supportive treatment with ITU.

Original disease now affecting the lung

- Often inflammation or fibrosis
- Usually more indolent presentation, with dry cough and dyspnoea, but can become acutely unwell with background of chronic lung disease
- Fine inspiratory crackles on auscultation
- Consider development of pulmonary hypertension in patients with systemic sclerosis.

New pulmonary pathology

- Unrelated to original condition, including pulmonary thromboembolic disease.

Drug side-effects

- Methotrexate—pneumonitis occurs in 5% of patients receiving methotrexate. Potentially life-threatening. Mortality 15–20%. Cough, fever, dyspnoea, widespread crackles, restrictive defect, and pulmonary infiltrates on CXR and CT. Peripheral eosinophilia in 50%. BAL lymphocytosis. Usually subacute onset, but may be sudden. Usually within 4 months of starting methotrexate. Non-specific histological findings. No more common in those with pre-existing lung disease. Treatment: stop the drug, commence steroids, and avoid methotrexate in the future. Can be reversible. Can also get mild intractable cough with methotrexate
- Gold—Alveolar opacities seen on HRCT, with associated fever and skin rash. BAL lymphocytosis. Treatment: stop the drug and commence steroids. Usually reversible
- Penicillamine—Causes obliterative bronchiolitis in rheumatoid arthritis. Can also cause a hypersensitivity pneumonitis and a pulmonary–renal syndrome causing alveolar haemorrhage. May respond to stopping the drug.

Standard tests to consider for the investigation of these patients

- Oxygen saturations and blood gas
- CXR ± HRCT
- Culture of respiratory secretions
- Pulmonary function tests, including KCO
- Bronchoscopy and bronchoalveolar lavage
- Transbronchial or open lung biopsies
- Autoantibody and inflammatory marker levels.

Rheumatoid arthritis (RA)

- Persistent deforming symmetrical peripheral arthropathy
- Pulmonary disease is commoner in men and occasionally occurs before the development of joint problems
- Pneumonia is a common terminal event, causing 15–20% of rheumatoid arthritis deaths.

Pleuritis Frequent, occurring in more than 30% of patients and usually mild. Pleuritic pain, with no obvious other cause.

Pleural effusion Usually asymptomatic. Fluid is typically exudative with a low glucose and low pH and usually a lymphocytosis. Need to exclude other causes for effusion, such as empyema or malignancy. If problematic, may require drainage and steroids. (See page 314.)

Pulmonary fibrosis Minor pulmonary fibrosis found in up to 60% of patients in lung biopsy studies, but CXR changes only seen in 1–5%. Hence symptomatic disease is unusual. Tends to occur in patients who have multisystem disease, including vasculitis, and those with nodules, seropositive disease, and high ANA titres. More common in men, and smoking is a risk factor for fibrosis development.

- *Presents* with progressive dyspnoea
- *Examination*: clubbing and bilateral basal crepitations
- *PFTs*: low kCO, restrictive pattern
- Radiologically and histologically similar to usual interstitial pneumonitis (UIP), with subpleural, basal reticular pattern, but can be like non-specific interstitial pneumonitis (NSIP)
- *Treatment* steroids or immunosuppressants do little to change the course, but should be tried.

Also can get acute pneumonitis, which presents with rapidly deteriorating dyspnoea and development of respiratory failure, or acute deterioration on background of chronic fibrosis. Acute pneumonitis tends to be more steroid-responsive.

Pulmonary nodules occur in less than 5% of patients with RA. Usually found incidentally on CXR. Only occur in seropositive disease and patients may have other nodules elsewhere, such as elbows and fingers. Single or multiple, may measure up to 7 cm. May cavitate and cause haemoptysis or pneumothorax. Mostly asymptomatic. Main differential diagnosis is lung cancer. Usually followed on CT to ensure they are of stable size. May need biopsy to exclude malignancy.

Bronchiectasis is often subtle with minimal clinical features, but may be found in 30%. May be seen in association with pulmonary fibrosis. Diagnosis made on HRCT.

Organizing pneumonia Clinical features of pneumonia, with fever, dyspnoea, and multifocal consolidation, that do not respond to antibiotics. Can be disease-or drug-induced (gold), or may have no obvious cause and is then known as cryptogenic (see page 450). Confirmed by transbronchial or open lung biopsy that shows acini filled with loose connective tissue and a variable inflammatory infiltrate. Often a dramatic response to steroids. May need long-term immunosuppression.

Obliterative bronchiolitis Rare. Terminal bronchioles progressively obliterated by inflammatory connective tissue.
- May present with dyspnoea and hyperinflated chest, with basal crepitations
- *PFTs:* irreversible obstructive pattern
- *CXR:* hyperinflation, no infiltrates
- *HRCT:* mosaic pattern
- *Biopsy* shows destruction of terminal bronchiolar wall by granulation tissue, effacement of the lumen, and replacement of the bronchiole by fibrous tissue. Irreversible pathology, usually unresponsive to treatment
- May be rapidly progressive
- Can give trial of oral steroids, continuing with high-dose inhaled steroids if any response. Consider transplant. Penicillamine was thought to be a causative factor, but the evidence for this is now weaker.

Vasculitis and rarely pulmonary haemorrhage.

Cricoarytenoid arthritis Seen in studies in up to 75% of patients with rheumatoid arthritis by fibre-optic laryngoscopy and HRCT, but rarely symptomatic. Unrelated to lung fibrosis. Can cause sore throat, hoarse voice, or upper airways obstruction with stridor. Flow volume loop may be abnormal. This may need tracheostomy and steroids—oral and joint injection.

Caplan's syndrome Rheumatoid arthritis, single or multiple chest nodules, and coal-workers' pneumoconiosis.

Systemic lupus erythematosus (SLE)

- Multiorgan autoimmune disease, mainly affecting women
- Double-stranded DNA antibodies present in high titres and these may be the causative agent
- Can also get a drug-induced lupus syndrome, which improves when the drug is stopped
- Pulmonary disease often seen and may be a presenting feature of the disease.

Pleural disease Most common manifestation of pulmonary disease. Often asymptomatic, but may have pain due to pleuritis. Can get pleural effusions in 50% of patients, which cause breathlessness. These are often bilateral and exudative, with a neutrophilia or a lymphocytosis if the effusion is chronic. Can be haemorrhagic. Pleural biopsy findings are non-specific. Need to exclude other causes for effusion, such as empyema or malignancy. If symptomatic, may need treatment with nonsteroidal anti-inflammatory drugs or steroids.

Atelectasis associated with pleurisy or effusion.

Diffuse lung disease Occurs in up to 70% of patients, but usually mild and asymptomatic. Radiologically similar to rheumatoid lung fibrosis. Only 5% develop clinical disease similar to UIP with dyspnoea, cough, and basal crackles. May be associated with pleuritic pain. PFTs show restrictive defect with reduced kCO. Rarely progressive and severe.

Acute lupus pneumonitis In <2%, severe illness with high mortality rate of over 50%. Cough, dyspnoea, fever, pleuritic pain, hypoxia. Widespread crackles. CXR shows infiltrates, which may be widespread. Histologically non-specific. Need to exclude infection, pulmonary oedema. Treatment with steroids and cytotoxic drugs may be necessary and may have dramatic response. Can progress to chronic interstitial pneumonitis.

Bronchiolitis obliterans See page 466.

Pulmonary nodules

Pulmonary hypertension due to pulmonary vasoconstriction, rather than pulmonary vasculitis. Commoner in those with Raynaud's phenomenon. Associated with poorer prognosis: 50% 2-year mortality. Diagnosed on echocardiography. Need to exclude pulmonary emboli as a cause, especially in those with antiphospholipid antibodies. Treatment as for primary pulmonary hypertension (see page 398).

Pulmonary emboli Commoner in the 20–30% with antiphospholipid antibodies.

Shrinking lung syndrome Dyspnoea caused by reduced lung volumes and poor respiratory reserve, due to diaphragmatic muscle weakness. Small lungs on CXR. Normal lung parenchyma on CT. Restrictive lung function tests, with high kCO. May improve with steroids.

Alveolar haemorrhage Rare. May be life-threatening. Can have associated glomerulonephritis. Acute dyspnoea with infiltrates on CXR. Raised KCO. Treat with high-dose steroids + cyclophosphamide.

Criteria of the American College of Rheumatology for the classification of SLE

SLE if 4 or more criteria present, serially or simultaneously, during any interval

- Malar rash
- Discoid rash
- Photosensitivity
- Oral ulcers
- Arthritis
- Serositis
- Pleuritis or pericarditis
- Renal disorder: proteinuria > 0.5 g/24 hrs or 3+ persistently, or cellular casts
- Neurological disorder: seizures, or psychosis (having excluded drugs or other causes)
- Haematological disorder: haemolytic anaemia, or leucopenia ($<4.0 \times 10^9$/l on two or more occasions), lymphopenia (1.5×10^9/l on two or more occasions), thrombocytopenia ($<100 \times 10^9$/l)
- Immunological disorder: raised anti-dsDNA antibody, anti-Sm antibody, positive finding of antiphospholipid antibodies
- Antinuclear antibody in raised titre (in the absence of drugs known to be associated with drug-induced lupus).

Drug-induced lupus: causative drugs include
- Isoniazid
- Procainamide
- Hydralazine
- Minocycline
- Penicillamine
- Anticonvulsants.

Further information

Pleuropulmonary manifestations of SLE, Rare diseases 7. Keane M, Lynch J *Thorax* 2000; **55**: 159–66

Polymyositis and dermatomyositis

Two separate disorders:
- Polymyositis is an inflammatory myopathy, causing symmetrical proximal muscle weakness
- Dermatomyositis is an inflammatory myopathy with a characteristic rash.

Creatine kinase levels raised up to 50 times normal. Antinuclear and myositis specific antibodies positive (Jo-1). Dermatomyositis is frequently associated with underlying malignancy, including lung, oesophagus, breast, colon, and ovary, so therefore needs thorough investigation. Pulmonary complications are a common and frequent cause of death.

Pulmonary fibrosis in 20–30%. Patients present with dyspnoea. Mostly there is basal fibrosis—usually similar to UIP, but can develop a more acute pneumonitis resembling acute interstitial pneumonia (page 452).
- *HRCT* shows patchy consolidation and peripheral reticular pattern
- *Histology* may show features of organizing pneumonia and fibrosing alveolitis and therefore may have better response to treatment
- Lung involvement frequently associated with antisynthetase antibodies
- May require treatment with steroids or cyclophosphamide.

Ventilatory failure due to intercostal and diaphragmatic muscle weakness. Restrictive defect on PFTs.

Organizing pneumonia Poorer prognosis if associated with features of fibrosis.

Pulmonary hypertension secondary to lung disease.

Pulmonary vasculitis Causing haemoptysis or, rarely, alveolar haemorrhage.

Aspiration pneumonia in 20%, associated with marked increase in mortality. Caused by dysphagia and pharyngeal muscle weakness and regurgitation.

Criteria for diagnosis of poly/dermatomyositis

- Symmetrical proximal muscle weakness developing over weeks or months
- Elevated serum muscle enzymes, creatine kinase, and aldolase
- Typical EMG findings:
  - Myopathic potentials (low amplitude, short duration, polyphasic)
  - Fibrillation
  - Complex repetitive discharges
  - Typical muscle biopsy findings—endomysial inflammation.
- Dermatological features of dermatomyositis:
  - Gottron's papules, involving fingers, elbows, knees, and medial malleoli
  - Heliotrope sign around the eyes
  - Erythematous rash around back, shoulders, upper chest and face.

Systemic sclerosis

This disease affects women more than men (4:1), and often presents in the fifth decade. It is a clinical diagnosis and there are 4 types:

- **Limited cutaneous** (formerly known as CREST). Accounts for 60% of systemic sclerosis cases. Patients often have longstanding Raynaud's, and develop non-pitting oedema of the fingers, which become 'sausage-shaped'. After a few weeks to months, they develop thickened shiny skin. Later they can develop skin changes on the hands, face, and neck, microstomia, digital and facial telangectasias, intra- and subcutaneous calcification, and oesophageal dysmotility (74%). Patients can also develop pulmonary fibrosis (26%), pulmonary hypertension (21%), cardiac (9%) and renal disease (8%), but less commonly than in diffuse cutaneous disease

- **Diffuse cutaneous** Abrupt onset disease, with widespread symmetrical itchy painful swelling of fingers, arms, feet, legs, and face, and associated constitutional symptoms. There is oedema, which is replaced by tight shiny skin, bound to underlying structures, within a few months. There is cutaneous thickening, as well as hypo- or hyperpigmentation. Raynaud's phenomenon is present, as well as skin sclerosis on the trunk and upper arms, arthropathy, renal disease (18%), pulmonary fibrosis (41%), pulmonary hypertension (17%), and cardiac (12%) and GI disease (68%)

- **Overlap syndromes,** or mixed connective tissue disease, have features of systemic sclerosis together with those of at least one other autoimmune rheumatic disease, such as SLE, rheumatoid arthritis, polymyositis. Over time they may develop other organ involvement and evolve into a more defined disease

- **Systemic sclerosis sine scleroderma** Vascular or fibrotic visceral features without skin scleroderma. May or may not have Raynaud's phenomenon. May develop interstitial lung disease, oesophagitis, arrhythmias, malabsorption, pseudo-obstruction, renal failure. Less than 2% of cases.

Systemic sclerosis pulmonary disease is the most common cause of death in patients with systemic sclerosis.

Pulmonary fibrosis is seen at post-mortem in up to 75% of patients. Antinuclear antibody is positive in 60%, of speckled or nucleolar type. Pulmonary involvement is seen particularly if Scl 70 antibody is present. Anticentromere antibodies, however, are associated with reduced risk.

- *Present with* dyspnoea and a history of Raynaud's
- *Examination:* signs of systemic sclerosis, fine bibasal crepitations
- *PFTs* show restrictive defect and reduced kCO. Rapidly falling kCO is a poor prognostic sign. *HRCT* is performed if PFTs are abnormal. Mostly non-specific interstitial pneumonitis (NSIP) pattern on HRCT, but can be UIP pattern. May need open lung biopsy to confirm diagnosis
- *Treatment* with steroids and cyclophosphamide
- *Prognosis:* Systemic sclerosis associated interstitial lung disease has better prognosis than pure UIP. This may be related to slower disease progression, rather than any greater response to immunosuppressive treatment. 15% of patients have progressive and severe disease. Associated increased risk of lung cancer.

Pulmonary hypertension May be isolated or secondary to interstitial lung disease. Isolated pulmonary hypertension is characteristic of limited cutaneous disease, especially in those with cutaneous telangectasias and anticentromere antibodies. Pathologically similar to primary pulmonary hypertension. Sub-intimal cell proliferation, endothelial hyperplasia, and the obliteration of small intrapulmonary vessels.

- *Present with* dyspnoea, right ventricular hypertrophy, and right heart failure
- *Diagnosis* by echocardiography
- *Treatment* as for PPH (see page 398). May respond to prostacyclin infusions, or may need transplant
- *Prognosis* better than for those with PPH.

Chest wall limitation by skin scleroderma over chest ('hide-bound chest').

Organizing pneumonia

Aspiration pneumonia Uncommon and due to oesophageal dysmotility.

Sjögren's syndrome

- Inflammation and destruction of primarily the salivary and lachrymal glands
- Keratoconjunctivitis sicca or xerostomia (dry eyes and dry mouth) is evidence of primary disease but, when associated with connective tissue disease, especially rheumatoid arthritis, is secondary Sjögren's
- Classical Sicca syndrome includes dry eyes and mouth and parotid or salivary gland enlargement
- Pulmonary involvement occurs in about 25%.

Pleurisy

Airways inflammation Bronchial hyperresponsiveness, chronic bronchitis, and small airways disease. Mild abnormalities on PFTs, rarely significant.

Dry cough Atrophy of mucus gland in trachea and bronchi and lymphoplasmocytic infiltrate (xerotrachea). Possibly a higher incidence of chest infections. Treatment: nebulized saline, physiotherapy.

Organizing pneumonia Rare.

Diffuse lung disease Often asymptomatic, but may have cough, dyspnoea, and crackles on examination. PFTs show a restrictive defect and lymphocytic interstitial pneumonia (LIP) or UIP pattern on CT.

Lymphoma Unusual, but is 40 times more common in Sjögren's syndrome, especially in patients with high levels of immunoglobulins, autoantibodies, and cryoglobulins. Usually B-cell lymphoma. Can mimic organizing pneumonia.

Ankylosing spondylitis

- Chronic inflammatory disease causing spinal ankylosis with sacroiliac joint involvement
- 90% of Caucasian patients are HLA B27 positive.

Pulmonary fibrosis occurs in 2%, especially those with advanced disease. Typically bilaterally in the upper lobes. May develop cysts/cavities and become colonized with Aspergillus, which can require treatment.

Pleural involvement Pleuritis and apical pleural thickening.

Restrictive defect due to fixed deformity of thorax, limiting breathing.

Autoantibodies: disease associations

Antinuclear antibody (ANA)	+ve in
SLE	99%
Rheumatoid arthritis	32%
Juvenile rheumatoid arthritis	76%
Chronic active hepatitis	75%
Sjögren's syndrome	68%
Systemic sclerosis	64%
Polymyositis	
Polyarteritis nodosa	
Myasthenia gravis	
Autoimmune thyroid disease	
Extensive burns	
Normal controls	0–2%

Extractable nuclear antigen (ENA)	(done by lab if ANA positive)

Anti-double stranded DNA—SLE
Anti Sm—SLE
Antitopoisomerase 1—diffuse scleroderma
Anticentromere—limited scleroderma
Anti Scl-70—pulmonary fibrosis in scleroderma
Anti Jo-1—myositis
Anti Ro—Sjögren's, SLE, fetal heart block
Anti RNP—SLE, scleroderma, myositis, mixed connective tissue disease, and rheumatoid arthritis

Rheumatoid factor	+ve in
Rheumatoid arthritis	70–80%
Sjögren's syndrome	<100%
Felty's syndrome	<100%
Systemic sclerosis	30%
Still's disease	Rarely positive
Infective endocarditis	<50%
SLE	<40%
Normal controls	5–10%

Also: Neoplasms after radio- or chemotherapy
   Hyerglobulinaemic states
   Dermatomyositis

Vasculitis and the lung

Classification

These are rare conditions, but are often seen in the specialist chest clinic. Clinical features can be non-specific and similar to those seen in other diseases and diagnosis can therefore be difficult. Vasculitides are great 'mimickers' of other diseases, such as lung cancer or ARDS, and have a high untreated mortality, so must be considered. There is considerable overlap between the different vasculitides, which can make definitive diagnosis difficult.

Suspect a diagnosis of vasculitis if:
- Weight loss
- Low-grade fever
- Raised inflammatory markers
- Chest disease is not improving or responding to treatment as expected:
  - Unexplained dyspnoea
  - Hypoxia
  - Unexplained desaturation on exercise
  - Haemoptysis
  - Sinus or nasal disease
  - Wheeze
  - CXR abnormalities / infiltrates
  - Abnormal KCO
- Associated renal impairment or positive urine dip for blood or protein
- Raised autoantibodies
- No other clear diagnosis.

The primary pathology in vasculitis is inflammation and necrosis of differing sized blood vessels. The pulmonary vessels are involved as part of a multi-systemic vasculitis process.

Small vessel vasculitides are the most common to involve the lung. Arterioles, capillaries, and venules located within the lung interstitium are affected. Neutrophil infiltration and subsequent fibrinoid necrosis causes vessel wall destruction. Necrotizing pulmonary capillaritis can also occur: a marked neutrophilic infiltration of the interstitium. Interstitial capillaries become damaged, allowing red blood cells to enter the alveolus; thus alveolar haemorrhage is a feature of many of the small vessel vasculitides.

Further information

Small vessel vasculitis of the lung. Rare diseases 10, Schwarz M, Brown K *Thorax* 2000; **55**: 502–10

Classification of vasculitis, based on the Chapel Hill International Consensus, 1992

Primary vasculitis	Lung involvement	ANCA
SMALL VESSEL		
Wegener's granulomatosis	Frequent	c-ANCA in 75%, p-ANCA in 15%
Churg–Strauss	Frequent	p-ANCA in 70%
Microscopic polyangiitis	Frequent	c/p-ANCA
Goodpasture's disease	Frequent	p-ANCA in 10–20%
MEDIUM SIZE VESSEL		
Polyarteritis nodosa	Rare	Negative
LARGE VESSEL		
Giant cell arteritis	Rare	Negative
Takayasu arteritis	Frequent	Negative

ANCA

Anti-neutrophil cytoplasmic antibodies react with cytoplasmic granule enzymes in neutrophils and stain them in one of two ways:
- Diffusely cytoplasmic pattern or **c-ANCA**
- Perinuclear pattern or **p-ANCA**.

These autoantibodies may have a direct role in pathogenesis as well as being disease markers.

ANCA have 2 major specificities:
- Antiproteinase 3 antibodies (anti-PR3)—associated with c-ANCA pattern
- Antimyeloperoxidase antibodies (anti-MPO)—associated with p-ANCA pattern.

c-ANCA (anti-PR3) targets proteinase 3 and may suggest Wegener's granulomatosis (75% of cases are c-ANCA positive). Levels correlate with disease activity. Also found in patients with microscopic polyangiitis (45% of those with clinical disease will be c-ANCA positive).

p-ANCA (anti-MPO) targets myeloperoxidase and has a wider range of disease associations, including other vasculitides and autoimmune diseases, HIV, lung cancer, pulmonary fibrosis, and pulmonary emboli.

Wegener's granulomatosis: presentation and diagnosis

Definition and epidemiology Necrotizing vasculitis affecting small and medium size vessels, especially in the upper and lower respiratory tract and also the kidneys. Associated granulomata.

- Unknown cause
- Male = female
- 3/100,000, 80–97% Caucasian
- Any age, but most common between 40 and 55 years.

Clinical features

- **ENT** In 90%, upper airways involvement will be the first presenting sign. Nasal congestion and epistaxis, with inflamed, crusty, ulcerated nasal mucosa. Nasal septum perforation. Late sign is a saddle nose deformity. Sinusitis is common and may be painful. Otitis media. Subglottic stenosis, causing upper airway obstruction, dyspnoea, voice change, and cough. Abnormal flow-volume loops
- **Lung** Affected in 85–90% of patients. Haemoptysis, cough, dyspnoea. Pleuritic chest pain
- **Kidney** Affected in 77% of patients. Haematuria, proteinuria, and red cell casts. Only 10% have renal impairment initially, but 80% will have involvement during their disease course. Characteristic progressive deterioration of renal function
- **Systemic** Fever and weight loss
- **Other organ systems (skin, eyes, joints, CNS)** Vasculitic skin rash with granulomatous involvement in 46%. Muscle and joint pains. Conjunctivitis, scleritis, proptosis, eye pain, visual loss. Mononeuritis multiplex and CNS disease.

Investigations

Consider:

- *CXR* Flitting cavitating pulmonary nodules, consolidation, or pulmonary infiltrates, alveolar haemorrhage, parenchymal distortion, large and small airway disease, pleural effusion, bronchiectasis. Can look like neoplasms, infection, or fluid overload
- *HRCT* of chest
- *Oxygen saturations*
- *FBC, U&E, CRP, ESR*
- *Serum ANCA*, especially c-ANCA, is sensitive and fairly specific. Present in 90% of patients with extensive Wegener's and 75% with limited. p-ANCA positive in 5–10% of patients with Wegener's. Combining indirect immunofluorescence with specific immunoassays for antibodies to PR3 and MPO increases sensitivity and specificity for Wegner's and microscopic polyangiitis to over 90%. **Remember ANCA can be negative, especially in disease confined to the respiratory tract.** ANCA titres rise prior to a relapse and are higher when disease is active, and this can act as a guide to starting treatment. However, high

ANCA levels in the absence of clinical symptoms or signs may not represent active disease, and therefore ANCA levels should not be used in isolation to determine treatment

- **Urine dipstick and microscopy** Red cell casts
- **Pulmonary function tests, including kCO**
- **Image sinuses** Bony destruction makes Wegener's likely
- **Bronchoscopy** May show inflammation and ulceration of larynx, trachea, and bronchi. Scarring and stenosis may be seen. BAL is neutrophilic, also with eosinophils and lymphocytes. Transbronchial biopsy is unlikely to be diagnostic
- **Biopsy** *Respiratory tract and nose*—granulomata in association with medium and small vessel necrotizing vasculitis and surrounding inflammation. Nasal biopsies are often non-specific and may not be diagnostic. *Renal biopsy*—focal segmental or diffuse necrotizing glomerulonephritis. Pauci-immune and granulomata rare. Not specific for Wegener's. *Skin biopsy*—leucocytoclastic vasculitis ± granulomata.

Diagnosis Biopsy and ANCA are key to diagnosis. Biopsy whichever site is affected. May be nasal, lung (open or thoracoscopic), skin, or renal. If there is evidence on urine dip of renal vasculitis, this may be the best and easiest biopsy site. Disease may be patchy in nature, requiring repeat biopsies if the first is negative. High c-ANCA and anti-proteinase 3 (PR3) highly suggestive of Wegener's.

Differential diagnosis of Wegener's granulomatosis

Malignancy, TB, sarcoidosis, allergic bronchopulmonary aspergillosis, Goodpasture's disease (anti-glomerular basement membrane disease with pulmonary haemorrhage and nephritis), SLE, microscopic polyangiitis, connective tissue disease.

Wegener's granulomatosis: management

- Involve the renal team and share care of the patient
- Standard regimen for active/progressive pulmonary or renal disease or CNS disease:
  - Oral prednisolone (1 mg/kg/day) for 1 month, decreased over 6–12 months
  - Combined with cyclophosphamide orally (2 mg/kg/day, up to 200 mg/day) for 6–12 months
  - Aiming to prevent irreversible tissue necrosis. There is good evidence that this regime gives improvement in 91% of patients
  - Restart the regime if the patient relapses—this may occur in 50%
- For patients who are unwell, with rapidly progressive renal failure or massive pulmonary haemorrhage:
  - Plasma exchange/plasmapheresis has been shown to be more effective than methylprednisolone in the treatment of Wegener's granulomatosis. In patients with severe pulmonary haemorrhage it is also effective and can be given along with fresh frozen plasma
  - Combined pulsed methyl prednisolone (500–1000 mg/day depending on body weight for 3 days) and intravenous cyclophosphamide (600 mg/m^2) may be required
  - Dialysis for renal failure
- Immunosuppression is recommended to continue for at least 1 year, as relapses are common
- PCP prophylaxis with co-trimoxazole is recommended (960 mg 3 x/week). There is some evidence that co-trimoxazole alone may be effective in the treatment of especially limited Wegener's, although the reasons are not clear. It is thought to be due to the suppression of *Staphylococcus aureus*
- Bone protection should be considered
- Low-dose methotrexate can be used in patients who cannot tolerate cyclophosphamide and have less aggressive disease. It can also be used to maintain remission in patients who have had cyclophosphamide initially. NB. Methotrexate is contraindicated in patients with renal failure
- **If isolated sinusitis:** can use antibiotics and nasal steroids initially, moving to oral steroids only if this fails
- **Follow-up:** Regularly, with monitoring of FBC, U&E, CRP, LFT, ANCA, CXR, and kCO
- 75–90% of patients can be brought into remission with treatment. Long-term follow-up is necessary as relapses occur in 50%.

Prognosis *Limited disease* with pulmonary but no renal involvement and an often negative c-ANCA test has a better prognosis. However, this can progress over time to *extensive disease*, with classical destructive sinusitis, nephritis, and vasculitis and strong c-ANCA positivity, and is associated with higher mortality. Untreated, 80% of people with extensive Wegener's will die in 1 year.

Microscopic polyangiitis

At least as common as Wegener's and may be hard to distinguish. Managed in the same way.

- **Incidence** Male = female, mean age 50, mainly Caucasians
- **Kidneys** Main organ affected by a small vessel necrotizing vasculitis, causing proteinuria, and haematuria. Renal biopsy shows focal segmental glomerulonephritis with fibrinoid necrosis and sparse immune deposits
- **Pulmonary involvement** occurs in 30–50% of patients, with pleurisy, asthma, haemoptysis, and pulmonary haemorrhage. CXR may be suggestive of pulmonary haemorrhage
- **p-ANCA** positive, often c-ANCA also.

Treatment with immunosuppression: steroids and cyclophosphamide.

Further information
Wegener's granulomatosis. Rare Diseases 3, Langford C, Hoffman G *Thorax* 1999; **54**: 629–63

Goodpasture's disease

Definition and epidemiology Linear deposition of IgG on the basement membranes of alveoli and glomeruli, which damages collagen and in the lungs allows leakage of blood.

- Anti-glomerular basement membrane antibodies are detectable in blood
- Alveolar haemorrhage and glomerulonephritis
- Important differential diagnosis of pulmonary–renal syndrome
- Annual incidence of 1 case per million
- Male:female = 4:1
- Commonest age 20–30 years
- Second peak when women in their late 60s are affected by glomerulonephritis alone
- Cause unknown. Often a preceding viral infection. Smokers at greater risk of pulmonary haemorrhage, but not of Goodpasture's disease
- HLA DR2 association in 60–70%.

Clinical features

- Haemoptysis in 80–90%—more common in smokers
- Cough, dyspnoea, fatigue, and weakness
- Examination: inspiratory crackles common.

Investigations

- **Serum electrolytes** show renal disturbance and often renal failure
- **FBC** Iron deficiency anaemia
- **Urine dip and microscopy** Haematuria, proteinuria, granular and typically red blood cell casts. Occasionally macroscopic haematuria
- **Anti-GBM** and autoantibody screen
- **CXR ± CT** Diffuse bilateral patchy air space shadowing in mid and lower zones. May see air bronchograms
- **PFTs** Restrictive defect with raised kCO if alveolar haemorrhage present.

Diagnosis Renal biopsy usually shows diffuse crescentic glomerulonephritis. Linear IgG deposition detected by immunofluorescence or immunoperoxidase. Lung biopsy shows active intra-alveolar haemorrhage with collections of haemosiderin laden macrophages. These are not specific changes, but may also show linear immunofluorescence staining of IgG.

Differential diagnosis Wegener's granulomatosis, other pulmonary renal syndromes

Management

- Involve the renal team and share care of the patient
- Plasma exchange improves the speed of response to immunosuppression
- High-dose steroids and cyclophosphamide

- May need dialysis. Renal function may not improve and renal transplant is only an option later if anti-GBM antibody levels become low
- Recurrence is uncommon once disease is controlled. It usually responds to further immunosuppression. Residual defects in PFTs frequent.

Prognosis Rapidly progressive pulmonary haemorrhage and renal failure. Usually fatal if not treated.

Churg–Strauss syndrome

Definition and epidemiology Asthma, blood eosinophilia, and an eosinophilic granulomatous inflammation of the respiratory tract, with necrotizing vasculitis affecting small and medium sized vessels.
- Rare, 2.4 per million population, but 64 per million of an asthmatic population (who may have been misdiagnosed with asthma)
- Middle-aged adults
- 2 male:1 female
- Unknown cause. Montelukast was postulated as a possible cause, but this is now thought unlikely. Development of Churg–Strauss syndrome in people on montelukast probably related to their decreased steroid dose 'unmasking' Churg–Strauss syndrome.

Clinical features A diagnosis of Churg–Strauss syndrome can be made if 4 of the following 6 criteria are present:
- Asthma—may have had for years, often maturity onset, difficult to control, associated with rhinitis and nasal polyps
- Blood eosinophilia >10%
- Vasculitic neuropathy, such as mononeuritis multiplex (occurs in 75%)
- Pulmonary infiltrates
- Sinus disease
- Extravascular eosinophils on biopsy findings (American College of Rheumatology criteria, 1990)
- Also may have:
  • Myositis and cardiac failure, cardiomyopathy, coronary artery inflammation, pericardial effusion
  • Eosinophilic infiltration of mesenteric vessels causing GI disturbance
  • Alveolar haemorrhage
  • Rarely, proteinuria caused by renal disease with focal segmental glomerulonephritis. Renal failure is rare
  • Skin nodules and purpura
  • Myalgia and arthralgia
  • Fever and weight loss.

Typical pattern of disease has three phases: beginning with asthma, then developing blood and tissue eosinophilia, then going on to systemic vasculitis. The asthma precedes the vasculitis, often by years (mean 8 years).

Investigations
- *CXR* Fleeting peripheral pulmonary infiltrates and bilateral multifocal consolidation
- *HRCT* Ground-glass inflammation, pulmonary nodules, bronchial wall thickening, or alveolar haemorrhage
- *Bronchoscopy* BAL: marked eosinophilia
- *Pathology* Extravascular tissue eosinophilia, necrotizing angiitis, granulomata
- *Serum markers* Peripheral blood eosinophilia. p-ANCA and anti-MPO positive in two-thirds. ANCA levels may not correlate with disease activity, but blood eosinophilia is a good guide.

Diagnosis Predominantly a clinical diagnosis. Pathological confirmation of eosinophilic tissue infiltration or vasculitis desirable. Biopsy easiest site affected, such as skin, kidney, or by open or thorascopic lung biopsy.

Differential diagnosis Allergic bronchopulmonary aspergillosis, sarcoidosis, drug and parasitic causes of eosinophilic pneumonias, hypersensitivity pneumonitis, hypereosinophilic syndrome.

Management Depends on severity of disease at presentation.
- *If isolated pulmonary disease*, oral prednisolone 1 mg/kg (max 60mg/day) for 1 month or until no evidence of disease, then slowly decrease over 1 year, with increases if symptoms recur
- *If unwell, or with alveolar haemorrhage*, pulsed methyl prednisolone IV for 3 days, followed by high-dose oral steroids, with or without cyclophosphamide
- *In cardiac or GI disease, relapse, or life-threatening situations*, such as requiring organ support, cyclophosphamide should be added
- Plasma exchange is of no benefit
- Treatment is aimed at reversing organ damage and reducing relapse rate
- *To maintain remission*, prednisolone and one other immunosuppressant drug are usually required. Cyclophosphamide is often changed to azathioprine after 4 to 6 months
- Prophylactic co-trimoxazole should be given (960 mg 3 x/week) and consider bone protection for steroids
- *Follow-up:* regularly, with checks on FBC and eosinophil count, CXR.

Prognosis Good prognosis if isolated pulmonary disease. Good response to steroids. May continue to have asthma despite control of vasculitis, which can be severe and difficult to control. Poor prognosis associated with cardiac disease and severe gastrointestinal disease, causing bleeding, perforation or necrosis. Untreated, 5-year survival rate is 25%. Also associated with worse prognosis: proteinuria >1 g/24 hrs, renal insufficiency, CNS involvement. Cardiac disease is the main cause of death.

Further information
Churg–Strauss syndrome. Noth I *et al. Lancet* 2003; **361**: 587–94

www.vasculitis.org

Rare pulmonary vasculitic diseases

Polyarteritis nodosa
- Similar to microscopic polyangiitis, but affecting medium-sized vessels
- May exist as an 'overlap' disorder with Wegener's or Churg–Strauss
- Lung involvement rare
- Sometimes associated with previous hepatitis B or rarely hepatitis C infection.

Takayasu's arteritis
- Predominantly young women, often Asian
- Vasculitis affecting the aorta and its major branches. Large- and medium-sized pulmonary vessels affected, but involvement is usually silent. Pulmonary artery stenosis and occlusion common, occasionally with mild pulmonary hypertension
- **Presents** with fevers and weight loss. Noted to have absent peripheral pulses, arterial bruits, and discrepancies in BP
- **Diagnosis** made by angiography
- **Treatment** Steroids may reduce symptoms, but do not affect mortality. Angioplasty and surgical procedures reduce the complications. Spontaneous remissions may occur.

Giant cell arteritis
- Commonest form of systemic vasculitis affecting large- and medium-sized vessels
- 24 cases per 100,000. Predominantly elderly females
- **Present with** non-specific symptoms of fever and weight loss, also headache, scalp tenderness, and jaw pain. Amaurosis fugax and visual loss due to optic neuritis
- **Pulmonary complications** occur in 9–25% of cases. They are relatively minor, with cough, sore throat, and hoarseness. Pulmonary function tests and CXR normal
- **Diagnosis** High ESR, temporal artery biopsy showing pan-arteritis and giant cell formation
- **Treatment** Good response to oral steroids. Continue for 1–2 years.

Gastrointestinal disease and the lung

Hepatic hydrothorax and hepatopulmonary syndrome

Hepatic hydrothorax Predominantly right-sided pleural effusion occurring in patients with liver disease and no cardiorespiratory disease, often with minimal ascites. The ascitic fluid accumulates in the chest as a result of diaphragmatic defects. Occurs in 5–12% of patients with cirrhosis and portal hypertension. Spontaneous bacterial empyema can occur and is associated with mortality of 20%. Diuretics are rarely effective. The definitive treatment is liver transplantation.

Hepatopulmonary syndrome (HPS) is the triad of:
- Chronic liver disease and portal hypertension
- Abnormal intrapulmonary peripheral vascular vasodilatation with decreased pulmonary vascular resistance (right to left shunt) and subsequent ventilation–perfusion abnormalities
- Arterial hypoxia.

It occurs in 4–29% of patients with chronic liver disease. The mechanism is thought to be related to the release of vasoactive mediators from portal hypertension causing altered bowel perfusion, which in turn leads to pulmonary vascular dilatation, with the formation of vascular spider naevi on the pleura. Patients with cirrhosis who develop hepatopulmonary syndrome have a worse prognosis.

Presentation is with progressive dyspnoea and cyanosis. Examination reveals clubbing and telangiectasia, with associated stigmata of chronic liver disease.

Diagnosis
- *Hypoxia* on blood gases <8.6 kPa on air, at rest and upright. Platypnoea and orthodeoxia are present, that is, breathlessness and desaturation on sitting upright, caused by preferential perfusion of basal pulmonary vasculature. Lying flat relieves this. These changes may be seen in other lung diseases but, in the presence of liver disease, is suggestive of HPS. Hypoxia is poorly reversed with 100% oxygen, due to the pulmonary shunting
- *Contrast-enhanced echocardiogram* is positive. Contrast/saline bubbles are injected peripherally, and are normally seen only in the right heart and are then filtered by the pulmonary bed. In the presence of intrapulmonary shunts, these are seen in the left ventricle. (False positive results occur if right-to-left cardiac shunt present, which can be excluded during echocardiogram)
- *Pulmonary technetium-99 perfusion scan* assesses the shunt fraction. Normally the radiolabelled albumin is trapped in the pulmonary capillary bed. In the presence of intrapulmonary or cardiac shunts, there is significant uptake of radiolabelled albumin in the brain or spleen. A shunt index fraction of >20% indicates severe hepatopulmonary syndrome
- *CT chest* is performed to rule out other pulmonary co-morbid disease.

Treatment
- Oxygen if PaO_2 < 8 kPa
- Avoid vasodilators. There is minimal evidence for pharmacological intervention
- Mainstay of treatment is liver transplantation, which reverses the condition. Hypoxia may take months to improve. Severe hypoxia (PaO_2 < 6 kpa) is associated with increased mortality post-transplant, as there is increased risk of hepatic ischaemia
- Transjugular intrahepatic portosystemic shunt (TIPS) is ineffective
- Coil embolization can be tried in selected cases with AV communications.

Prognosis is poor, with a mortality of 40% in 2.5 years.

Portopulmonary hypertension

Portopulmonary hypertension (POPH) is pulmonary artery hypertension occurring in association with portal hypertension. It occurs in an estimated 2–5% of patients with cirrhosis and is present in around 16% of those referred for liver transplant. The mechanism is unclear but probably relates to a hyperdynamic circulation, high cardiac output, cytokine release, and possible pulmonary emboli.

Defined as:

- Elevated pulmonary artery pressure (>25 mmHg at rest, >30 mmHg during exercise)
- Increased pulmonary vascular resistance due to pulmonary vasoconstriction and obliterative vascular remodelling (>120 dyne s^{-1} cm^{-5})
- Abnormal left ventricular end diastolic/wedge pressure (<15 mmHg)
- In the setting of portal hypertension (portal pressure > 10 mmHg).

Presentation Dyspnoea on exertion, possibly syncope, chest pain, fatigue, palpitations, haemoptysis, and orthopnoea. There may be signs of volume overload with raised JVP and pedal oedema. P2 may be loud, with pulmonary and tricuspid regurgitation, as well as stigmata of chronic liver disease. It is usually diagnosed 4–7 years after the diagnosis of portal hypertension.

Diagnosis

- **Hypoxia** on blood gases, but less so than in hepatopulmonary syndrome
- **CXR** may be normal or show prominent pulmonary arteries and enlarged right heart
- **ECG** shows RVH, RBBB, RAD, and sinus tachycardia
- **kCO** may be decreased
- **Echocardiography** is the main screening test and is diagnostic if the right ventricular pressure is >50 mmHg
- Exclude other causes of pulmonary hypertension
- **Right heart catheterization** with vasodilator studies is performed
- The changes in the vessels in POPH are the same histologically as those seen in PPH (see page 394).

Treatment Options are also the same as for patients with PPH, with vasodilators, prostacyclin and endothelin antagonists (see page 400). Avoid beta blockers, so manage varices with banding. Anticoagulation is not advised due to the risk of variceal bleeding. LTOT if PaO$_2$< 8 kPa. Liver transplantation may reverse mild to moderate POPH, although symptoms may take weeks to months to resolve. Severe POPH is not reversed and is associated with significant intra- and post-operative morbidity and mortality. A few cases of heart–lung–liver transplants have been reported.

Prognosis is poor in severe POPH, with a median survival after diagnosis of 6 months, without transplant.

Further information

Portopulmonary hypertension and hepatopulmonary syndrome. Hoeper M *et al. Lancet* 2004; **363**: 1461–8

Portopulmonary hypertension. A tale of two circulations. Budhiraja R, Hassoun P. *Chest* 2003; **123**: 562–76

Inflammatory bowel disease, coeliac disease, and pancreatitis

Inflammatory bowel disease (IBD) Pulmonary involvement tends to occur after the onset of the IBD, but can predate it. Pulmonary involvement is found in up to a quarter of patients, but this is usually subclinical. Patients can develop a variety of clinical syndromes, including: airway inflammation, subglottic stenosis, chronic bronchitis, bronchiectasis, and chronic bronchiolitis. Bronchoscopy may reveal inflammatory tissue within the large airway walls, which on biopsy shows mucosal ulceration, basal cell hyperplasia, basement membrane thickening, and submucosal inflammatory cell infiltration. IBD is also associated with the development of interstitial lung disease, such as cryptogenic organizing pneumonia (COP), pulmonary infiltrates with eosinophilia, or neutrophilic necrotic parenchymal nodules. Pulmonary involvement tends to be steroid-responsive. Inhaled steroids can be tried for chronic bronchitis, but oral or intravenous steroids may be required for worsening lung involvement. Note that drugs used in the treatment of IBD may also cause lung disease, such as sulphasalazine (alveolitis), mesalazine, or infliximab (both: pulmonary infiltrates and eosinophilia; infliximab: reactivation of latent TB).

Ulcerative colitis Pulmonary involvement is usually asymptomatic, or may be associated with dry cough. Minimal interstitial change may be suggested by abnormal pulmonary function tests. Restrictive, obstructive, or reduced kCO defects may be seen. Usually normal CXR and CT. No specific treatment indicated.

Crohn's disease Pulmonary involvement less common than in ulcerative colitis, but similar changes found.

Coeliac disease May be associated with idiopathic lung fibrosis, causing restrictive defect. Also may be at increased risk of asthma, bird fancier's lung, and haemosiderosis. Increased risk of lymphoma and malignancy in GI tract.

Pancreatitis Acute pancreatitis is frequently associated with exudative pleural effusion. Raised amylase in the pleural fluid is suggestive (see page 41). Adult respiratory distress syndrome (ARDS) may develop, which requires supportive care and mechanical ventilation (see page 522).

Further information

Clinical and radiological characteristics of lung disease in inflammatory bowel disease. Mahadeva *et al. Eur Respir J* 2000; **15**(1): 41–8

Acute respiratory distress syndrome

Pathophysiology and diagnosis

Definition and epidemiology ARDS (previously shock lung) is not a single entity but represents the severe end of a spectrum of acute lung injury due to many different insults. Essentially it is:

- Acute, persistent, lung inflammation, increased vascular permeability
- Bilateral and extensive infiltrates on the CXR
- Very poor oxygenation despite PEEP with variable ways of defining the severity of this, e.g. PaO_2/FiO_2 (≤1) ratio <27 kPa or <200 mmHg
- Not due to clinical left ventricular failure or associated with a wedge pressure of over 18 mmHg (non-cardiogenic)
- Most commonly seen on the ITU where about 10% of such patients will have ARDS depending on the definition.

The Murray lung injury score, grading ARDS, is based on plain CXR findings, oxygenation, PEEP level, and respiratory system compliance (see page 523).

Pathophysiology Inflammatory damage to the alveoli, either by locally produced pro-inflammatory mediators, or remotely produced and arriving via the pulmonary artery. The change in pulmonary capillary permeability allows fluid and protein leakage into the alveolar spaces with pulmonary infiltrates. The alveolar surfactant is diluted with loss of its stabilizing effect, resulting in diffuse alveolar collapse and stiff lungs. This leads to:

- Gross impairment of V/Q matching with shunting causing arterial hypoxia and very large A–a gradients. There are usually enough remaining functioning alveoli such that a degree of hyperventilation maintains CO_2 clearance; thus hypercapnia is infrequently a problem
- Pulmonary hypertension will develop secondary to the hypoxia but this is probably helpful (aids V/Q matching) rather than deleterious
- Reduced compliance (stiff lungs), due to loss of functioning alveoli (alveolar collapse, filled with fluid and protein), and hyperinflation of remaining alveoli to their limits of distension.

There are many causes of pro-inflammatory mediator release sufficient to cause ARDS, and there may be more than one present. Common causes in order of prevalence:

- Sepsis/pneumonia; secondary risk factors for developing ARDS, when septic, are alcoholism and cigarette smoking
- Gastric aspiration (even if on a proton pump inhibitor, indicating that a low pH is not the only damaging component)
- Trauma/burns, via sepsis, lung trauma, smoke inhalation, fat emboli, and possibly direct effects of large amounts of necrotic tissue.

Less common causes

- Blood transfusion, or other plasma-containing blood product (possibly due to HLA/white blood cell antibodies, older blood products, > 6 units); usually occurs within a few hours of transfusion
- Transplanted lung—worse if lung poorly preserved
- Post-bone marrow transplant as bone marrow recovers
- Drug overdose, e.g. tricyclic antidepressants, opiates, cocaine, aspirin
- Acute pancreatitis
- Near drowning

- Following upper airway obstruction; mechanism unclear
- Acute form of UIP/CFA. Also called AIP and used to be known as acute Hamman-Rich syndrome (page 452).

The course of ARDS is fairly characteristic:
Phase 1 is the early period of alveolar damage and hypoxaemia with pulmonary infiltration.
Phase 2 develops after a week or so as the pulmonary infiltrates resolve, and on histology seems to be associated with an increase in type II pneumocytes (surfactant producers), myofibroblasts, and early collagen formation.
Phase 3 if the patient survives, is the fibrotic stage that leaves the lung with cysts, deranged micro-architecture, and much fibrosis on histology.

Clinical features ARDS should be considered in any patient with a predisposing risk factor who develops severe hypoxaemia, stiff lungs, and a widespread diffuse pulmonary infiltrate. Approximately 1 to 2 days following the clinical presentation of the precipitating cause (sepsis, aspiration, etc.), there is rapidly worsening dyspnoea (± a dry cough) and hypoxaemia, requiring rapidly escalating amounts of supplemental oxygen up to 100% via a rebreathe system. There are coarse crackles in the chest. Intubation and ventilation are nearly always required, although initiating CPAP via a face-mask at 5–10 cmH$_2$O with 100% O$_2$ can improve oxygenation temporarily.

Diagnosis There are no specific tests that allow a confident diagnosis, and exclusion of other more specifically treatable diagnoses is required. The cause for the ARDS needs to be established and prevented from continuing or re-occurring if possible. The CXR or CT show diffuse alveolar infiltrates and air bronchograms, similar in appearance to cardiogenic pulmonary oedema or diffuse pulmonary haemorrhage. Left ventricular failure may be excluded on clinical grounds or by echocardiography, but confident exclusion requires a wedge pressure measurement less than 18 mmHg. Diffuse alveolar haemorrhage can occur in Goodpasture's, Wegener's, and SLE; clues will include a drop in haemoglobin, blood in the airways and pulmonary secretions, and other clinical features of one of these disorders. Some pulmonary infections (e.g. mycobacteria, legionella, PCP, viral pneumonia) may mimic ARDS and lavage fluid may reveal these. Some centres advocate lung biopsy to exclude alternatives, although the diagnostic yield is very low if a lavage is negative. Occasionally cancer and lymphangitis carcinomatosa can also mimic ARDS and these will show on a lung biopsy.

Management and complications

Management The essential aspects of management are to treat the precipitating cause, provide best supportive care with adequate oxygenation, and avoid further damage from barotrauma and nosocomial infections. Mechanical ventilation with PEEP is almost always required to maintain oxygenation, with high inflation pressures. There is some evidence that high inflation pressures may worsen ARDS directly (microbarotrauma); therefore try to maintain plateau pressures <30 mmHg.

Many special ventilation techniques have been tried to reduce the high inflation pressures that result from the stiff lungs (low compliance). For example, using low tidal volumes to reduce inflation pressures (6 ml/kg ideal body weight compared to 12 ml/kg) reduces mortality by 10%. Reducing the minute ventilation, and allowing the $PaCO_2$ to rise (permissive hypercapnia), also reduces the inflation pressures.

High-dose steroids are used but there is evidence of harm as well as benefit, and minimal evidence of overall improved survival. The timing of the steroids may be critical, with later use possibly beneficial if nosocomial infection rates are not increased.

Complications of ARDS include:
- The high ventilation pressures lead to barotrauma: pneumothorax, surgical emphysema, pneumomediastinum. Pneumothorax may be lethal but difficult to detect in the supine patient
- Nosocomial infections occur in about half the patients, making surveillance bronchoalveolar lavage important
- Myopathy associated with long-term neuromuscular blockade, high steroid doses, and poor glycaemic control
- Non-specific problems of venous thromboembolism, GI haemorrhage, inadequate nutrition.

Prognosis has improved over the last 20 years, probably due to improvements in supportive care rather than an ability to modify the inflammatory process and its subsequent repair. Prognosis is worse with pulmonary causes. Early deaths are usually due to the precipitating condition, and later deaths to complications. Over half the patients will survive with varying residual lung damage, although the pulmonary function tests often show only minor restrictive abnormalities (and reduced kCO) indicating the considerable capacity of the lung to recover.

Future developments The optimal level of PEEP in a particular patient is difficult to predict. Inadequate PEEP allows more atelectasis, but too high PEEP contributes to overdistension of remaining alveoli and further barotrauma. Ways to estimate the best PEEP are under investigation. High-frequency ventilation has been around a long while but its place in ARDS is still unclear. Prone ventilation has been tried in an attempt to improve V/Q matching and once again initial increases in PaO_2 are observed, but with no apparent effect on survival. Several different artificial surfactants to try and improve lung compliance have been tried, although good delivery to the abnormal areas is unlikely. Although effective in animal models, the mixed results have not been as impressive in humans. More recently, liquid ventilation with perfluorocarbons has been tried. These dense oxygen-carrying liquids reduce the heterogeneity of ventilation by nullifying the requirement for surfactant, thus recruiting the collapsed alveoli. There are improvements in oxygenation but no evidence yet of increased long-term survival.

Nitric oxide (NO) has been tried with clear improvements in oxygenation but very little effect on survival. The mode of action is not clear and may be more than just vasodilatation. Inhaled prostacyclin is similarly unconvincing. Anti-inflammatory and anti-oxidant therapies are still very much in the experimental phase.

Extracorporeal oxygenation/CO_2 removal will buy time and allow the lung to 'rest', but these techniques are very expensive and it is difficult to demonstrate any long-term benefit.

Further information

Murray ARDS score calculation, *www.clinicalschool.swan.ac.uk/wics/itugl/ali.htm*

Upper airway diseases

Acute upper airway obstruction

Presentation Sudden respiratory distress with cyanosis and aphonia. Airway obstruction can occur at any level within the airway. Partial airway obstruction leads to noisy breathing, with stridor, gurgling, or snoring. Complete airway obstruction is associated with distress and marked respiratory effort, with paradoxical chest and abdominal movement ('see-saw breathing'), and use of accessory muscles of respiration. This may be followed by collapse with loss of consciousness, and progress to cardiorespiratory arrest. Look for chest and abdominal movements and listen and feel for airflow at the nose and mouth.

Causes

- Pharyngeal occlusion by tongue and other muscles, secondary to loss of muscle tone. This may be secondary to drugs, alcohol, a neurological event, or cardiorespiratory arrest
- Vomit or blood
- Inhaled foreign body, which may also cause laryngeal spasm
- Laryngeal obstruction due to oedema from burns, inflammation, or anaphylaxis
- Excessive bronchial secretions, mucosal oedema, bronchospasm may cause airway obstruction below the larynx
- Infection, such as epiglottitis
- Any cause of chronic airway obstruction, such as an airway tumour or extrinsic compression due to tumour or lymphadenopathy, may deteriorate precipitously.

Management

Call for senior anaesthetic help early

1. Open the airway with backwards head tilt, chin lift, and forward jaw thrust. In cases of trauma, do not tilt the head, but perform a jaw thrust only.

2. If unsuccessful at restoring normal respiration, visually inspect the mouth for obvious occlusion and remove it with a finger sweep. Leave well-fitting dentures in place.

3. If there is a witnessed history of choking, consider performing the Heimlich manoeuvre to dislodge the particle (firm and rapid pressure applied beneath the diaphragm in an upwards movement), or directly visualize the airway with a laryngoscope and use McGill's forceps to remove the particle, or with bronchoscope and the use of biopsy forceps.

4. If the patient is breathing, consider inserting an airway to maintain patency: oropharyngeal (Guedel) or nasopharyngeal. Maintain oxygenation, using mask with reservoir bag, delivering 10–15 l/min. If there is no spontaneous respiratory effort, insert a laryngeal mask or endotracheal tube and deliver oxygen via self-inflating bag with supplemental oxygen 10 l/min and reservoir bag. If they are not breathing and cannot be ventilated, a cricothyroidotomy may be necessary (page 663).

5. Suction out secretions.

6. Maintain circulation with cardiac compression if necessary.

7. Seek definitive treatment for the cause of airway obstruction, as appropriate.

Heliox Helium–oxygen mixtures have been used for patients with airway obstruction, often due to tumour compression or invasion. Helium has a lower density than nitrogen and can improve ventilation rapidly when used with oxygen. It can be used as an interim measure until more definitive management is available, such as radiotherapy, or to allow time for radiotherapy to take effect. The evidence relating to its use is mainly case studies, with no randomized control trials.

Nebulized adrenaline may also be helpful in upper airway obstruction, especially laryngeal oedema. This is only a stabilizing measure to buy time until definitive treatment is available.

Anaphylaxis

Causes IgE-mediated type 1 hypersensitivity reaction to allergen. Histamine release causes the clinical syndrome. Typical allergens include: bee or wasp sting, peanuts, fish, drugs, foods, latex, contrast media, muscle relaxants, anaesthetic agents.

Presentation Varying severity of:
- Angiooedema
- Urticaria
- Dyspnoea
- Wheeze
- Stridor
- Hypotension
- Arrhythmias
- Also: rhinitis, abdominal pain, vomiting, diarrhoea, sense of impending doom
- May have had previous episodes of severe allergic-type reactions.

Management

This is a potentially life-threatening medical emergency. Call for help
- Remove likely allergen
- Cardiopulmonary resuscitation if necessary
- *Airway and breathing* Administer high-flow oxygen through non-rebreathable mask. If airway obstruction present, consider tracheal intubation. Airway swelling may make this difficult and cricothyroidotomy may need to be performed (see page 663)
- *Circulation* Give adrenaline (epinephrine) IM 1:1000 solution 0.5 ml (500 μg). Repeat after 5 minutes if no improvement or deterioration
- In those with profound shock and immediately life-threatening anaphylaxis, such as during anaesthesia, or those with no pulse, IV adrenaline can be given slowly, 100 μg per minute or 1 ml of 1:10,000 solution per minute. Stop as soon as there is a response. This can be hazardous and needs cardiac monitoring
- IV fluids if hypotension persists: 1–2 l rapidly infused
- Antihistamines, such as chlorpheniramine 10–20 mg IV
- Consider steroids: 100–500 mg hydrocortisone IV
- Consider nebulized salbutamol or adrenaline if bronchospasm
- On discharge, provide an Epipen (IM self-administered adrenaline) and advice on future episodes, medic alert bracelet, and card
- Consider immunology referral if allergen unknown.

Future developments Allergen immunotherapy aiming to desensitize to the allergen. Useful in those who cannot avoid allergen exposure. Small amounts of the allergen are injected usually weekly, with slowly increasing dose strengths until the maximum dose of the allergen is administered, which can take up to 12 months. Mechanism unknown, but probably related to increased IgG binding to the allergen, falling allergen-specific IgE levels, and decreased amount of circulating inflammatory cytokines. Can protect against anaphylaxis for 3–5 years, but 'top-up' doses necessary.

Effective for dust, grass, tree, and weed pollen, mould spores, latex, and insect venom as well as some animal allergens. Side-effects of administration: anaphylaxis, bronchoconstriction, local reaction. Some centres may not perform in people with chronic asthma because of the risk of death.

Further information

Allergen immunotherapy for asthma. Abramson M, Puy R et al. Cochrane Database Syst Rev 2003; **4**: CD001186

Advanced Life Support Provider Manual, 4th edition 2000. Resuscitation Council UK

Upper respiratory tract infections 1

Acute upper respiratory tract infections (URTIs) include rhinitis, pharyngitis, tonsillitis, and sinusitis.

Upper respiratory tract infections are the commonest cause of people taking time off work in the United Kingdom. The majority are managed by general practitioners, and will not reach a respiratory specialist. They are usually self-limiting, and often do not require specific treatment.

Acute rhinitis Nasal congestion with rhinorrhea, mild malaise, and sneezing. Most commonly due to viral infection (the common cold).

Topical decongestants may be useful. There is no evidence for the use of antibiotics or antihistamines.

Candidiasis Oral candida infection is common in those who have received antibiotics, are immunosuppressed, or on oral or inhaled steroids. Seen as white plaque-like lesions on the tongue and pharyngeal mucosa. Treat with oral nystatin or amphotericin lozenges, and with oral hygiene. Severe infection can be debilitating, leading to difficulties with eating, especially in the elderly. Exclude underlying immunocompromise (e.g. HIV, leukaemia) in those with persisting infection despite treatment.

Acute epiglottitis (supraglottitis) is infection mainly localized to the epiglottis and surrounding supraglottic structures. It is commoner in children than adults, but a mortality of up to 7% is reported in adults. This is due to upper airways obstruction from grossly oedematous upper airway tissue.

- *Haemophilus influenza, Streptococci,* and *Staphylococci* are causative organisms
- Acute epiglottitis typically presents with a sore throat and dysphagia. Inspiratory stridor is less common, but it can also present with acute upper airway obstruction and CXR infiltrates consistent with pulmonary oedema (due to high negative intrathoracic pressure)
- May need airway protection with an endotracheal tube or tracheostomy: liaise with ENT/anaesthetic colleagues early
- In severe infection, epiglottic swabs may be of diagnostic use, but beware of precipitating airway obstruction. Treat with third-generation cephalosporin for 2 weeks (to cover β-lactam producing *H. influenzae*). Change to amoxycillin if sensitive.

Sinusitis The sinuses are normally sterile. The paranasal sinuses communicate with the nose, and are therefore susceptible to infection from this route. All the sinuses drain by means of the mucociliary escalator. Blockage of free sinus drainage is a predisposing factor for bacterial infection. Sinusitis is a common cause of persistent cough. Dental sepsis may lead to maxillary sinusitis, by direct spread.

Acute sinusitis complicates 1 in 200 upper respiratory tract infections and usually presents with fever and sinus pain, which is worse on leaning forward. It may be associated with systemic upset. Respiratory viral infection interrupts normal defences of the mucosal lining, producing mucous exudates, with secondary bacterial infection. *S. pneumoniae* and *H. influenzae* are the commonest pathogens. *S. aureus* and *S. pyogenes* are also causes, with *Pseudomonas* in cystic fibrosis. Mixed infections with anaerobes are seen in 10%. Specific diagnostic tests are not usually needed.

Chronic sinusitis by definition, if present for >3 months. The ciliated epithelial sinus lining is replaced by thickened stratified squamous lining, with absent cilia, due to repeated infection. Anaerobic infection is more common. Fungal infection is more common in atopic people with nasal polyps. Sinus mycetoma is a rare complication, in neutropenic patients, diabetics, and in the immunocompromised.

Presents with frontal headache (frontal sinusitis), maxillary pain, pain over bridge of nose (ethmoidal sinusitis), retro-orbital headache (sphenoidal sinusitis), with purulent nasal discharge and blockage. Wegener's granulomatosis may mimic the symptoms of sinusitis.

Investigations are not usually warranted, but a sinus radiograph may show an air-fluid level, with thickened mucosal lining, or sinus opacification. CT is more sensitive, but not usually warranted, unless surgical intervention planned, or malignant disease suspected.

Treatment Analgesia, topical decongestants, antibiotics if severe infection (amoxycillin first line, trimethoprim if penicillin allergic).

Surgery may be warranted if prolonged infection, anatomical abnormality, or other complications, e.g. if infection has spread to the cranial cavity or orbit. Spreading infection is uncommon if there has been prior antibiotic treatment.

Upper respiratory tract infections 2

Acute pharyngitis and tonsillitis 80–90% are caused by viruses, most commonly adenoviruses, coronaviruses, rhinoviruses, and influenza viruses. Group B streptococci, *Streptococcus pneumoniae*, and *Haemophilus influenzae* may cause secondary infection. Mycoplasma and chlamydia are seen less commonly.

- Pharyngitis and tonsillitis presents with a sore throat, which is usually self-limiting. May be associated with fever, malaise, lymphadenopathy, conjunctivitis, headache, nausea, and vomiting
- Infectious mononucleosis (EBV) is associated with pharyngitis in 80% of cases. Diagnose with Paul Bunnell test for heterophil antibodies, and atypical mononuclear cells in peripheral blood
- Coxsackie A and herpes simplex cause 'herpangina syndrome'— ulcerating vesicles on the tonsils and palate
- CMV can also cause pharyngitis associated with lymphadenopathy and splenomegaly
- Lemierre's syndrome (jugular vein suppurative thrombophlebitis) is a rare anaerobic pharyngeal infection (see page 202).

Other causative agents

- *Corynebacterium diptheriae* in unvaccinated populations. A pharyngeal membrane may form, with systemic symptoms, and 'bull neck' due to cervical lymphadenopathy. Low-grade fever, with a relatively high pulse rate. Treat urgently with diphtheria antitoxin
- Vincent's angina is anaerobic infection in those with poor mouth hygiene. Caused by Gram-negative *Borrelia vincenti* and other anaerobic infections. Treat with penicillin
- Group A streptococcus may cause a more unpleasant illness, with systemic upset, and dysphagia due to pharyngotonsillar oedema.

Treatment is usually supportive, but anti-streptococcal antibiotics may be warranted if there is severe infection. There is no evidence that antibiotics reduce the duration of symptoms, but they may reduce complications (e.g. sinusitis, quinsy, and rheumatic fever, which is rare in the Western world). Oral penicillin is the first-line treatment (or a macrolide if penicillin allergic). Amoxycillin can cause a rash in infectious mononucleosis and so should be avoided. Throat swabs for group A streptococcus may be helpful in directing treatment.

Complications of untreated infection include peritonsillar abscess (quinsy), retropharyngeal abscess, and cervical abscess. Treat with appropriate antibiotics. Surgical drainage is occasionally required.

Laryngitis This is usually part of a generalized upper respiratory tract infection. *M. cataharalis* is the causative agent in up to 50%. It may cause a hoarse voice or aphonia.

Other causes include inhaled steroids, occupational exposure to inhaled chemicals, and gastro-oesophageal reflux disease. If a hoarse voice persists in a smoker, a laryngeal or lung cancer (with recurrent laryngeal nerve involvement) must be excluded. Other causes include tuberculous infection, HSV, CMV, diphtheria, fungal infections, and actinomycoses.

Treatment Usually no specific treatment is required, as the illness is typically self-limiting.

Acute bronchitis, tracheitis, and tracheobronchitis Inflammation due to infection can occur in any part of the tracheobronchial tree, and is termed tracheitis, tracheobronchitis, or bronchitis depending on the anatomical site. It usually follows viral infection, especially of the common cold type, and is commoner during influenza epidemics. Secondary bacterial infection is common, with *H. influenza* and *S. pneumoniae* commonest. There is increased prevalence in the winter months.

Presents with a productive cough, small volume streaky haemoptysis, and fever. Breathlessness and hypoxia are uncommon unless there is coexistent cardiorespiratory disease, or a concomitant pneumonia. Retrosternal chest pain is common in tracheitis. Examination is often normal.

Diagnosis is usually on the basis of the history. A persisting cough, especially in a smoker, may warrant further investigation.

Treatment is usually symptomatic, particularly in the previously well. Use antibiotics for persistent cough productive of mucopurulent sputum, or if there is coexistent cardiopulmonary disease.

Hyperventilation syndrome

Definition Poorly defined, and the term is falling into disfavour. Most respiratory physicians use the term to describe breathlessness and over-breathing associated with fear, stress, and anxiety, in the absence of any demonstrable physiological abnormality.

It is usually part of a spectrum of physical symptoms (e.g. chest pain, palpitations/tachycardia, fatigue, dizziness, parasthesiae, headache, diarrhoea, inappropriate sweating, etc.) that occur as part of an anxiety syndrome or panic disorder. Other specialties may have been consulted due to the mixed symptomatology.

Pathophysiology Hyperventilation syndrome can occur *de novo*, or follow a respiratory disorder that has resolved—such as an attack of mild asthma. It appears to be based on a heightened awareness of breathing, and concerns as to what the shortness of breath signifies. The $PaCO_2$ is intermittently low, with a respiratory alkalosis. Recordings of breathing pattern often show a rather chaotic pattern.

Clinical features
- Intermittent episodes of breathlessness largely unrelated to exercise, although can be worsened by exercise
- May be associated with symptoms of respiratory alkalosis such as numbness, tingling of the extremities, feelings of impending doom, and light-headedness, occasionally to the point of losing consciousness (cerebral vasoconstriction due to the hypocapnia)
- Sensation of not being able to take a satisfactory breath
- No history suggestive of an alternative current respiratory disorder, although there may have been one previously
- History of some stressful situation in the patient's life
- Previous episodes.

Diagnosis is essentially one of exclusion, but with additional confirmatory findings.
- No evidence of a cardiac cause for the breathlessness
- No evidence of a respiratory cause, i.e. normal lung function, normal CXR, and normal SaO_2 at rest and on exercise to the point of breathlessness (SaO_2 may even rise on exercise)
- No evidence of pulmonary hypertension
- No evidence to support pulmonary emboli
- No evidence of hyperthyroidism
- Low $PaCO_2$, raised pH, on blood gases (and no A–a gradient)
- Unresolved psychological issues, or social phobia/agoraphobia.

Differential diagnosis The most important pathological causes to exclude are:
- Subtle interstitial lung disease with a normal CXR: consider HRCT
- Mild asthma with normal basic PFTs: consider PEFR monitoring, exercise provocation, or bronchial reactivity testing
- Pulmonary hypertension/thromboembolic disease: consider cardiac echo or CTPA
- Hyperthyroidism.

Management It is important not to dismiss the patient's symptoms, implying it is 'all in the mind'. The patient has a real symptom, which requires a real explanation. There are no controlled trials of management, but most clinicians will offer an explanation based on an 'over awareness' of respiratory sensations, heightened by anxiety. It is important to explain that the associated symptoms of tingling and light-headedness are well recognized and harmless.

Old recommendations to rebreathe into a paper bag have not stood the test of time and are rather impractical in the middle of a supermarket. Because cold peripheries often accompany an episode (vasoconstriction), placing the palms on to the cheeks can help suppress the desire to breathe, thought to be related to the diving reflex: again this is an untested remedy.

Careful explanation may be enough. A short period on an anxiolytic (e.g. diazepam 2–5 mg bd) may be helpful, to demonstrate that the symptoms can be controlled. Management of the psychological problem may be possible. Some respiratory physiotherapists can help patients control their breathing, but sometimes concentrating on their breathing in this way can make it all worse.

Failure to respond should always prompt a reconsideration of whether an underlying disorder is gradually progressing to the point where an investigation becomes abnormal. On the other hand, repeated investigations will confirm the patient's concern that the 'doctors think there is something wrong.'

Prognosis Some patients improve quickly with explanation. Some tend to relapse at times of stress. Some prove resistant to any treatment and probably should be seen in the clinic regularly, but infrequently, to reduce their likelihood of involving other medical services with another pointless round of investigations.

Unusual conditions/BOLD

British Orphan Lung Disease (BOLD) project

The British Orphan Lung Disease (BOLD) register was set up by the British Thoracic Society in 2001, to facilitate research into rare lung diseases and improve clinicians' knowledge of these conditions. It also aimed to help establish patient support groups.

In continental Europe there have been registers of rare lung diseases for many years. The term 'orphan' lung disease was coined because of the feeling that these diseases have, in the past, tended to be neglected because of their rarity, the limited knowledge of the conditions, and the limited available data on which to base practice.

The reporting system works via a web-based registration form, where consultants are encouraged to enter details of patients with any of the listed conditions. The data is anonymized, and the patient must sign a form (found on the BTS website at www.brit-thoracic.org.uk in the members only section), consenting for their details to be held on a central database. Interested parties are invited to submit research proposals, for which the collected data will be used.

The BOLD register collects data on:

- Alveolar proteinosis
- Churg–Strauss syndrome
- Ciliary dyskinesia
- Cryptogenic organizing pneumonia
- Langerhans' cell histiocytosis (histiocytosis x)
- Lymphangioleiomyomatosis
- Neurofibromatosis with lung disease
- Primary pulmonary hypertension
- Primary tracheal tumours
- Pulmonary arteriovenous malformations (including HHT)
- Tracheo/bronchial/pulmonary amyloidosis.

Rare lung disease patient support groups:

- Lymphangioleiomyomatosis Action—*www.lamaction.org*
- UK Histiocytosis Family Support Association—email ajes954836@aol.com
- Pulmonary Hypertension Association UK—*www.pha-uk.com*
- Churg–Strauss syndrome—*www.vasculitis-uk.org*
- Pulmonary Alveolar Proteinosis—*health.groups.yahoo.com/group/pulmonarypap/?s.*
- Primary Ciliary Dyskinesia Family Support Group—*www.webnautics.co.uk/pcd*
- Alpha-1 Antitrypsin Deficiency—*www.alpha1.org.uk.*

Alveolar microlithiasis

This is a rare interstitial lung disease of unknown aetiology, characterized by the accumulation of numerous and diffuse calcified microliths (calcium and phosphate hydroxyapatite bodies) in the alveolar space. There is no identifiable abnormality of calcium metabolism. Microliths are occasionally identified in the sputum. At post mortem the lungs are heavy and rock hard, often needing a saw to cut them. Fewer than 200 cases are reported.

Clinical features
- Typically presents in young adults, most commonly in the third and fourth decades of life
- May be an incidental CXR finding in asymptomatic patients
- Familial tendency—probable autosomal recessive inheritance
- Equal sex distribution in sporadic cases, 2:1 female preponderance in familial cases
- Usually slowly progressive, with progressive breathlessness, hypoxia, respiratory failure, and death
- CXR and chest CT show fine micronodular lung calcification, predominantly basally or around the hila. It may produce complete radiographic opacification. There is no associated lymph node enlargement. Progressive lung infiltration causes restriction of lung movement and impairs gas exchange, leading to progressive respiratory failure.

Treatment
- There is no effective medical treatment
- Lung transplantation has been successful.

Pulmonary alveolar proteinosis (PAP): pathophysiology and clinical features

Pulmonary alveolar proteinosis (PAP), also referred to as alveolar lipo-proteinosis, is a rare alveolar filling defect affecting around 3 per million people. There is a limited published literature-5 reported case series of ≥10 cases, and only 410 total cases reported.

Pathophysiology PAP is due to failure of alveolar macrophages to clear spent surfactant, leading to the filling of alveoli with a phospholipid proteinaeous material. It is thought that the defect has an autoimmune basis, due to the presence of antibodies to granulocyte–macrophage colony–stimulating factor (GM-CSF), which cause inhibition of normal alveolar macrophage function, leading to abnormalities of surfactant homeostasis. Defects in GM-CSF signalling have been identified in animal models. Congenital disease is thought to be due to mutations in surfactant gene proteins. Other mechanisms for surfactant accumulation have also been identified:

- **Heavy dust exposure** leads to surfactant hypersecretion, which exceed the lungs' normal clearance mechanism. Animal models have shown that this condition develops from endogenous lipoid pneumonia, with the accumulation of lipid-laden macrophages, which break down to release surfactant
- **Amphiphilic drugs**, e.g. amiodarone, chlorphenetermine
- **Lymphoma, leukaemia, and immunosuppression** The mechanism is uncertain, but it is thought that the lipoprotein may be generated from degenerating alveolar cells.

Appearances similar to alveolar lipoproteinosis may also be seen in endogenous lipoid pneumonia resulting from bronchial obstruction, and are described in surfactant-secreting alveolar cell carcinoma.

Histology The alveoli are filled with a granular acellular eosinophilic PAS (periodic acid Schiff) positive deposit. Cholesterol clefts and large foamy macrophages may also be seen. The alveolar architecture is usually well preserved. Surfactant protein can be identified using immunohistochemistry. Electron microscopy shows multiple osmiophilic bodies consistent with denatured surfactant.

Epidemiology
- Presents aged 30–50 (case reports in children and the elderly)
- Male to female ratio of 4:1
- Increased incidence in smokers
- Rare familial cases reported.

Clinical features
- Typically presents with breathlessness and a non-productive cough. Examination may be normal, or crackles may be heard on auscultation. Clubbing in one-third

- May present with superadded infection, causing an apparent acute onset of symptoms in association with fever
- Median duration of symptoms before diagnosis is 7 months
- Opportunistic infection is the major complication, most commonly *Nocardia* species, fungi, and mycobacteria. This occurs due to impaired macrophage function and impaired host defence, due to surfactant accumulation.

PAP: diagnosis and treatment

Diagnosis is usually made on the basis of a characteristic CT appearance, although other tests may also be useful.
- Raised serum LDH
- **ABGs** Hypoxia and increased alveolar–arterial (A–a) gradient
- **PFTs** Restrictive defect, with reduced lung volumes and transfer factor
- **CXR** Bilateral consolidation with thickened interlobular septa. Usually bilateral. The pattern is very variable, and in up to 50% may be perihilar (bat's-wing appearance)
- Characteristic **CT** appearance is of airspace shadowing in a geographical distribution, alternating with areas of normal lung, the so-called 'crazy paving' pattern. This CT appearance is not specific to alveolar proteinosis, but is also seen in lipoid pneumonia and bronchoalveolar cell carcinoma
- **BAL** reveals milky washings. Identification of antibodies to granulocyte-macrophage colony-stimulating factor in BAL washings is diagnostic. Cytological examination shows a granular extracellular deposit with foamy macrophages and cellular debris
- **Transbronchial/open lung biopsies** are occasionally needed, if the CT is not characteristic.

Treatment of choice is repeated therapeutic whole lung lavage, which should be performed at a specialist centre. There are no randomized controlled trials of this treatment, but there is evidence of efficacy in terms of subsequent improvement of symptoms, physiology, and radiology.
- The indication for whole lung lavage is usually breathlessness limiting activities of daily living
- The procedure is done under general anaesthesia using 100% oxygen, and one lung ventilation using a double lumen tube. Repeated warm saline lavage using a closed circuit continues until the bronchial washing returns are clear—this may take up to 40 litres lavage. One or both lungs may be treated at a time
- The response is variable—some patients need only one treatment, others may need multiple treatments, and about 10% fail to respond
- May be done on bypass if the patient is very hypoxic
- Characteristic milky lavage fluid is obtained.

Granulocyte colony-stimulating factor (subcutaneous injections) is a novel treatment option (only phase II studies, no RCT yet) that may prevent progression of disease.

There is no benefit from treatment with steroids, and they may exacerbate opportunistic infections.

Prognosis with whole lung lavage is generally good. Spontaneous remission occurs in 1/3, 1/3 remain stable, and 1/3 progress to respiratory failure and death. There are reports of progression to pulmonary fibrosis (which may be a coincidental occurrence).

Further information

Pulmonary alveolar proteinosis: clinical aspects and current concepts on pathogenesis. Shah P et al. *Thorax* 2000; **55**: 67–77

Pulmonary alveolar proteinosis: progress in the first 44 years. Seymour JF, Presneill JJ *Am. J. Respir. Crit. Care Med.* 2002; **166**: 215–35

Amyloidosis: pathophysiology and classification

Definition Amyloidosis is the extracellular deposition of low molecular weight protein molecules as insoluble fibrils. More than 20 such proteins have been described in different diseases and circumstances.

Pathophysiology The disease is one of abnormal protein folding, and classified by the origin of the precursor proteins that form the amyloid. For example, AL amyloid forms from the light chains of immunoglobulins. In familial forms, genetic missense mutations produce abnormal folding of the protein. Little is known of the specific genetic and environmental factors that lead to the development of this abnormal folding. Despite their different origins, these protein molecules fold into alternative forms that are very similar to each other: in the classic 'β-pleated sheet' structure, fibrils form in an ordered fashion, with uniformity of fibril structure within the sheet. Substitutions of particular amino acids at specific positions in the light chain variable region lead to destabilization of the light chains, increasing the chance of fibrillogenesis. In certain models, this abnormal folding can be initiated by the addition of 'amyloid enhancing factor', rather like the initiation of crystal formation in a supersaturated solution. Amyloid deposits accumulate in the extracellular space, disrupting normal tissue architecture, and leading to organ dysfunction, both directly, and having space-occupying effects. The fibrils may be directly cytotoxic (possibly by promoting apoptosis). The subdivisions of amyloid are largely based on the origin of the amyloid protein and shown in the box opposite.

Epidemiology The epidemiology of the disease is difficult to define accurately as the disease is often un- or misdiagnosed. The age-adjusted incidence is estimated to be 5.1 to 12.8 per million person years.

Future developments Anti-amyloid drugs are under investigation, including drugs to stabilize the amyloid precursor proteins in their normal configuration, and enhance fibril degradation.

Further Information

Systemic amyloidosis. Falk RH, Raymond L *et al*. *NEJM* 1997; **337**: 898–908

www.acor.org/amyloid.html is an online support and discussion group for patients.

Classification of amyloidosis

- Primary/light chain amyloid (AL), from immunoglobulin light chain fragments (λ or κ), usually monoclonal due to a plasma cell dyscrasia (a subtype of lymphoproliferative disorders)
  - 1 in 5000 deaths due to this type of amyloid
  - Median survival is 6–15 months
  - Frank myeloma is present in 20%, and a subtle monoclonal gammopathy in 70% (MGUS)
  - Systemic form due to circulating monoclonal light chains, widespread organ involvement, particularly heart, liver, and kidneys
  - Localized amyloid production by local clonal B cells; hence heterogeneous organ involvement is seen, commonly in the upper respiratory tract, orbit, with urogenital and gastrointestinal involvement—virtually any organ (except the brain) can be involved.
- Secondary amyloid (AA)
  - A complication of chronic disease with ongoing/recurring inflammation, e.g. rheumatoid, chronic infections
  - The fibrils are fragments of acute phase reactant, serum amyloid A
  - Commonly renal, hepatic, and lower GI involvement, rarely neurological, lung, and cardiac involvement
  - Median survival 5 years
  - Only a small number of patients with chronic inflammation will develop AA amyloidosis, and the time period for the development of the disease is very variable.
- Dialysis-related (DA), due to fibrils derived from beta-2 microglobulin that accumulate in dialysis patients
- Inherited amyloidosis, e.g. due to abnormal pre-albumin (transthyretin, TTR), damaging neural and cardiac tissue
- Organ-specific amyloid, such as Alzheimer's disease, plaques of the beta protein derived from the larger amyloid precursor protein (APP). Protein presumed to be generated locally.

Amyloidosis: lung involvement

Clinically significant respiratory tract disease is almost always AL in type, though the presence of a strong family history or chronic inflammatory disease may suggest other types.

Laryngeal amyloidosis Amyloid causes up to 1% of benign laryngeal disease. May present as discrete nodules or diffuse infiltration, and is usually localized, though can be a rare manifestation of systemic (AL) amyloid. Deposits are seen most commonly in the supraglottic larynx (presenting with hoarse voice or stridor). May present with choking and exertional dyspnoea that can be progressive or recurrent.

Tracheobronchial amyloid is rare (67 worldwide cases reported by the mid-1980s). Macroscopically is either diffusely infiltrative or 'tumour-like'. It is associated with tracheobronchopathia osteoplastica (a disorder characterized by the deposition of calcified submucosal airway nodules). It presents after the fifth decade with dyspnoea, cough, and rarely haemoptysis. Airway narrowing can lead to atelectasis or recurrent pneumonia; solitary nodules may lead to investigation for presumed lung cancer. Symptomatic disease is usually localized.

Parenchymal amyloid is the most frequently diagnosed amyloid respiratory disease. It is usually divided radiologically into solitary/multiple pulmonary nodules (usually localized AL amyloid) or a diffuse alveolar pattern (usually a manifestation of systemic AL amyloid). Parenchymal amyloid lung nodules are usually peripheral and subpleural, they may be bilateral, and are more common in the lower lobes, ranging in diameter from 0.4 cm to 15 cm. They may cavitate or calcify. Clinical signs are non-diagnostic, PFTs may show a restrictive defect with reduced transfer factor. The differential diagnosis usually includes fibrosis. Cardiac amyloid may coexist, and distinguishing the contribution to the symptoms of the pulmonary and cardiac disease can be difficult. Median survival with clinically overt lung disease is about 16 months (similar to that of systemic amyloid).

Mediastinal and hilar amyloidosis are rarely associated with localized pulmonary amyloidosis, and their diagnosis should lead to a search for a systemic cause of amyloid. Amyloid lymphadenopathy can also represent localized AL deposition in association with B cell lymphoma.

Other rare reports of:
• Ventilatory failure due to diaphragm or other respiratory muscle involvement
• Sleep apnoea from macroglossia due to amyloid
• Exudative pleural effusions.

Clinical features
• Dyspnoea and cough
• None—parenchymal disease may be an incidental finding on routine radiography
• Consider the diagnosis particularly in patients with odd upper airway symptoms and parenchymal involvement, or those with unexplained CCF or nephrotic syndrome.

Diagnosis Histological conformation is usually required. Congo red stain producing 'apple green' birefringence in crossed polarized light is the gold standard. Positive histology must lead to immunohistochemistry to determine the fibril type.

Histology Transbronchial biopsy or occasionally open or VATS biopsy (more likely if investigation for solitary pulmonary nodule).

I^{123} labelled scintigraphy Radiolabelled serum amyloid P (SAP) localizes to amyloid deposits, in proportion to the quantity of amyloid present, therefore allowing identification of the distribution and burden of disease. It is most sensitive for solid organ disease, though in lung disease is useful for determining the extent of disease in other organs. It is, however, expensive and carries an infectious risk, as the serum amyloid P component is currently obtained from blood donors.

HRCT may show nodules or parenchymal disease.

Laryngoscopy and bronchoscopy may be needed to obtain samples for histology, depending on the clinical presentation.

PFT to assess effect of disease on respiratory function. May show reduced transfer factor and a restrictive pattern. Tracheobronchial involvement may lead to abnormal flow volume loops due to larger airway obstruction.

Systemic disease
- FBC, biochemistry, and urinalysis (? renal involvement)
- Investigate for underlying blood cell dyscrasia, e.g. myeloma, Waldenstrom's macroglobulinaemia (bone marrow examination, and search for urine and serum monoclonal protein by immunofixation—the clonal proliferation underlying systemic AL amyloid is usually very subtle, and its identification may be difficult)
- Echo for associated cardiac involvement (when CCF is present, survival is 4 to 6 months)
- Thyroid/adrenal function are impaired in up to 10%.

Treatment There are limited clinical trials with which to guide management of respiratory tract amyloid. Management decisions are therefore often made empirically.
- No treatment may be needed
- Local measures may be warranted for endobronchial disease, e.g. symptomatic laryngeal disease—endoscopic excision, carbon dioxide laser evaporation (useful for small recurrent lesions), stenting. Steroids have no effect on laryngeal amyloid
- Tracheobronchial amyloid—management depends on symptoms and treatment may involve repeated endoscopic resection, YAG (yttrium–aluminium–garnet) laser therapy, and surgical resection. Repeated endoscopic procedures are thought to be safer than repeated open surgery
- Chemotherapy may be warranted for diffuse parenchymal amyloid if there is objectively measurable disease (prednisolone and melphalan, to suppress the underlying blood cell dyscrasia). More intensive chemotherapy has a better clinical response, but there are few trials.

Amyloidosis and the respiratory tract. Gillmore JD, Hawkins PN. In: Rare Diseases. *Thorax* 1999; **54**: 444–51

Idiopathic pulmonary haemosiderosis

A rare disease of undetermined aetiology, characterized by recurrent episodes of alveolar haemorrhage and haemoptysis (in the absence of renal disease), usually leading to iron deficiency anaemia.

Pathophysiology The alveolar space and interstitium contain haemosiderin-laden macrophages, with variable degrees of interstitial fibrosis and degeneration of alveolar, interstitial, and vascular elastic fibres, depending on the chronicity of the condition. Electron microscopy shows damage to the endothelial and basement membranes, but no consistent or diagnostic features have been recognized.

No antibodies have been identified, though serum IgA levels are sometimes raised. With recurrent alveolar haemorrhage, the alveolar blood provokes a fibrotic reaction, with the development of diffuse pulmonary fibrosis.

Iron turnover studies show that the accompanying iron-deficient anaemia is due to loss of iron into the lung through haemorrhage.

Aetiology is uncertain, but likely to be multifactorial. Possible associations include toxic insecticides (epidemiological studies in rural Greece) and premature birth. The disease has an equal sex incidence in childhood, with twice as many men affected in adulthood.

Most patients present in childhood, with 85% of cases having onset of symptoms before 16 years. The actual prevalence is unknown, but a Swedish children cohort study in the 1960s described an incidence of 0.24 per million children.

Pulmonary haemosiderosis is associated with rheumatoid arthritis, thyrotoxicosis, coeliac disease, and autoimmune haemolytic anaemia, suggesting a potential autoimmune mechanism.

Clinical features The clinical course is very variable, and ranges from continuous low level bleeding to massive pulmonary haemorrhage. The latter may be fatal, but is fortunately rare.
- Continuous mild pulmonary haemorrhage leads to a chronic non-productive cough with haemoptysis, malaise, lethargy, and failure to thrive in children
- Iron deficiency anaemia is common, as are positive faecal occult blood tests (due to swallowed blood)
- Generalized lymphadenopathy and hepatosplenomegaly are recognized.
- With an acute bleed, cough and haemoptysis may worsen, and dyspnoea, chest tightness, and pyrexia may develop
- Chronic bleeding leads to chronic disabling dyspnoea, chronic anaemia, and clubbing (in 25%). Cor pulmonale secondary to pulmonary fibrosis and hypoxaemia may develop.

Examination may be normal. Clubbing, basal crepitations, and cor pulmonale are all recognized, depending on the severity of the resulting lung disease.

Investigations The diagnosis is one of exclusion, with no evidence of other organ involvement. The main differential diagnosis is Goodpasture's syndrome, Wegener's granulomatosis, SLE, and microscopic polyarteritis.

- **Blood tests** Microcytic, hypochromic anaemia, with low iron levels. ANCA, dsDNA, and anti-GBM antibodies should be negative
- **CXR** May show transient patchy infiltrates, which worsen during an acute bleed. The apices are usually spared. Progressive disease leads to the development of reticulonodular infiltrates, and a ground-glass appearance that is typically perihilar or in the lower zones. Hilar lymphadenopathy may be seen
- **PFTs** kCO is transiently elevated during bleeding episodes ($\geq 130\%$ is abnormal), but this is only useful acutely. A restrictive defect with reduced kCO may develop with chronic disease
- **CT chest** The changes seen are fairly non-specific, showing a diffuse bilateral infiltrate, with patchy ground-glass change
- **BAL samples** (if done) contain haemosiderin-laden macrophages.

Management There is no specific treatment.

- Steroids and immunosuppressive drugs may be of benefit during acute bleeding episodes, but do not appear to affect the long-term outcome. There is no published data to guide the optimal timing of treatment during the course of disease
- The iron deficiency anaemia responds to replacement therapy, and blood transfusion may be needed in severe bleeds.

At routine clinic appointments

- Check spirometry
- Measure haemoglobin and serum iron levels
- Ask about increases in SOB or haemoptysis.

Prognosis The prognosis is very variable, with some patients showing spontaneous remission. The duration of disease in the literature ranges from death within days following an acute severe illness, to survival with cor pulmonale associated with chronic disease after 20 years.

Pulmonary Langerhans' cell histiocytosis

Definition Pulmonary Langerhans' cell histiocytosis (LCH; previously termed pulmonary histiocytosis X or pulmonary eosinophilic granuloma) is a rare condition characterized by infiltration of the lung with histiocytes (Langerhans' cells). Pulmonary LCH overlaps with a number of other conditions with similar pathological findings but diverse clinical features. These range from localized infiltration of a single organ (e.g. eosinophilic granuloma of bone) to systemic diseases affecting multiple organs (Letterer–Siwe disease, a multiorgan disease affecting infants and elderly, associated with poor prognosis; also Hand–Schueller–Christian syndrome). Although the isolated pulmonary form most commonly presents to chest physicians, pulmonary manifestations also commonly occur in the systemic forms of the disease.

Epidemiology Rare, it tends to affect young adults aged 20–40 years. The vast majority of cases occur in current smokers, usually heavy smokers. May be more common in men, who tend to present at a younger age than women.

Pathogenesis Langerhans' cells are involved in antigen presentation, and are characterized by the presence of well-demarcated cytoplasmic organelles called Birbeck granules on electron microscopy. The Langerhans' cells seen in LCH appear to be monoclonal, although it is unclear if this represents a true neoplastic process. The antigen stimulus for activating Langerhans' cells in the lung is unknown, although cigarette smoke is a possible candidate. Langerhans' cells are typically organized into granulomata that are located in bronchiolar walls, and subsequently enlarge and invade adjacent structures. This results in the radiological appearance of nodules that at first cavitate and then become cystic.

Clinical features Typically exertional breathlessness and cough, sometimes with systemic symptoms (e.g. fever, weight loss). Pneumothorax occurs in at least 10% of patients and may be the presenting feature. Rib lesions may also give rise to chest pain. Around 25% of patients are asymptomatic. Examination is usually normal.

Investigations
- **CXR** Typically diffuse reticulonodular shadowing, sometimes with cystic change; upper and middle lobe predominance. May be normal
- **HRCT** Diffuse centrilobular nodules, sometimes with cavitation, and thin-and thick-walled cystic lesions, reflecting lesions of varying age. These are interspersed with normal lung. Upper and middle lobe predominance; costophrenic angles are typically spared. Purely nodular or purely cystic appearances may occur. Unusual manifestations such as single nodules or large airways involvement are also described
- **PFTs** variable, ranging from normal to obstructive, restricted or mixed patterns. Reduced gas transfer and exertional hypoxia are common
- **TBB** may yield diagnostic material, although is often unhelpful; risk of pneumothorax is unknown although may be increased. Surgical lung biopsy is often preferable

- *BAL* Increased total cell counts and pigmented macrophages, reflecting simply the presence of cigarette smoking. Use of antibodies (e.g. OKT6) to detect Langerhans' cells in BAL fluid is limited by poor sensitivity
- *Extrathoracic tissue biopsy* of involved sites (e.g. bone) may be diagnostic.

Diagnosis Usually based on the combination of clinical and HRCT findings: typically a young adult smoker with cysts and nodules on HRCT. Confirmation by surgical lung biopsy may be considered in atypical presentations, such as the finding of solely nodular or cystic disease on HRCT. The appearance of purely cystic disease on HRCT may be confused with emphysema (where cysts lack walls) or lymphangioleiomyomatosis (where cysts are present uniformly in all regions of lung, including the costophrenic angles).

Associations
- Severe pulmonary hypertension—may be seen in the absence of significant parenchymal lung involvement; direct disease involvement of pulmonary vessels has been described
- Manifestations of systemic LCH—particularly diabetes insipidus from pituitary disease, skin involvement, lytic bony lesions, and rarely cardiac or gastrointestinal disease
- Lymphoma—may precede, complicate, or coexist with pulmonary LCH
- Lung cancer—more common, probably as a result of cigarette smoking.

Management Treatment other than smoking cessation is often not required. Oral corticosteroids may be tried in symptomatic disease, although there is little evidence to support their use; they are usually administered for at least 6 months. Lung transplantation should be considered in patients with severe respiratory failure or pulmonary hypertension. Pulmonary LCH may recur in transplanted lungs. Experimental treatments such as the use of IL-2 and anti-TNFα may be of benefit in the systemic forms of LCH seen in children.

Prognosis is variable. Spontaneous improvement is common, although later reactivation of disease may occur. A minority of patients deteriorate rapidly with respiratory failure and death within months. Overall life expectancy is reduced, with median survival 12–13 years from diagnosis. Death is most commonly due to respiratory failure. Poor prognostic factors include reduced FEV_1, increased residual volume, and reduced gas transfer.

Further Information

Pulmonary Langerhans cell histiocytosis. Sundar KM *et al. Chest* 2003; **123**: 1673–83

Lymphangioleiomyomatosis (LAM): clinical features

Definition and aetiology A rare disorder characterized by abnormal proliferation of smooth muscle cells, affecting women of child-bearing age, usually in their 30s. The disease is hormone-dependent, so can occur in post-menopausal women on oestrogen replacement therapy.
- Incidence of 1 in 1.1 million population
- Unknown cause
- Not hereditary
- 40% of adult women with tuberous sclerosis (learning difficulties, seizures, facial angiofibromas, autosomal dominant inheritance) develop pulmonary changes identical to those of LAM.

Pathology Abnormal proliferation of atypical smooth muscle cells (LAM cells) throughout lung, airways, blood vessels, and lymphatics. There is nodular infiltration, which is initially subtle. Progressive growth causes lymphatic and airway obstruction, leading to cyst formation throughout the lungs.

Clinical features

Common
- Secondary pneumothorax (in two-thirds of patients; occurs due to lung cystic change; recurrence is common)
- Dyspnoea (in 42%)
- Cough (in 20%)
- Haemoptysis (in 14%)
- Chylothorax (in 12%, thoracic duct leakage as a result of lymphatic obstruction by LAM cells, may be bilateral).

Less common
- Pleural effusion
- Chest pain
- Pulmonary haemorrhage (due to blocked blood vessels and increased intraluminal pressure).

Other organs affected

Kidney Angiomyolipoma, a benign tumour, occurs in 50% of LAM patients. Usually diagnosed on CT, these are mostly small and single, but can be multiple and larger in tuberous sclerosis. Smaller tumours are usually asymptomatic, but larger ones can cause flank pain and bleeding into the renal tract. Treatment options include tumour resection or embolization. Nephrectomy is not usually required. Screening for these lesions is important as it allows careful treatment planning in case they become symptomatic.

Abdomen Lymphadenopathy due to lymphatic blockage. Occurs in one-third of patients and is usually asymptomatic.

Pelvis Lymphangioleiomyoma—a cystic mass that enlarges during the day and causes fullness and bloating.

Chylous ascites can occur in the absence of chylothorax.

Skin Cutaneous swellings, likely due to localized oedema.

Examination May be normal. There may be pulmonary crepitations or signs of pleural effusion. Palpable abdominal masses may be present.

Investigations

- *PFTs* may be normal, or show a predominantly obstructive pattern. Rarely restrictive. Decreased TLCO, with a normal or increased TLC
- *CXR* may be normal. Lungs may appear hyperinflated, with reticular shadowing and septal lines due to obstructed lymphatics. There may also be a diffuse interstitial infiltrate
- *HRCT* shows a characteristic appearance, with multiple cysts throughout the lung of varying size, which are usually small (<1 cm) and thin-walled. The adjoining lung parenchyma is normal. There may be pleural effusions.

LAM: diagnosis and management

Diagnosis Consider particularly in young or middle-aged women with:
- Recurrent pneumothoraces, especially those with pre-existing dyspnoea or haemoptysis
- Cystic lung disease, airflow obstruction, or chylous pleural effusions
- Angiomyolipomas or other retroperitoneal tumours
- Tuberous sclerosis and respiratory symptoms

The disease is easily missed in its early stages. The diagnosis can be made on the characteristic CT appearances, or with open lung biopsy. Transbronchial biopsies may not be diagnostic. Large retroperitoneal abdominal lymph nodes can also be biopsied.

Management
- There are no controlled trials of treatment
- The course of LAM is variable. Treatment should be aimed at those who are symptomatic and declining
- *Diet* Low fat diet with medium chain triglyceride supplementation may prevent chylothorax recurrence, but there is not strong evidence for this. The diet is difficult to adhere to
- *Bronchodilators* may improve airflow obstruction
- *Hormonal manipulation* with progesterone has been tried. It may be beneficial in reducing the decline in FEV_1 and TLCO, particularly in patients with progressive disease, but there are no large studies. Tamoxifen and oophrectomy have also been tried
- *Avoid oestrogens* i.e. the oral contraceptive pill and hormone replacement therapy
- *Contraception* An increase in symptoms and accelerated disease decline are reported in pregnancy. Use the progesterone-only pill
- *Pleural aspiration* when required for pleural effusions. For recurrent effusions or chylothoraces, thoracic duct ligation or pleurectomy may be effective. Pleurodesis can be performed, but this is relatively contra-indicated if future lung transplant is an option
- *Recurrent pneumothoraces* Advise regarding flying and diving. Thoracic surgery may be necessary
- *Avoid air travel* if possible due to risk of pneumothorax
- *Transplant* Single or double lung, or heart–lung. LAM can recur in the transplanted lung
- *Stop smoking* as this accelerates the rate of decline
- Influenza vaccine
- Liaise with a specialist centre if required (this is Nottingham City Hospital in the UK).

Prognosis is very variable. The condition usually slowly progresses to respiratory failure. At 10 years 55% of patients have MRC grade 3 dyspnoea, 23% are on LTOT, and 10% are housebound. Survival: 70% of patients are alive at 10 years, 33% are alive at 15 years, and 25% are alive at 20 years.

Future developments Rapamycin may switch off the defect in LAM cells and prevent their proliferation. Studies are ongoing.

Further information

Clinical experience of LAM in the UK. Johnson SR, Tattersfield AE. *Thorax* 2000; **55**: 1052–7

LAM: A review. Sullivan EJ. *Chest* 1998; **114**: 1689–703

Chylothorax in LAM. Ryu JH *et al. Chest* 2003; **123**(2): 623–7

LAM Action (UK), *www.lamaction.org*

LAM Foundation (USA), *lam.uc.edu*

Recurrent respiratory papillomatosis

These are essentially warts of the upper respiratory tract, caused by the human papilloma virus (HPV 6 or 11). The virus infects epithelial cells and mucous membranes, similar to that seen in cutaneous and anogenital infection. The infection is most commonly acquired during ororespiratory exposure from the mother during vaginal delivery, and typically presents in childhood from 6 months onwards, with signs and symptoms of upper respiratory tract infection. It may also present for the first time in adulthood. It is associated with HLA DR3, and with sexual transmission in adults. Recurrent respiratory papillomatosis is rare (2 per 100,000), but oral HPV infection is common.

Clinical course

This is variable
- May remit spontaneously
- Progressive voice loss and airway obstruction
- Most cases are confined to the larynx, although up to 25% of patients subsequently develop extralaryngeal spread to the bronchial tree
- 1% have malignant change to squamous cell carcinomas.

Management

- Surgical excision to maintain airway patency
- Laser therapy—but potential problems of thermal injury, stricture formation, and spread of papillomas
- Photodynamic therapy reduces recurrence rate, using oral or intravenous photosensitizing agent, then a laser to destroy photosensitive tissue
- Microdebrider is now used more commonly
- Medical treatment—interferon, acyclovir, ribovarin, isoretinoin, and methotrexate have all been tried
  - *Interferon*-α as a daily subcutaneous injection leads to complete remission in 30–50%, and partial resolution in 30%. One-third recur when treatment is stopped. Adverse reactions are common: flu-like symptoms, deranged LFTs, leucopenia, and alopecia
  - *Cidofovir* is a nucleoside monophosphate analogue and inhibits viral polymerase. It is given as an intralesional injection. Potential side-effects include nephrotoxicity and neutropenia.

Pulmonary arteriovenous malformations (PAVMs): aetiology and diagnosis

Aetiology

- Pulmonary arteriovenous malformations (PAVMs) are abnormal blood vessels replacing normal capillaries, making a direct, low-resistance connection between the pulmonary arterial and systemic venous circulations. They vary in size from tiny clusters of vessels (telangiectasia) to larger, more complex aneurysmal-type sacs
- The disorder is rare, affecting 1 in 15,000 to 24,000
- Several genetic susceptibility loci have been identified on chromosomes 9 and 12. One identified mutation is in the endoglin gene. This modulates signalling via the transforming growth factor-beta family of growth factors. This gene is also implicated in the development of primary pulmonary hypertension
- Subjects with significant PAVMs have low pulmonary vascular resistance, a low mean PAP, and a high cardiac output—due to longstanding adaptive mechanisms to the effects of the shunt, in addition to vascular remodelling effects
- Most patients present post-puberty, as AVMs probably develop at this time. They probably grow throughout life, especially during puberty and in pregnancy. They may rarely regress spontaneously.

Diagnosis

- Most patients present with an abnormal **CXR**, classically showing a smooth, rounded intrapulmonary mass, with draining or feeding vessels
- Mild **hypoxaemia**. An AVM is a direct communication between the pulmonary artery and pulmonary vein. Blood therefore bypasses the pulmonary capillary bed, with reduced oxygenation, which poorly corrects with supplementary oxygen
- **Orthodeoxia** is desaturation on standing, due to an increase in blood flow in the dependent lung areas. 70% of PAVMs are basal; hence the desaturation seen
- **CT** identifies all AVMS, and can determine those suitable for embolization. Contrast is not required
- Patients may present with the complications of a PAVM, particularly bleeding or peripheral abscess formation. The absence of a normal filtering capillary bed means small particles can reach the systemic circulation, leading to sequelae, particularly in the cerebral circulation—strokes and cerebral abscesses. These abnormal vessels are also at risk of rupture.

Shunt quantification

- **100% oxygen rebreathing study**, a non-invasive method of shunt quantification
- **99mTC perfusion scan**, a tracer study; the size of the shunt can be assessed from the proportion of radiolabelled macroaggregates reaching the systemic circulation, compared to the total number injected. In a normal study, aggregates accumulate in the kidneys

- *Contrast echocardiogram* to measure the circulatory transit time of injected echocontrast
- *Angiography* at specialist centre only
- In normal individuals the anatomical shunt is < 2–3.5 % of the cardiac output (due to post-pulmonary drainage of bronchial veins into pulmonary vein, and drainage into the left atrium).

Clinical features
- Asymptomatic (50%)
- Dyspnoea
- Haemoptysis (10%), probably due to additional bronchial telangiectasia, which can also cause haemorrhage into bronchi or the pleural cavity
- Chest pain (12%); aetiology is uncertain
- Clubbing
- Cyanosis
- Orthodeoxia
- Vascular bruits
- Telangiectasia; 80% of PAVM patients have hereditary haemorrhagic telangiectasia (HHT), and their families should be screened because of the risk of stroke (see page 565)
- May present with acute stroke, with focal neurological signs.

PAVMs: management and complications

Management

Embolization is usually done with coils, which generate local thrombin, leading to cessation of blood flow in AVM feeding vessels. This results in a reduction in the right–left shunt and improvement in hypoxaemia, and should be done by an expert in a specialist centre only. The small risk of neurological sequelae and angina/arrythmias is reduced with operator experience.

60–70% of patients are left with a small persisting shunt following treatment, and retain a small risk of abscess formation. Patients are therefore given prophylactic antibiotics for dental and surgical procedures (ensure the patient has a medic alert card).

Surgical resection may be more appropriate than embolization in some cases.

Anti-platelet therapy (rarely) in individual cases, if ongoing transient ischaemic attacks.

Transplantation is not advised as there is no increased survival benefit over medical treatment.

Screening The majority of patients with PAVMs have HHT, and so screening of family members is important.

Follow-up All patients need regular follow-up with shunt assessment post-surgical resection or embolization, as removal of one shunt may unmask or provoke the development of others.

Female patients should be advised to defer pregnancy until completion of formal assessment, because of the risks of growth and rupture of PAVMs in pregnancy (see below).

Complications

- PAVM patients never die of respiratory failure in the absence of additional respiratory disease
- All patients are at risk of stroke and cerebral abscesses
- Transient ischaemic attack/stroke (in 25%), due to rupture of abnormal capillaries in aneurysms
- Abscess (in 10%), due to paradoxical emboli through the right to left shunt, and the absence of a filtering capillary bed.

Pregnancy is associated with an increase in size of AVMs, and new ones may develop, with potentially catastrophic consequences. Careful shunt assessment is therefore needed prior to pregnancy, with contraceptive advice prior to specialist assessment. Close liaison between the specialist centre and obstetric team is paramount. AVMs may need embolization in the third trimester to allow safe delivery.

Hereditary haemorrhagic telangiectasia

(HHT; also referred to as Osler–Weber–Rendu syndrome) Prevalence: 1 in 5–8000.

Definition

An autosomal dominant disorder characterized by the development of abnormal, dilated vessels in the systemic circulation, which may bleed leading to:

- Recurrent epistaxis
- Gastrointestinal bleeding
- Iron deficiency anaemia
- Other organ involvement, e.g. hepatic (in 30%, commonly asymptomatic), renal, pulmonary, and spinal AVMs.

Screening Careful questioning of family members (does anyone in the family have frequent nose bleeds?) and examination for telangiectasia should reveal those in whom screening should occur.

All those with HHT should be screened for PAVMs, and all of their off-spring post-puberty and pre-pregnancy. There is increasing penetrance with increasing age (62% at age 16, 95% at age 40). Similarly, the detection of PAVMs in a patient should lead to screening for HHT in family members.

There is no consensus regarding the best screening method, but a combination of the following tests may be used:

- CXR
- Supine and erect oximetry
- CT chest
- Shunt quantification techniques, e.g. contrast echocardiogram, 100% oxygen rebreathing.

Screening should continue throughout life (every 5 to 10 years) and during times of enlargement or development of AVMs—post-puberty and pre-pregnancy.

Management

- Usually involves liaison with ENT and gastroenterological colleagues for symptomatic treatment
- Iron replacement, transfusions
- Asymptomatic hepatic AVMs—no treatment usually required
- Cerebral AVMs (in 15% of HHT patients)—some specialists argue these should be treated prophylactically, due to the risk of rupture and bleeding (2% per year, often fatal).

Further information

Shovlin CL, Letarte M. *Thorax* 1999; **54**: 714–39

A website for patients and their relatives, *www.hht.orga*

Telangiectasia Self Help Group website, *www.telangiectasia.co.uk*

Primary ciliary dyskinesia (PCD)

A rare, genetic cause of chronic respiratory disease, usually encountered in adult respiratory clinics as a cause of bronchiectasis. Cilia are found in:
- The whole length of the upper respiratory tract
- Brain ventricles
- Fallopian tube/ductus epididymis.

They are made up of dynein arms, with outer and inner connecting rings, and beat at 14 beats/second. Many gene defects have been identified in PCD, causing a number of cilial abnormalities.

Abnormal cilia do not beat normally, leading to reduced mucociliary clearance, microbiological colonization (which further inhibits cilial action), chronic infection, and the development of bronchiectasis.

The main aim following diagnosis in childhood is the prevention of chronic respiratory disease and bronchiectasis.

Clinical features
- Autosomal recessive
- May present with neonatal respiratory distress
- Situs inversus (in about 30%, as cilia determine the side of the organs. Random organ siding occurs with cilial dysfunction, hence the situs inversus of Kartagener's syndrome)
- Nasal blockage/rhinitis
- Persistent wet cough in childhood
- Hearing problems/history of glue ear/grommets in childhood
- Clubbing and signs of chest disease are rare in childhood
- Wheeze in 20%
- Infertility due to low sperm count in men
- In adults the disease usually presents with the clinical signs of bronchiectasis: cough productive of purulent sputum, recurrent chest infections, intermittent haemoptysis.

Diagnosis Saccharin test (see page 357). Cilial biopsy via the nasal route. Cilia are examined by high-speed digital video, where their beat frequency and pattern can be assessed. Most cases of PCD are diagnosed in childhood. There is an increased frequency in the children of consanguineous marriages.

Consider the diagnosis in:
- Bronchiectasis
- Situs inversus
- Persistent upper and lower respiratory infection from early childhood
- Infertility—males may present in infertility clinics.

Management
In adults this involves the treatment of secondary bronchiectasis (see page 358), with:
- Antibiotics
- Physiotherapy
- Vaccinations
- Management of haemoptysis.

Chapter 47

Flying, altitude, and diving

Lung disease and flying

Problems Flying presents problems for three reasons:
- Extra hypoxia
- Volume changes in gas compartments
- Closed environment and disease transmission.

Extra hypoxia Modern aeroplanes are pressurized to the equivalent of about 5000 ft (1500 m). This gives an atmospheric pressure of about 85 kPa and an FiO_2 of about 18 kPa compared to 21 kPa at sea level. In normal subjects this causes an inconsequential fall in PaO_2 and SaO_2.

Some companies pressurize less to save money, e.g. 8000 ft (2400 m), FiO_2 16 kPa, and even in normal subjects the SaO_2 may fall to 92% or so.

Patients with lung disease and a degree of hypoxia will be nearer the steep part of the haemoglobin dissociation curve and will experience bigger proportional falls in oxygen carriage by the blood. The estimated PaO_2 at 8000 feet (the lowest cabin pressurisation likely to be encountered) is estimated by this formula:

Estimated PaO_2 at 8000 ft = (0.24 x PaO_2 at sea level) + (2.7 x FEV_1/VC) + 3
e.g. sea level PaO_2 = 8 kPa, FEV_1/VC = 0.40, estimated PaO_2 = 6 kPa

This is only an approximation, and will vary considerably patient to patient, particularly due to differences in hypoxic drive. An alternative is to give the patient an hypoxic mixture to breathe and measure the PaO_2/SaO_2. This is most easily achieved by feeding a 35% Venturi mask with 100% nitrogen (17% O_2, simulating 6500 ft), and a 40% Venturi mask simulates 8000 ft (equivalent to 16% O_2). Even this will not necessarily predict that a patient will or will not run into trouble. Empirically oxygen is often prescribed if the in-flight PaO_2 at 8000 ft, estimated from the above equation or by experimentation, is less than 7 kPa or 86% SaO_2. This is not evidence-based, so a simple recommendation based on sea level oximetry measurements is likely to be as valid.

Simple recommendations for oxygen when flying	
SaO_2 > 92%	No oxygen required
SaO_2 90–92%	Perform challenge test
SaO_2 < 90%	Recommend oxygen

These are not quite the same as the BTS guidelines, which are more complex and consider co-morbidities. Two litres/minute via nasal cannulae, or 28% Venturi mask, are usually sufficient to raise the SaO_2 to sea level equivalent. Airlines vary as to whether they charge for this and at least a month should be allowed to arrange it.

Volume changes in gas compartments Ascent to the equivalent of 5000 ft will increase gas in trapped compartments by 20%, and ascent to 8000 ft by nearly 40%. A pneumothorax, or bullae, will therefore increase by this amount. Therefore it is advised that patients with current pneumothoraces should not fly. In addition they are advised not to fly within 6 weeks of a pneumothorax because of the higher chance of a recurrence and the lack of adequate emergency medical treatment on board. The same arguments are applied to patients having had recent thoracic surgery (for whatever reason) who are advised not to fly for 6 weeks after surgery, although some airlines allow 2 weeks. None of this is evidence-based and the risks of ignoring these guidelines are not known. It is probable that the risk of a second pneumothorax within this period is only significant in patients with pre-existing lung disease.

Closed environment Patients with infectious diseases such as TB should not fly. There seems to be a significant risk of infecting others.

Further information

Aircraft cabin pressures. Cottrell JJ *Chest* 1988; **98**: 81

British Thoracic Society guidelines, *www.brit-thoracic.org.uk/docs/flyingguidelines.pdf*

British Lung Foundation patient leaflet on flying with a lung condition, *www.britishlungfoundation.org/docs/info_sheets/btsair.doc*

Altitude sickness

Definitions of acute mountain sickness, or high altitude sickness, are not precise, but include several symptoms provoked by the hypoxia.

Pathophysiology Some of the pathophysiology is well understood and explains some of the symptoms and signs. These largely fall into two categories, minor and major.

Minor, due to hyperventilation provoked by the hypoxia, and include:
- Light-headedness/fatigue
- Numbness/tingling of extremities
- Nausea/vomiting and anorexia
- Headache
- Insomnia/sleep disturbance
- Periodic ventilation during sleep.

These symptoms are common, develop over 6–12 hours after arrival, and affect about 1/4 of those flying to Colorado for a skiing holiday (altitude 2400–3400 m, ~10,000 ft, barometric pressure 70 kPa, inspired oxygen tension 14.5 kPa, average SaO_2 on arrival 89–90%). Most of the symptoms are due to a respiratory hypocapnic alkalosis and resolve as the kidney retains $[H^+]$ and excretes $[HCO_3^-]$, returning pH towards normal. This allows further hyperventilation and the rise in SaO_2 helps resolve any symptoms due to the hypoxia itself. This scenario tends to be common in those with a higher hypoxic drive (measured at sea level, as it encourages greater hypocapnia and alkalosis). These symptoms may also indicate the early development of the more major category.

Major, those due to the hypoxia itself. These are more serious, can develop rapidly, and tend to occur more in those with a lower hypoxic drive. There is also a genetic component influencing susceptibility, related to the ACE gene. In *high altitude pulmonary oedema* (**HAPE**) the hypoxia provokes a *non-uniform* pulmonary vasoconstriction, raising pulmonary artery pressure (PAP); hence some pulmonary capillaries are unprotected and receive the full rise in PAP. Fluid leakage into alveoli, pulmonary oedema, and capillary damage (with pulmonary haemorrhage) produce clinically apparent disease. The dominant symptoms/signs are:
- Extra breathlessness/cough
- Cyanosis
- Blood tinged frothy sputum
- Crackles on auscultation/raised JVP.

In *high altitude cerebral oedema* (**HACE**) hypoxia can also cause increased cerebral blood flow and cerebral oedema, with retinal haemorrhage, cerebral thrombosis, and petechial haemorrhage. The dominant symptoms are:
- Ataxia (may be the first sign)
- Confusion/disorientation/hallucinations/behavioural change
- Severe headache/reduced conscious level
- Papilloedema.

Both HAPE and HACE are potentially fatal.

Management Risk factors are mainly the rate and degree of altitude attained. Keep ascent to ≤300 m/day and rest every third day. The minor form of altitude sickness is likely to resolve spontaneously over a few days with simple symptomatic treatment, analgesics, and plenty of hydration. However, prophylaxis, or early treatment on symptom appearance, with acetazolamide, is very effective, as are limiting further ascent and encouraging descent. *Acetazolamide* provokes a mild metabolic acidosis (by reducing $[H^+]$ availability for excretion in the distal tubule) and 'pre-acclimatizes' the subject to allow greater hyperventilation in response to hypoxia without the usual alkalosis. It is recommended when rapid ascent to altitudes ≥2500 metres is unavoidable (such as a package ski trip to Aspen). 500 mg per day (slow release–Diamox) two days prior to ascent is probably adequate for most subjects (or as treatment after symptoms develop). The commonest side-effect is a harmless and reversible tingling of the extremities. *Temazepam* has been shown to reduce the periodic breathing at night (by reducing the arousals that help maintain the periodicity) and does not appear to worsen the hypoxia.

The management of the more severe forms of altitude sickness that tend to occur with rapid ascent to over 4000 m, pulmonary and cerebral oedema, is urgent.

Management of severe altitude sickness
- Increase inspired oxygen tension, either by rapid descent, extra inspired oxygen, or a local pressurized environment (e.g. a portable hyperbaric chamber such as the Gamow bag).

HAPE
- Sit upright and keep warm
- Nifedipine (20 mg bd up to qds + loading dose, 10 mg sublingually) to reduce PAP.

HACE
- Dexamethasone (4 mg qds + loading dose, 8 mg) to reduce cerebral oedema.

Improvement is usually rapid once the inspiratory oxygen tension is raised. Prophylaxis for this more severe form of altitude sickness is more controversial but graded ascent is important, acetazolamide probably helps, and nifedipine is used by some, particularly if there is a history of a previous episode.

Further information

Information for patients, *www.thebmc.co.uk/world/mm/mm1.htm*

Information for patients, *familydoctor.org/247.xml*

Information for patients and doctors, *www.high-altitude-medicine.com*

Diving

Problems Increased recreational diving has raised the awareness of respiratory problems at depth. These can essentially be divided into four.
- Barotrauma, e.g. ruptured bullae and pneumothorax
- Worsening of pre-existing disorder whilst at depth, e.g. asthma
- Nitrogen gas evolved from solution in body fluids
- Breath-hold diving and ascent hypoxia.

Pathophysiology

Barotrauma (*second commonest cause of death in SCUBA divers after drowning*). During descent, any air-containing cavity in the body will be compressed by the rise in external pressure. If there is any communication with the airways (e.g. middle ear, lung bullae) then gas will slowly move into the air space. On ascent the airspace will expand and, if air cannot escape quickly enough, may lead to rupture, of the eardrum or the bullae for example. *A tension pneumothorax can be rapidly fatal in this situation.* Obstructive lung diseases in general can predispose to ruptured alveoli. In addition to pneumothoraces, the escaped air can produce a pneumomediastinum, causing chest pain, and a radiolucent band (air in the pericardium) along the cardiac border on CXR. Breathing 100% O_2 will clear the air more quickly. Air emboli can also occur and produce a wide range of symptoms; hyperbaric oxygen may be required.

Pre-existing lung disease The onset of asthma during a dive can be disastrous and may be provoked by the dry gases breathed from SCUBA gear (self-contained underwater breathing apparatus). *See BSAC recommendations on asthma and diving opposite.* Many lung diseases such as cystic fibrosis, COPD (FEV_1 < 80% predicted), fibrotic lung disease, previous pneumothorax (with no pleurodesis), and lung bullae are considered contraindications to diving.

The bends or caisson disease (caisson are underwater air chambers in which people work). During periods of high pressure, extra nitrogen dissolves into the blood and other tissue fluids. This takes many minutes. On ascent this nitrogen literally bubbles off. If the amount coming out of solution is too great, nitrogen bubbles act as emboli and limit blood flow. This produces microinfarction with activation of inflammatory and clotting cascades and damage to several organs, e.g. joints, spinal cord, brain. Limited diving times and slow ascents reduce this problem, as do breathing mixtures containing helium rather than oxygen. Severe cases require treatment in hyperbaric chambers.

Breath-hold diving During a breath-hold dive, the increased pressure on the chest elevates the alveolar PO_2 and thus the arterial PO_2. This extends the breath-hold time, particularly if prior hyperventilation to reduce the $PaCO_2$ has been practised. During the dive, oxygen is used and the alveolar PO_2 falls. On ascent, with rarefaction of the thoracic gas, the PO_2 falls precipitously with possible loss of consciousness and drowning.

British sub aqua club (BSAC) recommendations re asthma

- Asthma may predispose to air-trapping leading to pulmonary barotrauma and air embolism, which may be fatal. An acute asthma attack can also cause severe dyspnoea that may be hazardous or fatal during diving
- These theoretical risks should be explained fully to the asthmatic diver. There is little, if any, evidence that the mild, controlled, asthmatic that follows the guidelines below is at more risk
- Asthmatics may dive if they have allergic asthma but not if they have cold-, exercise-, or emotion-induced asthma
- All asthmatics should be managed in accordance with British Thoracic Society Guidelines
- Only well-controlled asthmatics may dive
- Asthmatics should not dive if he/she has needed a *therapeutic* bronchodilator in the last 48 hours, or has had any other chest symptoms.

Control of asthma

- The asthmatic should not need more than occasional bronchodilators, i.e. daily usage would be a disqualifying factor, but inhaled steroids/cromoglycate/nedocromil are permissible
- During the diving season he/she should take bd peak flows. A deviation of 10% from best values should exclude diving until within 10% of best values for at least 48 hours before diving
- The medical examiner should perform an exercise test such as the 18 in (43 cm) step test for three minutes, or running outside (not a bicycle ergometer) to increase the heart rate to 80% (210 minus age). A decrease in PEFR of 15% at three minutes post-exercise should be taken as evidence of exercise-induced bronchoconstriction and hence disbars. The patient should be off all bronchodilators for 24 hours before the test
- A β_2 agonist may be taken pre-diving as a *preventative* but not to relieve bronchospasm at the time.

Further information

Aberdeen emergency number for hyperbaric chambers, *www.hyperchamber.com* 07831 151523.

British Thoracic Society guidelines, *www.brit-thoracic.org.uk/docs/diving.pdf*

Diving and medical conditions, *www.bsac.org/medical/index.htm*

Diving and pneumothorax, *www.bsac.org/medical/r_pneumo.htm*

Diving, medical forms and certificates, *www.bsac.org/medical/index.html*

Plymouth Diving Disease Research Centre, *www.ddrc.org/docs/contact.htm* (24hr help line and register of hyperbaric chambers) 01752 209999

Toxic agents

Drug-induced lung disease: clinical presentations

Introduction A vast number of drugs can damage the respiratory system, from nose to alveoli. The most complete and useful list (plus references) is kept at **www.pneumotox.com** and can be queried either by drug (or drug type), or by clinical/radiological presentation: all agents have equal prominence, but are coded with a star rating to indicate likely prevalence. This chapter describes the commoner drugs that produce respiratory problems.

Commoner presentations of drug-induced lung disease and examples of causative agents

- Interstitial lung disease, pneumonitis, fibrosis
  - Acute hypersensitivity pneumonitis (nitrofurantoin, methotrexate)
  - Interstitial pneumonitis ± eosinophilia (amiodarone, ACE inhibitors)
  - Chronic organizing pneumonia (amiodarone, bleomycin)
  - Pulmonary fibrosis (bleomycin, amiodarone, nitrofurantoin, β blockers)
- Airways disease
  - Bronchospasm (β blockers, contrast media)
  - Obliterative bronchiolitis (busulphan, penicillamine)
  - Cough (ACE inhibitors)
- Pleural changes
  - Pleural effusion/thickening (β blockers, nitrofurantoin, methotrexate, dopamine agonists)
  - Pneumothorax (bleomycin)
- Vascular changes
  - Thromboembolic disease (phenytoin)
  - Pulmonary hypertension (dexfenfluramine, other appetite suppressants)
  - Vasculitis (nitrofurantoin, L-tryptophan)
- Mediastinal changes
  - Node enlargement (bleomycin, phenytoin)
  - Sclerosing mediastinitis (ergot)
- Pulmonary oedema (methotrexate, contrast media)
- Pulmonary haemorrhage (methotrexate, nitrofurantoin, penicillamine, contrast media).

Drug-induced lung disease: examples 1

Amiodarone Iodinated benzofuran used to suppress supra- and ventricular tachycardias. Lung toxicity correlates loosely with total dose and therefore usually occurs after a variable number of months. Seen in 10% of subjects on >400 mg/day. Rare if <300 mg/day.

Risk factors
- Daily dose >400 mg
- Increasing age of patient
- Use for more than 2 months
- Pre-existing lung disease (although not a contraindication to its use)
- Recent surgical intervention or lung infection.

Diagnosis is usually one of exclusion, and response to cessation of drug (which can take months). Infiltrative lung disease varying from acute respiratory distress (rare) through to COP (cough, pleuritic pain, fever, dyspnoea, asymmetric patchy infiltrates, effusion), and the most indolent, chronic interstitial pneumonitis (cough, dyspnoea, weight loss, diffuse and/or focal opacities).

On *CT* the liver, thyroid, and lungs will usually show increased attenuation, indicating a significant amiodarone load. A baseline CXR is useful.

Lung biopsies exclude other diagnoses and provide compatible findings, but there is dissent as to how diagnostic they are (except for the finding of foamy macrophages in the airspaces, filled with amiodarone–phospholipid complexes, but may occur in absence of lung toxicity). Mechanisms of toxicity are unclear, and there are features to suggest hypersensitivity and direct toxic damage.

Treatment Steroids are effective and required in severe disease. The half-life of amiodarone in the tissues is in excess of a month and response to stopping the drug may be slow. Prognosis is good in the majority.

Azathioprine Extensively used as an immunosuppressant but has remarkably little pulmonary toxicity other than via opportunistic lung infection. Case reports of pneumonitis only.

Bleomycin DNA-damaging glycopeptide used in the treatment of lymphomas, germ cell tumours, squamous carcinomas (cervix, head, neck, and oesphagus). Pulmonary fibrosis occurs in about 10%.

Risk factors
- Older age
- Those receiving total dose of >400 mg (1 mg ≈ 1000 units [1 old unit])
- Increased FiO_2 (even for some time after drug administration), probably via increased superoxide/free radical formation
- Pulmonary irradiation, not just in the irradiated field
- Renal failure decreases drug elimination and thus toxicity
- Associated use of cyclophosphamide.

Symptoms (cough, dyspnoea, chest pain, fever) develop 1–6 months after bleomycin. There is hypoxia and a restrictive defect. Progressive basal subpleural shadowing, small lungs, and blunting of costophrenic angles.

Histology shows a dominant subpleural distribution of damage and repair with fibrosis; this appearance is non-diagnostic and common to many drugs/disorders. Toxicity is probably due to DNA damage or oxidative injury, with interindividual variation occurring due to differing activity of the enzyme bleomycin hydrolase; only low levels of this enzyme exist in the lung (and skin). A rare acute hypersensitivity form comes on within days of administration.

Treatment
- Bleomycin must be stopped on suspicion of damage, and some units use lung function tests (kCO) to detect early damage
- Steroids are used, but there is little evidence they alter long-term prognosis (in the acute hypersensitivity subgroup there is a clear beneficial effect)
- Use the minimum FiO_2 to maintain an adequate SaO_2
- Over 50% may experience a relentless decline in lung function.

Busulphan DNA alkylating, myelosuppressive, agent mainly used to treat chronic myeloid leukaemia, and prior to bone marrow transplantation, with a low rate of lung toxicity (4–10%) due to fibrosis.

Risk factors
- Cumulative doses over 500 mg (mostly over 120 days)
- Concurrent administration of other alkylating agents
- Pulmonary irradiation.

Presents with cough and progressive SOB, often years after exposure (usually about 4). CXR is typically unremarkable. Reduced kCO and restrictive defect. Diagnosis is usually by exclusion. The place of steroids is unproven.

Chlorambucil DNA alkylating agent mainly used to treat chronic lymphocytic leukaemia, lymphomas, and ovarian cancer. It has additional immunosuppressive actions, and is also used in conditions such as rheumatoid arthritis. Low risk (1%) of pulmonary toxicity and confined to those who have received >2 grams. Similarly to busulphan, presentation may be many years later. Presents with cough, dyspnoea, weight loss, and basal crackles. CXR shows diffuse basal reticular shadowing. Non-specific histology. On suspicion, chlorambucil should be stopped; use of steroids is unproven. Prognosis is poor (50% fatal).

Drug-induced lung disease: examples 2

Cyclophosphamide DNA alkylating agent mainly used to treat chronic lymphocytic leukaemia, small cell lung cancer, and other solid tumours. Particularly useful as an immunosuppressive agent in certain vasculitides and nephropathies. Lung toxicity is rare.

Risk factors
- Pulmonary irradiation
- Oxygen therapy
- Concurrent drugs causing pulmonary toxicity, e.g. bleomycin.

Clinical presentation is usually within 6 months, with a short duration of fever, cough, and fatigue. Reticular shadowing with ground-glass appearance on CT. Later onset progressive pulmonary fibrosis can also develop insidiously in those on therapy for many months with progressive SOB and dry cough. The histology of the more acute type can be similar to any of the acute interstitial pneumonias (e.g. COP, diffuse alveolar damage), whereas the more chronic form is indistinguishable from UIP. Cyclophosphamide is not itself toxic to the lung, but its metabolites are. There appears to be genetic variation to susceptibility, as there is no obvious dose–response relationship. Cessation of drug and steroid therapy is used successfully in the acute form, but the chronic form seems to progress inexorably, in a similar manner to UIP. Lung transplantation is an option.

Gold Used in rheumatoid arthritis, >500 mg cumulative dose can produce pneumonitis (possibly COP, obliterative bronchiolitis) with cough, dyspnoea, and basal crackles. Rare (1%), but associated with certain HLA types and distinctive histological feature of alveolar septal inflammation. Good prognosis following drug cessation; poor evidence for steroids.

Infliximab Anti-TNF agents represent a large step forward in the treatment of rheumatoid arthritis and Crohn's disease. However, there is a small but important risk of reactivating TB. See page 252.

Methotrexate Folic acid derivative, inhibiting cell division by blocking dihydrofolate reductase and nucleic acid production. Mainly used in leukaemia and as an immunosuppressive, e.g. rheumatoid arthritis and psoriasis. Commonly (4–10%) causes a variety of lung pathologies, not associated with folic acid deficiency.

Risk factors
- Hypoalbuminaemia
- Diabetes
- Previous use of drugs that modify disease progress in rheumatoid
- Rheumatoid or other lung/pleural disease
- Not particularly dose-related; can occur at doses of <20 mg per week
- Daily rather than intermittent (weekly) therapy
- >60 years.

Presents both acutely (interstitial pneumonitis, fever, and eosinophilia) and over very long time periods; however, the subacute form (within a year, dyspnoea, fever, cough, hypoxia, basal crackles, restrictive defect, and reduced kCO) is commoner. Bilateral diffuse pulmonary infiltrates or mixed pattern with alveolar shadowing on CXR, occasional effusions.

Histology is more useful than in other drug toxicities, showing alveolitis, interstitial pneumonitis, epithelial cell hyperplasia, eosinophilic infiltration, and granuloma formation in the more acute, hypersensitivity, form, and more UIP-like changes in the indolent form. Mechanism of damage is unknown but likely to be multifactorial.

Treatment consists of drug withdrawal and the unproven use of steroids. Anecdotal reports support the use of steroids in the more acute, hypersensitivity form.

Other methotrexate-related lung diseases include opportunistic lung infection and non-Hodgkin's B-cell lymphoma, which may regress with drug withdrawal, and may be associated with Epstein–Barr virus.

Nitrofurantoin is used commonly for long-term prophylaxis against urinary tract infections (UTIs). Acutely nitrofurantoin causes a hypersensitivity vasculitis, and, much less frequently, a chronic interstitial fibrosis. Most patients are women due to their much higher prevalence of chronic UTIs. The acute form presents abruptly with fever, dyspnoea, dry cough, rash, chest pain, hypoxia, crackles, and eosinophilia within a week or two of starting, and is dose-independent. Lower zone diffuse patchy infiltrates and sometimes unilateral effusions on CXR. Lung biopsy reveals vasculitis, eosinophilia, reactive type II pneumocytes, focal haemorrhage, and some interstitial inflammation. Treatment consists of discontinuation and improvement begins rapidly. Prognosis is good with or without steroids.

Oxygen Prolonged use of oxygen therapy at 80–100% can provoke lung damage.

Penicillamine Used in the treatment of rheumatoid arthritis, penicillamine may increase the prevalence of obliterative bronchiolitis. This is dose-related but rare, with a subacute onset (after several months) of dyspnoea and cough. There is a progressive obstructive pattern without bronchodilator response. 50% mortality.

Talc is commonly used for pleurodesis (page 692). Talc particles may be small enough to enter the circulation after intrapleural instillation, being found throughout the body at post mortem. They appear to provoke a systemic reaction with fever, raised inflammatory markers, and hypoxia suggestive of an ARDS-like pathology. Occasional deaths after talc pleurodesis have been reported. Refined talc with fewer smaller particles seems less toxic.

Paraquat poisoning

Definitions

Paraquat (Weedol, Pathclear, Gramoxone) and related bipyridyl compounds are used as contact herbicides. They kill plants by inhibiting NADP reduction during photosynthesis, which involves the production of superoxide radicals. The toxicity of paraquat in animals is also believed to be due to the production of damaging superoxides. Most cases of poisoning are deliberate, and the treatment should be commenced as soon as possible. Serious poisoning is usually by ingestion (although paraquat is absorbed through the skin and mucous membranes, including the conjunctiva and bronchial mucosa).

- More than 6 g is always fatal
- Less than 1.5 g is rarely fatal
- Between 1.5 and 6 g, the mortality is 60–70%
- A mouthful of 20% Gramoxone liquid (10 g/50 ml) is almost certainly fatal
- Less than 1 sachet of Weedol granules (1.4 g paraquat/57 g sachet) is unlikely to cause death
- Usually fatal if blood level >0.2 mg/ml at 24 h.

Clinical features

- Oral and oesophageal ulceration shortly after contact, with later formation of a pseudomembrane
- Renal failure (reversible) within a few days, but delayed excretion of paraquat prevents falls in blood levels
- Pulmonary oedema early on, evolving into 'acute respiratory distress syndrome'
- Death usually occurs within 1 to 2 weeks
- Pulmonary fibrosis if the patient survives, with varying degrees of recovery.

Management

- Gastric lavage with either Fuller's earth/bentonite/activated charcoal/sodium resonium to reduce absorption
- Haemoperfusion (haemodialysis less effective) to reduce blood levels
- Lowest inspired oxygen tension possible (high concentrations probably increase superoxide formation)
- Supportive measures which may require intubation and ventilation
- Other treatments (e.g. immunosuppression, NO) are experimental.

Inhalational lung injury 1

Definition Agents damaging the lung and airways through direct toxicity. Much of the acute damage is common to many toxic agents including pneumonitis/pulmonary oedema, mucosal damage/sloughing/airway debris. Secondary infection is common due to breached defences.

Management Following acute exposure, supportive therapy is critical.
- Look for respiratory failure, stridor, or distress; may occur hours later
- CXR (poor sensitivity until pulmonary oedema develops)
- May need intubating/tracheostomy to bypass oedematous and sloughing upper airway mucosa
- Humidified oxygen,
  - Raise SaO_2 into low/mid 90s (higher levels may contribute to oxidative damage)
  - Raise PaO_2 as high as possible if CO poisoning suspected.
- Treat cyanide poisoning if suspected (dicobalt edetate, little evidence)
- Bronchodilators
- Nebulized dilute heparin/acetyl cysteine—variable opinions on value
- Steroids and prophylactic antibiotics—variable opinions on value
- Mechanical ventilation (low volume/pressure, permissive hypercapnia)
- Fluid replacement, but not excessive as encourages pulmonary oedema
- Enteral feeding.

Examples of toxic agents, listed alphabetically

Aldehydes (acetaldehyde, formaldehyde)
- Chemical and plastics industry, used for disinfection
- Highly irritant to mucosal membranes
- Acute damage
  - Pneumonitis and pulmonary oedema
- Chronic effects
  - Rhinitis/asthma.

Ammonia
- Fertilizer and plastics production, used in many chemical industries
- Highly irritant to mucosal membranes
- Acute damage
  - Upper airway obstruction from secretions and mucosal oedema
  - Lung damage and secondary infection
- Chronic effects
  - Airways obstruction and bronchiectasis described.

Chlorine
- Extensive use in the chemical industry, bleaching agent
- Acute damage
  - Overwhelming toxicity producing rapid hypoxia
  - Pneumonitis and pulmonary oedema
- Chronic effects (e.g. from repeated accidental exposure)
  - Airways obstruction; sometimes reversible.

Cocaine (when smoked)
- Pneumothorax/pneumomediastinum
- Pulmonary haemorrhage
- Pulmonary oedema
- Allergic responses (asthma, pulmonary eosinophilia, hypersensitivity pneumonitis).

Metals and metal compounds (as fumes or nebulized solutions)
- Mainly used in the chemical industry
- Acute damage
  - Mucosal irritation
  - Pulmonary oedema
- Chronic effects
  - Pneumoconiosis
- Some specific effects such as:
  - Sarcoid-like reaction to beryllium
  - Asthma/from cobalt, chromium, nickel, vanadium
  - Fibrosing alveolitis from cobalt and zinc fumes.

Methyl isocyanate (Bhopal disaster: 3800 dead, 170,000 injured)
- Chemical industry, carbamate pesticides
- Acute damage
  - Pneumonitis and pulmonary oedema
  - Secondary infection
- Chronic effects
  - Airways obstruction
  - Bronchiolitis obliterans
  - Pulmonary fibrosis.

Hydrocarbons/mineral oils
- Used as lubricant and cooling agent
- Acute damage
  - Pneumonitis
- Chronic effects
  - Pneumonitis
  - Fibrosis
  - Asthma.

Nitrogen dioxide
- Chemical industry (explosives)
- Agricultural silos
- Odourless and therefore high doses inhaled without knowing
- Acute damage (several hours after exposure)
  - Silo fillers lung (pneumonitis/pulmonary oedema)
- Later effects
  - Secondary pulmonary oedema 2–8 weeks after exposure
  - Steroid-responsive, needs 2 months therapy after exposure.

Inhalational lung injury 2

More examples of toxic agents

Ozone
- Bleaching agent
- Product of welding
- Similar to NO_2
- Both immediate and late effects of pneumonitis/pulmonary oedema.

Phosgene
- Chemical warfare, chemical industry, chlorination
- Released from heated methylene chloride (paint stripper)
- Acute damage
  - Pneumonitis and pulmonary oedema
  - Produces COHb; breath CO therefore reflects degree of exposure.

Smoke
- Most smoke injury is due to heat damage to upper airway
- Hypoxia, vaporized toxins (e.g. formaldehyde, chlorine), systemic agents (e.g. CO and cyanide)
- Acute damage
  - Mucosal oedema and sloughing with airway blockage
- Look out for:
  - Peri-oral burns
  - Black sputum
  - Altered voice
  - Respiratory distress
  - Stridor (rapid inspiration to accentuate)
  - Additional CO and/or cyanide poisoning.

Sulphur dioxide
- Used as a fumigant, and bleaching agent in the paper industry
- Very irritant as dissolves to form sulphuric acid
- Acute damage
  - Sloughing of airway mucosa
  - Pneumonitis and haemorrhagic pulmonary oedema
- Chronic effects
  - Airways obstruction.

Welding fumes
- Many agents released
- Specific examples:
  - Cadmium—pneumonitis
  - Zinc—'metal fume fever'
  - Several agents may cause airways obstruction/COPD
- Siderosis (welders lung) non-fibrogenic pneumoconiosis
  - Iron deposits in lung producing small rounded opacities.

Carbon monoxide poisoning

Definition and epidemiology

- Carbon monoxide is a colourless, odourless gas formed when carbon compounds burn in limited oxygen
- It accounts for about 75 deaths per year in the UK, approximately 10% of which are accidental
- Accidental poisonings are commoner in the winter when faulty heating systems are in use
- Non-accidental deaths are mainly from car exhaust fumes
- Methylene chloride (industrial solvent, paint remover) is converted to CO in the liver and may present as CO poisoning
- Up to one-third die following acute high level exposure and another third may be left with permanent neurological sequelae
- Chronic low grade CO exposure may present as non-specific ill health and may affect thousands of individuals.

Pathophysiology and related conditions

- Carbon monoxide competes avidly with O_2 (250 times greater) to bind with the iron in haemoglobin making it less available for oxygen carriage
- The haemoglobin molecule is also distorted by combination with CO that makes it bind more tightly to O_2, shifting the O_2 dissociation curve to the left. The PaO_2 at which the haemoglobin is 50% saturated (P50) moves from about 3.5 to 2 kPa
- This further reduces oxygen delivery to the tissues: a 50% carboxyhaemoglobin level is far more dangerous than a 50% anaemia
- CO also binds to extravascular molecules such as myoglobin and some of the cytochrome chain proteins interfering with energy production, and in this respect is like cyanide
- Normal levels of carboxyhaemoglobin can be up to 3%, and up to 15% in heavy smokers.

Methaemoblobin

- Methaemoglobin is due to oxidation of Fe^{2+} to Fe^{3+} thus preventing O_2 carriage. This is due either to inherited deficiencies of enzymes (cytochrome b5 reductase) that reduce the Fe^{3+} back to Fe^{2+}, or toxic agents (e.g. nitrites [in 'poppers'], chloroquine) that overwhelm this reversal mechanism
- Methaemoglobin is slightly left shifted, but a 40% methaemoglobinaemia may be asymptomatic apart from the typical grey/blue colour of the patient, often mistaken for cyanosis.

Clinical features of CO poisoning

Immediate

- Nausea, headache, malaise, weakness, and unsteadiness
- Loss of consciousness, seizures, cardiac abnormalities (ischaemia, arrhythmias, pulmonary oedema)
- No cyanosis, healthy looking 'cherry red' colour
- Suspect if several members of household present with these features.

Delayed (approximately 1 to 3 weeks, can be longer)
- Cognitive defects and personality changes
- Focal neurology and movement abnormalities.

Investigations
- Pulse oximetry will appear *normal* due to COHb having similar absorption spectra to oxyhaemoglobin
- Arterial PaO_2 levels may be *normal*
- COHb levels can be measured on a Co-Oximeter
- Breath CO measured with devices used for smoking cessation work
- Routine tests to rule out other diagnoses.

Management
- CO is only removed from the body through displacement by O_2; therefore use high concentrations of oxygen
- Raise the PaO_2 as high as possible, intubate and 100% O_2 if necessary
- The half-life of COHb breathing air is about 6 hours; breathing 100% O_2 it is about 1 hour
- Hyperbaric O_2 more rapidly displaces CO and increases dissolved O_2. Reduces the frequency of delayed neurological symptoms from 46% to 25% following significant exposure in one randomized controlled trial, but needs to be instituted early. Still controversial, recent Cochrane report equivocal, and facilities poorly available.

Future developments Isocapnic hyperpnoea may further raise the PaO_2. Alkalosis must be avoided though, to prevent further left shift of the Hb dissociation curve. Can be done voluntarily with 5% CO_2 in O_2 or during intubation. Can double rate of CO elimination.

Further information

Cochrane review of hyperbaric oxygen, www.cochrane.org/cochrane/revabstr/AB002041.htm

01752 209999. Plymouth Diving Disease Research Centre, 24hr helpline and register of hyperbaric chambers

Isocapnic hyperventilation. Kreck et al., ajrccm.atsjournals.org/cgi/reprint/163/2/458.pdf

Carbon monoxide poisoning. Blumenthal I. *J R Soc Med* 2001; **94**: 270–72

Carbon monoxide poisoning: undetected by both patients and their doctors. Harper A, Croft-Baker J. *Age and Ageing* 2004; **33**: 105–9

Paediatric lung disorders pertinent to adult practice

Chronic lung disease of prematurity and viral wheeze

This chapter concentrates on pulmonary conditions that occur in childhood and may become increasingly relevant to adult practice.

Chronic lung disease of prematurity (CLD), formerly known as bronchopulmonary dysplasia (BPD). Advances in neonatal medicine have led to the improved survival of premature babies with immature lungs and respiratory disease. Babies born at lower gestational ages are surviving into adulthood, due to therapy with antenatal steroids to prevent respiratory distress syndrome and the use of artificial surfactant to decrease the surface tension of the neonatal alveolar membrane. There have also been improvements in ventilatory techniques. CLD usually occurs in babies who have been mechanically ventilated.

Usually caused by barotrauma from prolonged ventilation, high-pressure ventilation, and/or ventilation with high oxygen concentrations.

Typical presentation is a premature baby who remains oxygen-dependent after 36 weeks postconceptional age. It is now infrequent in those born at 30+ weeks and weighing more than 1200 g. Mortality of 25–30% with severe CLD. May require prolonged home oxygen therapy, up to one year or beyond. 50% of infants with CLD will need hospital readmission during their first year with respiratory infection. Some may have significant pulmonary sequelae during childhood and adolescence, with chronic hypoxia and pulmonary hypertension, but the majority of children with CLD do not have significant ongoing respiratory symptoms. Children may have disabilities associated with prematurity, such as cerebral palsy or learning difficulties.

Pathology Cytokine-mediated scarring and repair. *Early inflammatory phase:* bronchial necrosis, alveolar destruction, capillary permeability, and associated obliterative bronchiolitis. *Subacute fibroproliferative phase:* type II pneumocyte hyperplasia, bronchial and bronchial smooth muscle hypertrophy, and interstitial and perialveolar fibrosis. *Chronic fibro-proliferative phase:* airway remodelling for up to one year. Prior to surfactant use, these changes were more severe.

PFTs Functional respiratory abnormalities persist with increased airway resistance and airway hyperresponsiveness. RV and RV/TLC are raised, indicative of air trapping. Air trapping improves over 3–4 years as lung growth occurs; however, small airway abnormalities persist, at least until the age of 10.

Chest radiology Persisting mild to moderate abnormalities, with multifocal areas of reduced lung attenuation and perfusion, bronchial wall thickening and decreased bronchus:pulmonary artery diameter ratios on CT. These radiological abnormalities correlate with physiological evidence of air trapping.

Adulthood There are few longitudinal studies beyond childhood and it is unclear what the significance of CLD of prematurity is to adult lung disease.

Viral wheeze and asthma A controversial area. Wheezing is common in infants and toddlers and is often due to viral respiratory tract infections, causing a viral-induced wheeze. This has been found to be associated with passive cigarette smoke exposure, contact with other children, and not being breast-fed. This transient early wheezing is distinct from childhood asthma. The children are not atopic and have no family history of such. The wheeze has resolved usually by the age of 3, although they may persist in having airway hyperactivity for many years. Children with asthma tend to have a family history of eczema with concomitant atopic dermatitis and develop their symptoms at any age, but usually slightly later (by the age of 5). Half of them have mild symptoms, which regress by puberty. Those with more severe disease, requiring regular inhaled steroids, often have disease that persists into adult life.

Congenital abnormalities

Tracheomalacia Floppy trachea, usually associated with oesophageal atresia. Rarely will require intubation or tracheostomy.

Congenital lobar emphysema Overinflation of a lobe due to localized bronchomalacia or bronchial obstruction. May cause wheeze or produce chest deformity. Often resolves spontaneously.

Diaphragmatic hernia A diaphragmatic defect, causing bowel to be present in the chest. This may cause respiratory distress soon after birth and may have been detected during the antenatal period by USS, or it may be completely asymptomatic and found incidentally on CXR, with bowel seen in the chest. There are two types. *Bochdalek hernia* is the congenital absence of posterolateral part of diaphragm, with associated hypoplastic lung due to bowel limiting growth. Treatment is with surgical repair of the diaphragmatic defect, but survival rate is only 50% due to underlying lung problems. *Morgagni hernia* is anteromedial herniation through the foramen of Morgagni, which more commonly is found in adulthood. It may be asymptomatic or cause symptoms of fullness, tightness, or pain in the anterior chest; it does not cause intestinal obstruction. CXR shows a cardiophrenic angle density. Surgical repair is difficult and is usually not necessary.

Cystic adenomatoid lung Excessive overgrowth of bronchioles with multiple cysts occurring in a section of lung. Commonly affects left lower lobe. Can be diagnosed antenatally. Can present in the same way as congenital lobar emphysema. May be mistaken for diaphragmatic hernia. Treatment is by resection of the affected lobe, but there may be space-occupying effects of the abnormal lobe that can cause morbidity and mortality, e.g. due to vena cava obstruction.

Pulmonary sequestration/sequestrated segment Segment of lung parenchyma with no bronchial connection that is unventilated. May be supplied by aberrant artery from the aorta and have anomalous pulmonary drainage to the right atrium. Can be intralobar, sharing pleura with the rest of the lung, or extralobar, which is separated from the lung by a lining of pleural tissue. Mostly left-sided; 75% are situated between the diaphragm and left lower lobe. Associated with other congenital abnormalities in 60% of cases. Can be a chance finding on CXR at any age, when cystic change may be seen in this area. Contrast CT or MRI may aid diagnosis. Surgical resection may be necessary if there is repeated infection in this segment.

MacLeod's syndrome Focal hyperlucency of lung or lobe, due to parenchymal and vascular maldevelopment, following a childhood bronchitis or bronchiolitis. Usually asymptomatic, and is diagnosed on CXR, which shows a hypertranslucent lung, with reduced vascular markings and a small pulmonary artery.

Supportive care

Non-invasive ventilation

Terminology

Ventilatory support may be invasive (via endotracheal tube or tracheostomy) or non-invasive (via facemask). Non-invasive ventilation may be subdivided into positive or negative pressure ventilation.

Positive pressure ventilators deliver volume or pressure support; many different types are available. Bilevel pressure support ventilators are used extensively, and provide pressure support between selected inspiratory and expiratory positive airway pressures (IPAP and EPAP). They function in several modes, including patient-triggered inspiratory support with provision of an underlying back-up rate that will cut in if the patient fails to breathe. Non-invasive positive pressure support may be provided by specialized portable ventilators, or by standard critical care ventilators.

Negative pressure ventilators assist inspiration by 'sucking out' the chest wall; expiration occurs through elastic recoil of the lungs. Includes devices such as tank ventilators and chest 'shell' ventilators. Other devices such as the rocking bed and 'pneumobelt' displace abdominal contents to aid diaphragmatic contraction. Used extensively in the polio epidemics of the 1950s; now only rarely used to manage chronic respiratory failure.

Continuous positive airway pressure (CPAP) supplies constant positive pressure during inspiration and expiration, and is therefore not generally considered a form of ventilatory support. It provides a 'splint' to open the upper airway and collapsed alveoli and improves V/Q matching. CPAP is used extensively in the community to treat obstructive sleep apnoea, but also has a role in improving oxygenation in selected patients with acute respiratory failure, e.g. patients with cardiogenic pulmonary oedema.

Abbreviations

NIV = non-invasive ventilation, also referred to as non-invasive mechanical ventilation (NIMV).
NIPPV = non-invasive positive pressure ventilation; confusingly it is also sometimes interpreted as nasal intermittent positive pressure ventilation, and sometimes referred to as 'NIPPY', after the name of a particular type of ventilator.
IPAP = inspiratory positive airways pressure.
EPAP = expiratory positive airways pressure, also referred to as positive end-expiratory pressure (PEEP).
BiPAP = bilevel positive airway pressure (IPAP is greater than EPAP).
CPAP = continuous positive airway pressure (IPAP is equal to EPAP).

Further information
Noninvasive ventilation. Mehta, Hill. *Am J Respir Crit Care Med* 2001; **163**: 540–77

Indications

NIV may be used in an attempt to avoid invasive ventilation and its complications (e.g. upper airway trauma, ventilator-acquired pneumonia); alternatively, NIV may represent the 'ceiling' of treatment in patients deemed unsuitable for intubation. NIV is not an alternative to invasive ventilation in patients who require this definitive treatment.

Acute exacerbation of COPD

- Consider NIV in patients with an acute exacerbation of COPD who have a respiratory acidosis (pH < 7.35) despite initial medical treatment and controlled oxygen therapy
- Benefits include reduced mortality and need for intubation, more rapid improvement in physiological outcomes (respiratory rate, pH), and symptomatic relief from breathlessness when compared with standard medical treatment
- Invasive ventilation, if deemed appropriate, should be considered particularly in patients with a severe respiratory acidosis (pH < 7.25), as this is associated with increased mortality and treatment failure with NIV.

Acute cardiogenic pulmonary oedema

- Use of CPAP via facemask is effective and should be considered in patients who fail to improve with medical management alone
- Bilevel NIV has not been shown to be superior to CPAP and there is a suggestion of increased myocardial infarction rates following its use. It may, however, have a role in patients who do not respond to CPAP.

Decompensated obstructive sleep apnoea

- Both NIV and nasal CPAP with supplementary oxygen are effective in the treatment of severe decompensated obstructive sleep apnoea (typically with associated obesity hypoventilation or COPD), although NIV is generally recommended when a respiratory acidosis is present.

Respiratory failure from neuromuscular weakness

- NIV is the treatment of choice for decompensated respiratory failure resulting from neuromuscular weakness or chest wall deformity.

Immunocompromised patients

- Immunocompromised patients who develop acute respiratory failure have an extremely high mortality following endotracheal intubation and ventilation
- In immunocompromised patients with pulmonary infiltrates, fever, and hypoxaemic acute respiratory failure, intermittent NIV results in lower intubation rates and hospital mortality when compared to standard treatment
- CPAP is effective in the treatment of PCP.

Community-acquired pneumonia

- Use of NIV may result in a reduction in need for intubation compared to standard medical treatment, although no significant differences in hospital mortality or length of hospitalization have been shown

- CPAP may have a role in improving oxygenation in severe pneumonia
- In patients who would potentially be candidates for intubation, use of NIV or CPAP should not inappropriately delay invasive ventilation and so should only be attempted in an ITU setting.

Other conditions

- There is no evidence to support the use of NIV in acute severe asthma
- There is no strong evidence to support the use of NIV in exacerbations of bronchiectasis and cystic fibrosis, although NIV may be useful as a 'ceiling' of treatment in patients with severe underlying disease who would not be considered suitable candidates for invasive ventilation
- Bilevel NIV or CPAP may have a role in improving gas exchange following trauma or surgery.

Contraindications

Relative contraindications to the use of NIV are listed below. They should be considered in the context of individual patients; for example, severe hypoxaemia may not be considered a contraindication for NIV in a patient who is unsuitable for invasive ventilation.

Contraindications to NIV

- Cardiac or respiratory arrest
- Impaired consciousness or confusion
- Severe hypoxaemia
- Copious respiratory secretions
- Haemodynamic instability
- Facial surgery, trauma, burns, or deformity
- Upper airway obstruction
- Tracheal injury
- Undrained pneumothorax
- Inability to cooperate or to protect the airway
- Vomiting, bowel obstruction, recent upper gastrointestinal tract surgery, oesophageal injury.

Further information

BTS guidelines on non-invasive ventilation in acute respiratory failure. *Thorax* 2002; **57**: 192–211

Early use of non-invasive ventilation for acute exacerbations of chronic obstructive pulmonary disease on general respiratory wards: a multicentre randomised controlled trial. Plant *et al.* *Lancet* 2000; **355**: 1931–5

NIV in acute respiratory failure: practical use

The decision to start NIV should follow a period of initial standard medical treatment including appropriate supplementary oxygen concentrations; a proportion of patients will improve and will no longer require ventilation. Prior to commencing NIV a senior doctor should make a decision with the patient and their family regarding suitability for invasive ventilation should NIV fail and document this clearly in the medical notes. *If the patient is a candidate for invasive ventilation, care must be taken to avoid inappropriate delays in intubation through the use of NIV or CPAP.* Liaise with ITU staff early.

Setting up NIV

1. Select an appropriate mask type and size for the patient. Masks may be nasal or oronasal (full face). Nasal masks require clear nasal passages and may permit mouth leaks, particularly in the acutely breathless patient, but they are more comfortable. Full-face masks avoid mouth leakage and are generally favoured for initial use in acute respiratory failure.

2. Allow the patient to hold the mask to their face prior to attaching the head straps—this may increase confidence and compliance. Mask adjustments are often necessary to minimize air leaks, although some leakage may have to be accepted. Avoid excessive strap tension; one or two fingers should be able to fit under the strap.

3. Set up the ventilator. Typical initial pressures for ventilating a patient with hypercapnic respiratory failure due to an exacerbation of chronic obstructive pulmonary disease (COPD) would be EPAP 4 cm H_2O and IPAP 12 cm H_2O, with a back-up rate of 15/minute and inspiratory: expiratory ratio of 1:3 in spontaneous/timed mode. Increase the IPAP in increments of 2 cm H_2O to a maximum of 20, as tolerated by the patient. Similar settings can be used for patients with hypercapnic respiratory failure resulting from neuromuscular weakness. Consider increasing the EPAP (e.g. to 8 or 10 cm) in obese patients with an 'overlap' syndrome of COPD and obstructive sleep apnoea.

   Pressure support ventilators can also be set to provide CPAP by equalizing the IPAP and EPAP; typical pressures range from 5 to 12.5 cm H_2O. CPAP may improve oxygenation in selected patients with cardiogenic pulmonary oedema or pneumonia.

4. Supplementary oxygen concentration (FiO_2) should be guided by the underlying disease process and by oximetry monitoring. For many hypercapnic patients with COPD, maintenance of oxygen saturations between 85% and 90% effectively balances the risks of hypoxia and hypercapnic respiratory acidosis.

5. Patient monitoring should involve assessment of comfort, respiratory rate, synchrony with the ventilator, mask leaks, pulse rate, blood pressure, and oxygen saturations.

6. Arterial or capillary blood gas analysis should be performed after 1 hour and again after 4 hours if there has been no improvement. Improvement in acidosis and decline in respiratory rate after 1 and

4 hours of treatment are associated with a better outcome. Repeat the blood gas analysis if the clinical condition changes.

7. Lack of response may be indicated by a worsening acidosis or persistently abnormal arterial blood gases, or by a reduced conscious level and clinical deterioration. Consider invasive ventilation, if appropriate. The decision to halt NIV depends on the circumstances of the individual patient, and should be made by a senior doctor.

8. Subsequent management depends on the patient's response. Optimal duration of NIV is unclear but it is typically administered for up to 3 days in acute respiratory failure. NIV does not need to be continuous, and the patient may have breaks for meals and nebulizers. Consider switching to a nasal mask after 24 hours to improve patient comfort.

Troubleshooting

Problem	Possible solution
Clinical deterioration or worsening respiratory failure	Ensure optimal medical therapy
	Consider complications, e.g. pneumothorax, aspiration, sputum retention
	Does the patient require intubation, if appropriate?
pCO_2 remains high (persistent respiratory acidosis)	Exclude inappropriately high FiO_2
	Check mask and circuit for leaks
	Check for patient–ventilator asynchrony
	Check expiration valve patent
	Consider increasing IPAP
pO_2 remains low (< 7 kPa)	Consider increasing FiO_2
	Consider increasing EPAP
Irritation or ulceration of nasal bridge	Adjust strap tension
	Try cushion dressing
	Change mask type
Dry nose or mouth	Consider humidifier
	Check for leaks
Dry sore eyes	Check mask fit
Nasal congestion	Decongestants
Hypotension	Reduce IPAP

NIV in chronic respiratory failure

Chest wall deformity and neuromuscular weakness (page 29)

- NIV has a well-established role in the management of chronic respiratory failure due to chest wall deformity or neuromuscular weakness, and has been shown to improve symptoms, gas exchange, and mortality
- Common underlying diagnoses include chest wall deformity and kyphoscoliosis, post-polio syndrome, motor neurone disease, spinal cord injury, neuropathies, myopathies, and muscular dystrophies. The nature of the underlying disease must influence the appropriateness of initiating ventilation: progressive conditions such as motor neurone disease often result in increasing dependence on the ventilator, and the patient and their care-givers should be made aware of this
- NIV is typically administered at home overnight and this is sufficient to improve daytime gas exchange. The mechanism for this is unclear: it probably resets the central respiratory drive hypercapnia threshold, although respiratory muscle rest and improved compliance may also play a part
- Small, portable positive pressure ventilators and nasal masks are used in the majority of cases; negative pressure or abdominal ventilators may have a role in patients who are intolerant of masks, although their use may be limited by upper airways obstruction
- The decision to introduce overnight NIV is difficult, and is based on both symptoms (morning headaches, hypersomnolence, fatigue, poor sleep quality) and evidence of respiratory failure (daytime hypercapnia [pCO_2 > 6.0 kPa] and/or nocturnal hypoventilation with O_2 saturations < 88% on overnight oximetry). Daytime respiratory failure however is often a late feature, and is typically preceded by hypercapnic hypoventilation during sleep. A recent study in patients with myopathies demonstrated supine inspiratory vital capacity to be an accurate predictor of respiratory reserve: supine IVC < 40% of predicted was significantly associated with hypercapnic hypoventilation, and such patients should be considered for treatment with NIV. Supine IVC < 20% was typically associated with daytime respiratory failure, whereas supine IVC > 60% indicated a minimal risk of respiratory complications. Other factors include signs of cor pulmonale or multiple hospital admissions with respiratory failure
- Patients with excessive secretions may not be suitable for non-invasive ventilation, although face-mask ventilation is possible even in the setting of severe bulbar weakness
- Regular follow-up of patients on overnight ventilation is important. Ask about symptoms and compliance, and repeat arterial blood gas analysis. Lack of improvement in gas exchange may reflect non-compliance, excessive air leakage, inadequate pressure support, or progression of underlying disease; consider repeating nocturnal oximetry monitoring. Patients with persisting severe hypoxia may benefit from long-term supplementary oxygen, although this may worsen CO_2 retention.

Obstructive sleep apnoea (page 338)
● Overnight NIV may have a role in patients with central hypoventilation, Cheyne–Stokes respiration, obesity hypoventilation, overlap syndromes of obstructive sleep apnoea with coexisting COPD, and in severe obstructive sleep apnoea unresponsive to nasal CPAP.

Cystic fibrosis (page 370)
● Overnight NIV may have a useful role as a 'bridge' to transplantation in patients with cystic fibrosis and chronic respiratory failure.

COPD (page 125)
● Use of NIV in the management of chronic, stable COPD is controversial. Trials have shown conflicting results, although possibly some benefit in patients with severe hypercapnia and nocturnal hypoventilation.

Further information

Clinical indications for noninvasive positive pressure ventilation in chronic respiratory failure due to restrictive lung disease, COPD, and nocturnal hypoventilation—a consensus conference report. *Chest* 1999; **116**: 521–34

Patterns and predictors of sleep disordered breathing in primary myopathies. Ragette R *et al.* *Thorax* 2002; **57**: 724–8

When to involve the intensive therapy unit (ITU)

Ideally communicate with ITU early, as it is much better that they know about a potentially sick patient who may need ITU input, than to find your patient (and you!) in difficulty later on, with no ITU bed.

Scoring systems for the early recognition of sick patients are in use in many hospitals, enabling doctors and nursing staff to readily assess a deteriorating patient. An example is shown on the opposite page.

The common situations in which ITU input may be required in relation to respiratory disease are principally those relating to decisions about formal ventilation. Most commonly these will be:

- Respiratory failure (either type I or type II)
  - Exacerbation of COPD (usually type II failure). Patients with COPD admitted to ITU have a hospital mortality of about 20–25%. Poor prognostic factors include low baseline FEV_1, long-term oxygen use, low sodium and albumin, low BMI, poor functional status, and co-morbid disease. Age does not add prognostic information
  - Pneumonia (to maintain an adequate pO_2—usually type I failure). In this situation, ITU input may not necessarily lead to intubation, as adequate oxygenation may be achieved by the proper use of a non-rebreathable mask or CPAP, with the additional benefits of one-to-one nursing. Altered mental state and difficulty clearing secretions may make invasive ventilation necessary
- Upper airway emergencies
- ≥ 1 organ failure (not necessarily with respiratory failure)
- Sepsis requiring organ support
- Inotropic support.

PAR (patient at risk) scoring system

This is an example of a ward-based patient illness severity scoring system. It is used to assist medical and nursing staff in identifying sick patients earlier, and to enable earlier and appropriate HDU/ITU liaison.

Score	3	2	1	0	1	2	3
Heart rate/min		≤40	41–50	51–100	101–110	111–130	≥131
SBP	≤70	71–80	80–100	101–199		≥200	
Resp rate/min		≤8		9–14	15–20	21–29	≥30
Temp/°C		≤35				≥39.5	
Conscious level				alert	drowsy/ confused	painful stimuli	unrespon-sive
Urine output					<60 ml in 2 h	<40 ml in 2 h	0 ml

Score 1–3: increase observations to 4 hourly.

Score 3 in one category: contact doctor for immediate review.

Score total ≥3: contact doctor for review within 30 minutes. SHO should consider senior review.

Score >6: patient needs immediate review, contact ITU outreach team if appropriate.

Respiratory rate is the most sensitive marker of illness severity.

Ethical issues

Background and COPD

Most ethical issues faced by doctors arise at the end of a patient's life. This particularly applies to respiratory physicians, where difficult decisions about the appropriateness of treatment and the prolongation of life in patients with chronic underlying lung disease may need to be made. In some situations artificial ventilation may prolong the dying process; life has a natural end and the potential to prolong life in the intensive care unit can sometimes cause dilemmas.

The General Medical Council (GMC) states that doctors have an obligation to respect human life, protect the health of their patients, and put their patients' best interests first. This means offering treatments where the benefits outweigh any risks, and avoiding treatments that carry no net gain to the patient. If a patient wishes to have a treatment that in the doctor's considered view is not indicated, the doctor and medical team are under no ethical or legal obligation to provide it (but the patient's right to a second opinion must be respected).

The discussion about resuscitation and formal ventilation is never an easy one, but should ideally be taken with nursing staff, the patient, and their next of kin, in advance of an emergency situation. In practical terms, clearly this is not always possible. Ideally all decisions regarding resuscitation and the ceiling of treatment (particularly relating to ventilation) should be documented in advance, and handed over to the on-call team. Most possible outcomes can be anticipated.

Where it has been decided that a treatment is not in the best interests of the patient, there is no ethical distinction between stopping the treatment, or not starting it in the first place (though the former may be more difficult to do), and this should not be used as an argument for failing to initiate the treatment in the first place.

Some clinical scenarios are more commonly encountered by the respiratory physician. These are discussed below and over the page:

COPD is the 4th commonest cause of death in America, and most patients die of respiratory failure during an exacerbation. A commonly encountered clinical situation is where a patient with COPD is admitted with an exacerbation, and is in type II respiratory failure. Standard treatment does not improve the respiratory acidosis, so non-invasive ventilation is commenced. Before starting NIV, a decision must be clearly documented as to whether or not NIV is the ceiling of treatment. It may be, especially if the patient has severe or end-stage COPD.

Formal ventilation in the intensive care unit may be appropriate in certain specific situations, for example: in a relatively young patient (i.e. < 65 years); a patient with a relatively new diagnosis of COPD, in whom the episode is the first or second admission; and in the patient in whom there is a very obviously potentially reversible cause for the exacerbation, e.g. pneumonia. Sometimes in this situation, a defined time period for intensive care input may be decided, e.g. ventilation for 48 hours (to allow treatments to work and to allow time to assess for any improvement), with extubation after that time period if no improvement has been made.

Decisions about formal ventilation and intensive care admission can only be made with knowledge of the patient's usual level of functioning and previous quality of life. The problem in this situation is that quality of life is a very subjective measure. Objective measures of usual functioning, such as measures of daily activity, usual exercise tolerance, and whether home care or assistance with activities of daily living is required are more useful in guiding the appropriateness of escalating therapy. With particular reference to the patient with COPD, the number of hospital admissions and exacerbations and the need for home oxygen or nebulizers will also be useful. Helpful information may be obtained from the GP, if the previous hospital notes are unavailable.

Neither the next of kin nor those with enduring power of attorney have the legal right to determine any treatment; the responsibility remains with the doctor and multidisciplinary team, occasionally involving the courts of law.

Where limited information is available about the patient, and therefore uncertainty exists about the appropriateness of ventilation, it should be started until a clearer assessment can be made. This may be relevant for a patient attending the accident and emergency department, in whom little information is available. The above point concerning the withdrawal of therapy, should it subsequently be found to be inappropriate, also holds.

There are downsides to invasive ventilation: the risk of pneumothorax is increased in those with end-stage emphysema, and the risk of ventilator-acquired pneumonia increases with time ventilated. Knowledge of the risk of these adverse events helps the medical team to balance the argument and make a decision about whether the risks of ventilation are likely to outweigh its benefits. The issue of limited resources should not influence a decision about formal ventilation or ITU admission.

The average length of intubation of patients with COPD admitted to ITU is 3.2 days. These patients have a 20–25% in-hospital mortality, with 50% of patients surviving 1 year post-ITU discharge. About 50% will be living independently 1 year post-hospital discharge. Clearly, only a very selected subgroup of patients are admitted to ITU, but concerns about prolonged periods of ventilation in this group of patients seem to be unfounded. Patients in whom a clear cause for the exacerbation can be identified (e.g. pneumonia) tend to do better, as there is a treatable cause for the exacerbation, and not just progression of the underlying disease.

Lung cancer and neurological disease

Lung cancer The use of antibiotic treatment for pneumonia in a patient with advanced lung malignancy may be inappropriate in some circumstances. The stage and extent of disease, response to other treatments (e.g. chemotherapy), and the patient's wishes and quality of life are all paramount. This is another situation in which it might be appropriate to define at the outset the treatments that are appropriate, e.g. 10 days total of intravenous and oral antibiotics. Note that treatments such as antibiotics can lead to improvement in symptoms (e.g. by reducing fever), without necessarily prolonging life, and it may be kinder to continue antibiotics in this situation.

Progressive neurological disease The decision about non-invasive ventilation in a patient with a progressive neuromuscular disease can be difficult. In this setting the clinical deterioration can usually be anticipated, and in most situations, discussion should have taken place early on (unless the patient presents in respiratory failure, for example, due to pneumonia, and subsequent ventilator weaning is difficult). Different centres, patients, and their relatives will have differing views as to whether life-prolonging NIV ventilation in the face of progressive neuromuscular disability is warranted. Some centres take the view that if the quality of life and higher mental functioning is good, and the respiratory muscles are affected early on (and other functions and mobility remain good), then NIV is warranted. Further decisions about withdrawal of treatment with progression of the underlying neurological disease of course will still be needed. In, for example, motor neurone disease with bulbar palsy, aspiration is a relative contraindication to non-invasive/mask ventilation. Aspiration in these patients is a poor prognostic sign, and often a sign of imminent death.

Advance directive documents the patient's wishes in the event of serious illness. It will usually include a decision about resuscitation and other potential life-prolonging treatments. The patient must understand the implications of his/her decision.

Further information
Withholding and withdrawing life-prolonging treatments: good practice in decision-making. General Medical Council 2002

Tracheostomy

Temporary tracheostomy is most often performed as an adjunct to assisted ventilation. Such patients are now often returned to respiratory wards for 'decannulation'.

Indications for tracheostomy on the ICU (no uniform agreement)
- Usually performed after a period of time following intubation with an endotracheal tube
- Improved patient communication (with appropriate cuff deflation and/or tube fenestration)
- Possible reduction in laryngeal damage. The evidence for this is very limited
- Nursing care potentially easier
- Facilitation of weaning.

(No evidence for a reduced incidence of aspiration and pneumonia.)

The usual practice is to convert from endotracheal tube to tracheostomy at 7 days if ventilation is likely to be needed beyond 14 days. Conversion beyond 14 days is considered best practice and certainly by 21 days.

Percutaneous versus surgical tracheostomy Percutaneous tracheostomy (PT) can be performed on the ICU immediately once the decision is made and is quicker than conventional tracheostomy. There are a variety of PT techniques: Griggs' guide wire with dilating forceps, and the Ciaglia multiple or single (Blue Rhino) dilator approach, preferably with endo-scopic verification of placement. In the Blue Rhino system a curved, cone-shaped dilator is slid over a guide wire and introduced into the tracheal lumen between the 2nd and 3rd tracheal rings, until the hole is large enough to accept the required tracheostomy tube. This technique requires con-trolled force and there is significant potential for traumatic damage. The fit of the tracheostomy tube is tight, with less stomal infection, less post-operative haemorrhage, and the long-term complications of the two techniques are similar. Humidification of the inspired gas is always required to prevent the build up of thick viscid mucus. Humidification can only be withdrawn in long-term tracheostomy patients after several weeks or months.

Decannulation Tracheostomy may still be required to administer inter-mittent ventilation, reduce ventilatory dead space, aid respiratory secretion clearance, limit aspiration (when cuffed), and bypass any upper airway obstruction. This is weighed against the consequences of a tracheostomy: increased tendency to aspirate (because of a reduced ability to swallow), the reduced ability to talk, and the increased infection brought about from a foreign body in the trachea and bypassing the upper airway. Thus decannu-lation should be carried out as soon as:
- Adequate clearance of secretions, i.e. good cough and thin secretions
- No upper airway obstruction
- No significant aspiration (can be checked by drinking methylene blue and then suctioning), although a small amount is not an absolute contraindication
- No need to continue ventilation for maintenance of gas exchange
- Conversion to non-invasive ventilation is possible, and has been demonstrated to work adequately.

The ability to cope adequately without the tracheostomy can be repeatedly determined (and for increasing periods) by capping the tube with the cuff fully deflated, and preferably with a fenestrated tube.

Once a tube has been removed, the stoma can close very quickly and make reinsertion difficult. Introducing a 'guidewire', over which the old tube is removed and the new can be inserted, is often useful (a suction tube with the connector cut off will suffice).

The final decision to decannulate is often delayed unnecessarily. Sooner rather than later is usually better.

Available tube options Tracheostomy tubes can be cuffed or uncuffed. If ventilation is not necessary, and aspiration is not a problem, cuffs are not required. Sometimes patients can be adequately ventilated even with the cuff down or no cuff at all: this is usually in patients with normal lungs where the compliance is good and inflation pressures therefore low.

Tracheostomy tubes can either be single, or double (with an inner and outer tube). Double tubes allow better cleaning and maintenance of the lumen, but the diameter of the lumen is of course less for a similar sized external diameter.

Tracheostomy tubes can be fenestrated to allow exhalation via the larynx to aid talking. The fenestration can be closed off with a non-fenestrated inner tube should intermittent ventilation still be required.

Further information

Commercial video of Blue Rhino insertion,
www.cookgroup.com/cook_critical_care/education/video/index.html

Inhalers and nebulizers

Background

Inhalers
- There are many different inhaler devices that deliver drugs directly to the airways
- Ideally patients should try a range of devices to choose the most appropriate for them
- Patients should receive advice on techniques for inhaler use. Technique should be checked regularly and, if patients cannot manage a particular device, they should be switched to another
- The percentage of a drug delivered to the airway varies for each device (from 15–60% according to the manufacturers), and depends on good technique
- Spacer devices improve this delivery and are particularly useful for the elderly, children, and those who find it difficult to coordinate inhaler administration with breathing
- Try to use the same inhaler device for all the drug classes used by a patient
- Advise the patient how to recognize when a device is empty: some have dose counters; others are shaken to hear if they still have contents
- Titrate inhaler doses with clinical response.

Nebulizers are used by patients who gain greater relief from nebulized therapy than from inhaled therapy. This may be during acute respiratory illnesses, because of disease severity, or because they are unable to use inhalers. Patients who are being considered for nebulizer therapy should be referred to a respiratory physician. If antibiotics are being nebulized, a more powerful nebulizer is required.

How to use: Open the nebule containing the drug solution and squirt the solution into the nebulizer chamber. Salbutamol and ipratropium bromide can be taken together, but nebulized budesonide or antibiotics should be used separately. If ipratropium bromide only is being used, this should be delivered via a mouthpiece, as it can lead to glaucoma if used via a mask. Reattach the chamber to the nebulizer mask or mouthpiece. Put the mask over nose and mouth, or position mouthpiece between the lips in the mouth. Switch the nebulizer machine on. Breathe slowly in and out. Continue until all the solution is gone. If this takes more than 10 minutes, the machine should be serviced. Switch off the machine. Rinse the nebulizer chamber with water after each use. If the patient is using oxygen, this can still be used during nebulization, either via nasal prongs under the nebulizer mask or by using oxygen tubing attached directly to the nebulizer chamber to drive the nebulization. Nebulizer machines should be serviced annually.

Different inhaler types and instructions for their use

Different inhaler types

Generic name of drug (with product names)	Mechanism of action	Inhaler colour
Salbutamol (Ventolin®, Asmasal®, Pulvinal® Salbutamol, Salamol®, Salbutamol Cyclocaps®, Airomir®, Asmasal Clickhaler®, Salamol Easi-Breathe®, Ventodisks®) **Terbutaline** (Bricanyl®)	Short-acting β_2 agonist Duration 3–5 hours	Blue
Salmeterol (Serevent®) **Formoterol** (Foradil®, Oxis®)	Long-acting β_2 agonist Duration 12 hours	Green Green/turquoise
Ipratropium bromide (Atrovent®) **Ipratropium and salbutamol** (Combivent®)	Short-acting anticholinergic	White/grey
Tiotropium (Spiriva®)	Long-acting anticholinergic	Grey Handihaler®
Beclometasone dipropionate (Becotide®, Becloforte®, Pulvinal® Beclometasone, Beclomethasone Cyclocaps®, AeroBec®, AerobecForte®, Asmabec Clickhaler®, Beclazone Easi-Breathe®, Beco-disks®, Qvar®)	Corticosteroid	Brown Red
Budesonide (Pulmicort®, Budesonide Cyclocaps®)		Brown
Fluticasone propionate (Flixotide®)		Red
Mometasone furoate (Asmanex®)		Red
Salmeterol and fluticasone (Seretide®) **Eformoterol and budesonide** (Symbicort®)	Combination steroid and bronchodilator	Purple Red and white
Sodium cromoglicate (Intal®, Cromogen Easi-Breathe®) **Neocromil sodium** (Tilade®)	Unknown, stabilize mast cells	Yellow and white

Immunosuppressive drugs

Patient advice and monitoring

Immunosuppressive drugs are used mainly in the management of pulmonary vasculitis, but also in asthma, sarcoidosis, and interstitial lung diseases. Centres differ in their use of these drugs and local guidelines are often available.

General advice for patients on immunosuppressive drugs

- Increased risk of infections and increased likelihood of severe infections. Check FBC if develop febrile illness
- May have atypical presentation of infections
- Avoid live vaccines, such as measles, mumps, rubella, BCG, yellow fever, oral typhoid, oral polio
- If never had varicella zoster:
  - Avoid contacts with chicken pox or shingles
  - Consider passive immunization
  - Immunoglobulin therapy if exposed
  - Hospital treatment with close monitoring if develop chicken pox
- Avoid measles exposure. Prophylaxis with immunoglobulins if exposed.

Summary of tests to perform before and during immunosuppressive drug treatment

Drug	Check before starting	Follow-up
Corticosteroids	BP, glucose. Consider bones/osteoporosis	BP, glucose if symptoms of diabetes.
Azathioprine	FBC, LFT	FBC every 2 weeks for 3 months, then monthly. LFT monthly.
Methotrexate	FBC, U&E, LFT CXR Folic acid	Bloods every 2 weeks for 3 months, then monthly.
Cyclophosphamide	FBC, U&E, LFT Urine dip Semen store	Check all every week for 1 month, then every 2 months.

Corticosteroids and azathioprine

Corticosteroids

- First-line treatment for suppressing inflammation. At high doses, also cause immunosuppression
- IV methylprednisolone (500–1000 mg/day) for 3–5 days can be used for aggressive induction of remission, e.g. Wegener's granulomatosis, followed by maintenance oral steroids (prednisolone 30–40 mg/day). Usually taken in the morning as they may disturb sleep
- Dose should be slowly reduced when control of the disease is achieved. Gastric and bone protection may be necessary as the patient will be on high doses for some months. Also ensure BP and glucose are controlled
- Ensure patients have steroid treatment card.

Side-effects include skin and hair thinning, obesity, cataracts, diabetes, and aseptic bone necrosis. Inform patient of these and document. PCP infection can occur secondary to steroid treatment, particularly with high doses for prolonged periods. Some centres therefore use PCP prophylaxis.

Steroids and osteoporosis

Current guidelines suggest patients being started on long-term steroids, with one other osteoporosis risk factor (such as being over 65, or having had a previous osteoporotic fracture), should also start on a bisphosphonate.

In other patients, bone mineral density should be checked via DEXA scan of hip and spine after 6 months treatment with 7.5 mg or more of prednisolone per day, and offer lifestyle advice and bisphosphonates if this is reduced.

(see Royal College of Physicians guidelines, www.rcplondon.ac.uk)

Azathioprine

- Mainly used as a steroid-sparing agent, or when vasculitis is under control to enable cyclophosphamide to be stopped
- Cytotoxic drug, less effective than cyclophosphamide. May be reasonable alternative if side effects of cyclophosphamide are unacceptable
- Maximal effect on disease may not be evident for 6–9 months, but can be used long-term
- For vasculitis, start with 2 mg per kg/day after cyclophosphamide. Maximum dose usually around 150–200 mg/day
- **Check FBC** every 2 weeks for 3 months, then monthly. **Check LFTs** monthly. Stop treatment if WCC < 3, platelets < 100, or ALP and transaminases 3× normal. Restart when they recover.

Side-effects include sore mouth, ulcers, nausea and vomiting, diarrhoea, skin rash, alopecia (rare). Most respond to stopping the drug and restarting at a lower dose. Interacts with allopurinol and leads to increased toxicity.

Methotrexate and cyclophosphamide

Methotrexate

- Can be used as a second-line treatment
- Dose: 7.5–20 mg once/week. Usual starting dose is 10 mg. Can increase after 6 weeks to 15 mg
- Baseline CXR. Monitor FBC, U&E, and LFTs every 2 weeks for 3 months then monthly. Give folic acid 5 mg 3–4 days after dose.

Side-effects include mouth ulcers, skin rashes, nausea, macrocytosis, myelosuppression, pneumonitis (dyspnoea and dry cough). Avoid if significant renal or hepatic impairment, or if pleural effusions or ascites, as it can accumulate in these fluids. Stop if WCC < 3, platelets < 100, transaminases $3 \times$ normal, pneumonitis.

Cyclophosphamide

- The primary cytotoxic drug used for treating systemic vasculitis. Used particularly if there are life- or organ-threatening features, such as requiring ventilation for lung vasculitis, systemic features, or renal involvement
- Causes immunosuppression without anti-inflammatory effects
- Takes 12–14 days to work; hence is combined with high-dose steroids at the beginning of treatment. When combined with steroids, it induces remission of vasculitis in 95% of patients
- Oral cyclophosphamide is used if possible in active vasculitis, at a dose of 2 mg/kg
- Pulsed intravenous cyclophosphamide is given if patients cannot take oral preparations, using doses of around $0.375–1 \text{ g/m}^2$ every 2–4 weeks. The lowest white cell count occurs 10 days after a pulse. Non-randomized studies have shown that pulsed doses give a lower cumulative dose than oral regimes, are as likely to induce remissions, and cause fewer adverse effects, but have a non-significantly higher vasculitis relapse rate
- If giving IV cyclophosphamide, patients should be well hydrated before and after, and given Mesna, which chelates with the urotoxic cyclophosphamide metabolite, acrolein. Dose varies according to the cyclophosphamide dose and is available on product literature. Give during cyclophosphamide infusion and also 4 and 8 hours after. Also prescribe anti-emetics. Dose may need reduction with renal failure
- Haemorrhagic cystitis is a potentially serious side-effect of cyclophosphamide therapy. Perform a baseline urine dip for blood prior to treatment (although note that microscopic haematuria is common with active vasculitis). Check routinely for macroscopic haematuria in patients receiving IV cyclophosphamide and, if it is present, stop drug and arrange cystoscopy (rare if Mesna is used, and rare with oral cyclophosphamide regimes)
- **Check blood counts** at least weekly for 4 weeks (FBC, U&E, LFT). Then check every 2 months and ensure results are seen. Withhold or reduce treatment if leucopenic, until bone marrow recovers

- Treatment likely to last for 6 months. Longer courses are no more effective and carry the risk of side-effects from the cumulative dose. Cyclophosphamide is not recommended for more than one year as total overall dose has cumulative side-effects. Induce remission with cyclophosphamide and prednisolone and maintain remission with prednisolone and another immunosuppressant.

Side-effects include nausea, vomiting, hair thinning or alopecia, bone marrow suppression (2%), leucopenia, haemorrhagic cystitis, transitional cell carcinoma of bladder, infertility, lymphoma (0.7%), and leukaemia, pulmonary and bladder fibrosis. Risks of cystitis and bladder cancer increase with increasing cumulative dose. Treat patient with minimum dose required to maintain remission. Semen storage for men prior to starting treatment.

Long-term oxygen therapy

Background and indications

Two landmark trials of long-term oxygen therapy (LTOT) were published in the 1980s: the British Medical Research Council (MRC) Working Party trial and the American Nocturnal Oxygen Therapy Trial (NOTT).

The **MRC trial** compared a group of COPD patients receiving oxygen for 15 hours per day, with a control group receiving no oxygen. The **NOTT trial** compared continuous daily oxygen (average 17.7 hours a day) with overnight oxygen (average 12 hours). The patients in the MRC trial were, on average, hypercapnic (mean $PaCO_2$ 7.3 kPa), whereas those in the NOTT trial were, on average, normocapnic (mean $PaCO_2$ 5.7 kPa). The main outcome in both trials was improved survival in those patients receiving oxygen for at least 15 hours a day, though this improved survival was not seen in the MRC trial until after a year of oxygen therapy.

The **NOTT trial** showed a reduced exercise pulmonary artery pressure (PAP) after 6 months of continuous or nocturnal oxygen therapy. The same group also showed that 8 year survival was related to the fall in mean PAP during the first 6 months of continuous oxygen use.

The **MRC trial** failed to show a fall in mean PAP with LTOT, but the mean annual increase in PAP (3 mmHg) in patients in the control arm was not seen in the oxygen treated group.

The reason for the improved survival with LTOT is not clear, and is unlikely to relate to the small changes in pulmonary haemodynamics seen.

COPD is the disease for which LTOT is most commonly prescribed, and the disease in which the original studies were completed. Subsequent oxygen studies have shown improved exercise endurance in COPD patients breathing supplemental oxygen, with improved walking distance and ability to perform daily activities. FEV_1 is the strongest predictor of survival in COPD; LTOT does not influence the decline in FEV_1.

Additional benefits of LTOT include

- Reduction of secondary polycythaemia
- Improved sleep quality, by reducing hypoxia-associated brain arousals
- Reduced cardiac arrthymias, and potentially reducing the risk of nocturnal sudden death
- Reduced sympathetic outflow, with increased salt and water excretion, leading to improved renal function.

Indications for LTOT in COPD patients

The criteria for the prescription of LTOT in the UK are based on the clinical parameters of the patients who showed improved survival in the original two LTOT trials.

- $PaO_2 < 7.3$ kPa (55 mmHg) breathing air (i.e. a saturation on air $\leq$ 88%), in a stable clinical state
- PaO_2 7.3–8 kPa (56–59 mmHg, SaO_2 89–90%) if pulmonary hypertension (i.e. symptoms and signs of cor pulmonale), polycythaemia, or additional nocturnal hypoxaemia ($SaO_2 \leq 90$ % for at least 30% of the night). There is no evidence that treating solely nocturnal hypoxaemia leads to improved survival
- Clinical stability is defined as the absence of an exacerbation for the previous 4 weeks. This is usually assessed twice, several weeks apart

to ensure stability, and ideally at least 6 weeks following an exacerbation
- LTOT is usually prescribed for those with an FEV_1 <1.5 l or <40% predicted. If the FEV_1 is higher, it suggests an additional cause for the hypoxaemia such as sleep apnoea, and further investigations may be indicated
- Medical management of the disease must be optimized prior to the prescription of LTOT
- $PaCO_2$ does not influence the prescription of LTOT for COPD. There is a small risk of precipitating worsening hypercapnia with LTOT in those who are already hypercapnic, if the patient has OSA, or is experiencing an exacerbation
- Blood gases should be checked on LTOT, to ensure the absence of worsening hypercapnia (if symptoms such as headache and confusion suggest that this has occurred), and to ensure a satisfactory increase in PO_2 has occurred. Aim for PaO_2 values of 8–9 kPa (60–65 mmHg, SaO_2 90–92%)
- Patients should have stopped smoking: the benefit of LTOT in continued smokers is limited, and there is an increased risk of fire. However most studies suggest that around 18% of patients on LTOT continue to smoke; they should be warned of the risks.

Indications for **LTOT** in non-COPD patients
- There is limited evidence to support the use of LTOT in these patient groups, and no data showing improved survival. Ensure optimal medical management first. Consider in:
  - Interstitial lung disease if PaO_2 < 8 kPa (SaO_2 90%)
  - Neuromuscular or skeletal disorders. Consider either oxygen alone, or in combination with ventilatory support (usually via a specialist centre)
  - Cystic fibrosis if PaO_2 < 8 kPa (SaO_2 90%)
  - Pulmonary hypertension with PaO_2 < 8 kPa, in the absence of parenchymal lung disease
  - Palliative care—for the dyspnoea of lung malignancy, or other causes of disabling dyspnoea due to terminal disease
  - Heart failure if PaO_2 < 7.5 kPa.

Practical use

- LTOT prescription in the UK will be by respiratory physicians only from 2005. Previously it was prescribed by a GP, following respiratory physician recommendation
- LTOT is best provided by an oxygen concentrator, set at 2–4 l/min depending on the arterial blood tensions. The concentrator contains a molecular sieve containing zeolite, which entraps gas molecules depending on their size and polarity. It can produce up to 96% oxygen, depending on the flow rate (the argon is also concentrated, to 4%)
- Patients can use nasal prongs or a fixed concentration mask (controlled or uncontrolled oxygen) depending on their preference. A back-up cylinder should be prescribed in case of power cuts. Oxygen humidification is possible
- LTOT should be used for a minimum of 15 hours per day in patients with COPD, though survival improves when used for more than this time period; therefore the number of hours it is used for should not be restricted
- Patient education in the use of LTOT, and machine maintenance are important. Specialist respiratory nurses may be involved with this
- If the patient is using more than 3 oxygen cylinders per week, an oxygen concentrator is more economical (even if the patient does not actually meet criteria for the prescription of LTOT).

How to organize LTOT

- GP writes the prescription (FP10 or WP10 in Wales), which needs to state:
  - the number of hours of oxygen use per day
  - the flow rate
  - face mask or nasal cannulae
  - also prescribes a back-up cylinder
- GP then phones the supplier for their area (see below)
- Supplier then phones the patient to arrange a date for installation
- The patient gives the prescription to the engineer who installs the concentrator
- Oxygen suppliers: see the BNF and GP Drug Tarrif. British Oxygen Company Medical (0800 136 603) supplies South London, the South-East, and South-West. De Vilbiss Medequip Ltd (0800 020 202) supplies North London, the Eastern Counties, the North-West, West Midlands, and North Wales. Oxygen Therapy Co Ltd (0800 373 580) supplies Central and South Wales, North Yorkshire, and Humberside.

Follow-up is needed to ensure:

- Compliance
- Confirm the ongoing requirement for LTOT. Some patients improve and no longer need LTOT
- Ideally yearly monitoring of arterial blood gas tensions (may be performed by specialist nurses).

Ambulatory oxygen is oxygen delivered by portable equipment, and may be suitable for:

- Patients on LTOT who are mobile
- Those with evidence of exercise desaturation, or those who show an improvement in exercise capacity or dyspnoea with oxygen-titrate oxygen for the exercise desaturation, aiming for $SaO_2 > 90\%$.

Liquid oxygen is not currently available on prescription.

Intermittent/short burst oxygen should be considered for patients with episodes of severe breathlessness due to hypoxia, not relieved by other means. This is best provided by using one or more oxygen cylinders placed strategically round the house. It is an expensive treatment, and some would argue there is a large placebo effect, due to the cooling effect of the oxygen on the face. A similar effect may be achieved by using a fan.

Portable oxygen cylinders

- DD—460 l. Lightweight and easily portable. Lasts 3 hours 50 minutes at 2 l/min
- F size—1360 l. Lasts approximately 11.5 hours at 2 l/min
- PD—300 l. Much smaller, but heavier than DD. Lasts 2.5 hours at 2 l/min
- E size—600 l. Lightweight and portable. Lasts 5 hours at 2 l/min. (Not available on the NHS.)

Further information

www.britishlungfoundation.org/docs/info_sheets/oxygen%20 suppliersis2.DOC

NICE COPD Guidelines, *www.nice.org.uk/pdf/CG012*

Pulmonary rehabilitation

Aims and patient selection

Pulmonary rehabilitation is a well-established, multidisciplinary programme of care for patients with chronic respiratory impairment. The programme is individually tailored for each patient. Pulmonary rehabilitation is not available yet in every centre, although it is probably the most cost-effective intervention in COPD.

Aims of rehabilitation

- To reduce disability and handicap in people with chronic lung disease
- To improve quality of life and restore independence
- To diminish the health care burden of disease.

Early studies measured pulmonary function tests and found there was no improvement after pulmonary rehabilitation. The first positive study of pulmonary rehabilitation measured functional status.

Meta-analysis of 14 RCTs using a variety of different style programmes has confirmed the benefit of rehabilitation, with improvements in functional exercise.

- Further UK RCT of patients with severe airflow obstruction showed improvements in exercise, health status, and health economic advantages
- Patients who had completed rehabilitation courses had no fewer hospital admissions for exacerbations than those who had not had rehabilitation, but hospital stays were shorter (10 days versus 21 days)
- Patients with COPD who have completed rehabilitation courses perform better than controls on walking tests and have less subjective dyspnoea
- Rehabilitation programmes containing lower-extremity training are better, when compared to controls, than those using just respiratory muscle training
- Short-term programmes achieve overall similar outcome benefits across the spectrum of patient disability. A minimum programme length of 6 weeks is recommended
- Decline in exercise tolerance and health status tends to occur between 6 and 12 months after completion of a course. Sustained improvement with ongoing rehabilitation sessions has yet to be evaluated.

Candidates

- Anyone with chronic lung disease causing functional impairment
- The majority of candidates will have COPD, but also asthma, pulmonary fibrosis, and bronchiectasis
- Any stage of a lung disease, when symptoms are affecting a patient's activity. Ideally receiving optimum medical treatment
- Well-motivated patients seem to benefit most
- Patients with poor lower limb mobility may benefit from upper limb exercise
- Oxygen therapy is not a contraindication to rehabilitation
- Stable ischaemic heart disease is not a contraindication to rehabilitation.

Candidates in whom rehabilitation may not be indicated
- Unstable ischaemic heart disease, severe valvular heart disease, cognitive impairment, locomotor difficulties
- Poorly motivated people with geographical or transport problems making attendance difficult tend to do less well.

Programme

Programmes are usually run on an out-patient basis, but can be done in the community, the home, or as an in-patient. They are run by a multi-professional team—physician, physiotherapist, occupational therapist, dietician, nurse, pharmacist, social worker, and psychologist. A minimum programme length of 6 weeks is recommended. Programmes should be regularly audited by the department.

- **Physical training** The main component of the programme, with aerobic exercise such as walking and cycling 2–3 times per week, with 2 supervised/class sessions. May include upper limb strength exercise with weights. Individually prescribed exercise programmes, designed for each patient to work to high intensity. Benefit increases with training intensity. Oxygen supplementation may be required if significant desaturation occurs during exercise to below 80%
- **Disease education**
- **Psychological and social intervention** with advice on anxiety and depression, smoking cessation, plus physiotherapy and occupational therapy input
- **Nutritional education** to optimize body weight and muscle mass.

Pre-rehabilitation assessment

- Optimize medical treatment
- Oxygen saturation on exercise
- ECG may be warranted, especially if history of cardiac disease.

Outcome assessment measures

- **Physical** Often with shuttle walk tests (SWT) or six-minute walk test (6MWT) to assess ability and progress (see opposite page)
- **Health status**
  - Disease-specific questionnaires
      Chronic Respiratory Questionnaire (CRQ)
      St George's Respiratory Questionnaire
  - Generic questionnaires
      Short Form-36 (SF-36)
      Hospital Anxiety and Depression scores (HADS) are measured, but are insensitive to change during pulmonary rehabilitation
- **Practical** Pulmonary Function Status–Dyspnoea Questionnaire (PFS-DQ) may be used to measure performance and satisfaction relating to activities of daily living.

Shuttle walk test (SWT)

10 metre course between two points. Walking speed determined by external audio-tape signals ('beeps'), and the patient should pace their walk to reach each point at a beep. The patient is required to incrementally increase their speed as the beeps occur more frequently. Test finishes when the patient needs to stop and distance achieved calculated.

6 minute walk test (6MWT)

30 metre course between two points on a hard flat surface. Patients do as many 60 metre laps as they can around the 2 points in 6 minutes. They determine their pace and intensity of exercise. They are allowed to rest in the time if they need to. Total distance walked in 6 minutes is counted. Results vary according to mood and encouragement.

Future developments
- Determining which components of rehabilitation are the most valuable to improvements in exercise: intensity of exercise programme, type of exercise
- How to optimally maintain the improvements following a rehabilitation programme
- Performance enhancement, using oxygen, steroids, nutrition, creatine.

Further information
Pulmonary Rehabilitation for COPD (Cochrane Review). Lacasse Y, Brosseau L et al. CD003793

Rehabilitation for patients with COPD: meta-analysis of RCTs. Salman et al. J Gen Int Med 2003 Mar; **18**(3): 213–21

BTS Statement on Pulmonary Rehabilitation. Thorax 2001; **56**: 827–34

Results at one year of outpatient multidisciplinary pulmonary rehabilitation: a randomised controlled trial. Griffiths et al. Lancet 2000; **355**: 362–68

American Thoracic Society. Pulmonary rehabilitation-1999. Am J Resp Crit Care Med 1999; **159**: 1666–82

Meta-analysis of Pulmonary Rehabilitation in COPD. Lancet 1996; **348**: 1115–19

Smoking cessation

Aims and nicotine replacement therapy

Smoking is the main cause of chronic obstructive pulmonary disease and lung cancer. The NHS spends £1.7 billion per year caring for people with smoking-related conditions. Government targets have been set to reduce the number of smokers in the UK and health authorities have been allocated funding for smoking cessation services.

- 31% of men and 29% of women in the UK smoke
- 82% of smokers start as teenagers
- The incidence of smoking is increasing in developing countries
- Smoking is also associated with bladder, oesophageal, cervical, and renal cancers, as well as cardiovascular and cerebrovascular disease
- Nicotine exerts its effects on the CNS and is very addictive
- Peak nicotine withdrawal time is 2–3 days
- 2% of smokers manage to stop each year
- Stopping smoking is associated with an average weight gain of 2 kg.

Aims of smoking cessation interventions In order to achieve the goal of sustained abstinence, the aim is to reduce short-term cravings for nicotine (nicotine and non-nicotine replacement therapy) and in the long term to modify behaviour (counselling, telephone or group support, buddy systems). It is vital that the smoker is motivated to stop, or attempts will fail. It is important as a health professional to address smoking cessation at all opportunities. Health professionals can trigger quit attempts by giving brief advice to all smokers. This can lead to 1–3 out of 100 people stopping smoking for 6 months. Doctor advice often has the strongest impact. People can be more receptive to smoking cessation messages during times of concern for their own or their families health. A guide to approaching the topic is:

- Ask how much a person smokes and document pack years
- Advise on risks of continued smoking and suggest possible treatments and the help available
- Assist by referring to a counsellor or providing nicotine replacement therapy
- Arrange follow-up.

Some hospitals or primary care trusts have smoking cessation counsellors. The best results in terms of quit rates are achieved by combining counselling with nicotine replacement therapy or bupropion, with regular support and follow-up. These can improve quit rates to around 25%. The National Institute of Clinical Excellence has issued guidance on the use of nicotine replacement therapy and bupropion for smoking cessation.

Nicotine replacement therapy (NRT) allows short- and medium-term nicotine withdrawal symptoms to be minimized, by replacing the nicotine. Should not be used whilst still smoking, as it is possible to overdose on nicotine (symptoms: agitation, confusion, restlessness, palpitations, hypertension, dilated pupils, SOB, abdominal cramps, vomiting). Can be bought over the counter or be prescribed by general practitioner. Cheaper than cigarettes! Most NRT products are contraindicated in pregnancy, breast-feeding mothers, and in children under 18, but are used under supervision.

- *Patches* Give small amounts of nicotine via transdermal patch to decrease cravings before they occur. Different strength patches according to how much is smoked. Use higher dose patch if 10+ cigarettes per day smoked. Convenient. Worn continuously throughout day, but often removed at night due to vivid nature of dreams. Can get localized irritation at patch site. Patches should be used for 6–8 weeks at the higher dose and then weaned to a lower dose for 2–4 weeks. Available to buy over the counter
- *Chewing gum* Different strengths of gum that release nicotine as they are chewed. Relieves cravings as they occur. When mouth tingles and has peppery taste, should stop chewing and 'park' the gum inside the cheek. Nicotine is then absorbed through the lining of the mouth. Should not chew continuously, or may become nauseated. Nicotine needs to be absorbed through mouth and not swallowed in saliva. Therefore don't drink with gum. Physical act of chewing can relieve craving. Can taste unpleasant and may need to use several packs of gum a day. Use high-dose gum if 20+ cigarettes per day are smoked. Use for 3 months and then reduce the strength and the amount of gum used. Available to buy over the counter
- *Sublingual tablets* used on demand to help with cravings. Useful for smokers wanting a discreet form of treatment. 1–2 tablets should be placed under the tongue every hour when needed. Dissolve over 30 minutes. Licensed for use in pregnancy (one tablet only). Use for 3 months and then gradually reduce the number of tablets used a day. Available on prescription
- *Lozenges* Available to buy over the counter
- *Inhaler* Cigarette style appliance giving small amounts of nicotine when used. Useful for people who are habitual or ritualistic in when they have a cigarette and want the 'hand to mouth' routine. Nicotine is absorbed through the lining of the mouth, not via the lungs. Use for 2 months, and then gradually reduce. Available on prescription
- *Nasal spray* provides rapid relief of craving. Faster absorption than other forms of NRT. May cause local irritation. Use for 2 months; then reduce. Available on prescription.

Non-nicotine replacement therapy

Drugs Bupropion (Zyban) is promoted as an aid to smoking cessation in combination with motivational support. It is an antidepressant that was found to reduce the desire to smoke, regardless of whether people were depressed or not. It weakly inhibits dopamine, serotonin, and noradrenaline reuptake in the CNS. It counteracts nicotine withdrawal symptoms by increasing these levels in the brain. It is suitable if people smoke 10 or more cigarettes a day. Liver metabolized. 20 hour half-life. Smokers start taking bupropion 1–2 weeks before their intended 'quit day'. Continue taking it for 7–9 weeks after. Improved abstinence rates compared to placebo or nicotine patch if associated with counselling (30% 12 month abstinence rate with bupropion, 16% with nicotine patch, 15% with placebo, 35% with patch and bupropion). Also thought to lessen weight gain associated with stopping smoking. Contraindicated in patients with epilepsy or at risk of fits, pregnancy, and those on monoamine oxidase inhibitors. Reduce dose if elderly or hepatic or renal impairment. Recognized adverse effects include dry mouth, hypersensitivity, insomnia, and seizures (1 in 1000 users) and death. Prescription only.

Hypnosis aims to improve will power in the subconscious state with therapeutic suggestion. Anecdotal success, but Cochrane review of trials showed no greater abstinence rate with hypnosis than any other treatment, or placebo treatment.

Acupuncture/acupressure No evidence in favour of it over placebo acupuncture.

Future developments
- Increasing and improving hospital-based smoking cessation services with links to community-based services
- Nicotine immunotherapy. Laboratory-based models to create a 'nicotine vaccine' to try and prevent abstinent smokers from re-starting are in progress. Induce specific nicotine antibodies to prevent inhaled nicotine from binding to nicotine receptors and causing neurological stimulation.

Further information

ABC of smoking cessation series. *BMJ* Feb-April 2004

Systematic review of the effectiveness of stage based interventions to promote smoking cessation. Riemsma RP *et al. BMJ* 2003; **326**: 1175

Smoking cessation guidelines for health professionals. West R *et al. Thorax* 2000; **55**: 987–99

A controlled trial of sustained-release bupropion, a nicotine patch or both for smoking cessation. Jorenby DE *et al. NEJM* 1999; **340**: 685–91

www.doh.gov.uk/tobacco

www.nosmokingday.org.uk

Quitline 0800 002200

Palliative care of the chest patient

Pain and dyspnoea

Palliative care is defined as the total care of patients whose disease is not responsive to curative treatment. It aims to provide the best possible quality of life for patients, their carers, and families. It includes control of pain and other physical symptoms, as well as care for psychological, social, and spiritual problems. Within chest medicine, palliative care is most commonly considered for patients with lung cancer and mesothelioma; many other patients with progressive, end-stage respiratory disease (such as COPD, CF, and UIP) also benefit from specific palliative interventions.

- Involve the specialist palliative care team early
- Recognize that delirium, dyspnoea, and decreased mobility often herald the terminal phase of cancer.

Pain

- Aim to determine cause, type, and site
- Start with simple analgesia and increase according to the WHO analgesic ladder, moving from non-opioid analgesia through weak opioids to strong opioids
- Prescribe analgesia as required for breakthrough pain
- Give drugs a chance to work at appropriate doses
- The addition of an anti-inflammatory drug can be effective for bony pain
- Treat drug side-effects, e.g. constipation, nausea. Prescribe prophylactic laxatives with morphine
- Consider radiotherapy for localized pain in the chest related to cancer
- Pain from bony metastases may be treated with bisphosphonates, e.g. 90 mg of pamidronate every 4 weeks
- Neuropathic pain can be treated with specific antidepressants (e.g. amitriptyline 10–50 mg) or anticonvulsants (e.g. carbamazepine or sodium valproate 200 mg/day)
- Consider referral to pain clinic for further intervention such as a nerve block, transcutaneous electrical nerve stimulation (TENS), or complementary therapies.

Dyspnoea

- Consider possible causes (see box). Dyspnoea may be due to the underlying lung disease, or due to an additional pathology
- Dyspnoea is made worse by anxiety and panic
- Lung cancer and pulmonary metastases are associated with the sensation of shortness of breath, often due to stimulation of receptors by malignant infiltration or lymphangitis carcinomatosis
- Optimize treatment of any underlying lung disease with bronchodilators and steroids if appropriate
- Treat concurrent chest infections
- Opioids (e.g. 2.5–5 mg oramorph 4 hourly) relieve the sensation of dyspnoea without affecting respiratory function
- Oxygen cylinders for intermittent use may help symptoms
- Consider the need for an airway stent in a patient with lung cancer experiencing dyspnoea due to bronchial obstruction or compression with tumour.

Causes of breathlessness in patients with lung cancer

- Pneumonia
- Underlying chronic lung disease (e.g. COPD, UIP)
- Lobar collapse
- Pleural effusion
- SVCO
- Upper airway obstruction
- Pulmonary emboli
- Lymphangitis carcinomatosis
- Pericardial effusion
- Anaemia
- Depression
- Anxiety and panic.

Other symptoms

Anxiety
- Leads to dyspnoea, which in turn worsens anxiety
- Benzodiazepines (such as short-acting lorazepam 0.5–1 mg sublingually 8–12 hourly) are effective for respiratory panic
- Acute panic may be helped by midazolam 2.5 mg IV, increased in steps of 1 mg, given in a controlled environment with oxygen
- Relaxation exercises and diaphragmatic breathing training may help some patients.

Cough
- Try simple or codeine linctus
- Methadone linctus 2–4 mg nocte or bd may be of benefit
- Nebulized saline may help expectoration
- Nebulized local anaesthetic often helps, e.g. 5 ml 2% lidocaine maximum tds (avoid in asthmatics, as it causes bronchospasm). Pharyngeal numbness is likely to occur, so avoid fluids for 1 hour after.

Pleural effusion
- Drain if symptomatic and pleurodese early if recurrent, although not if prognosis is poor (less than a few months)
- Consider an in-dwelling tunnelled catheter (such as Pleur$_x$) to drain fluid if effusion is symptomatic and pleurodesis has failed due to trapped lung.

Poor appetite
- Common symptom and may be primary due to cachexia–anorexia syndrome, or secondary, due to mouth problems such as candidiasis, nausea, hypercalcaemia, drugs, or depression
- May be improved in the short term (about 6 weeks) by a course of oral steroids, such as prednisolone 20 mg daily
- Cachexia leads to decreased respiratory muscle strength and increased shortness of breath
- Consider nutritional supplements.

Brain metastases
- Steroids relieve the cerebral oedema associated with brain metastases, e.g. dexamethasone 4 mg bd–qds initially and then decrease
- Avoid steroid dosing in the evening, as sleep is affected
- Radiotherapy may be considered if there is a good response to steroids.

Instructions for use of different inhaler types

Type of device	Instructions for use
Pressurized aerosol metered dose inhaler (MDI) Aerosol Evohaler®	Remove the mouthpiece and shake the inhaler well. Hold the inhaler upright with the thumb on the base below the mouthpiece and the first finger on the metal canister. Breathe out as far as is comfortable then place the mouth piece between the teeth and close lips around it. Do not bite it. As you start to breathe in through the mouth, press on the top of the inhaler to release the medication whilst still breathing in steadily and deeply. Hold your breath, take the inhaler from your mouth and continue holding your breath for up to 10 seconds if possible. Wait 30 seconds prior to taking second puff. Use with spacer device to improve drug delivery. CFC-free inhalers need device washing every 2–3 weeks, as they can block.
Spacer Nebuhaler® Volumatic® Aero Chamber® Able Spacer®	Ensure spacer is compatible with patient's inhaler. Remove cap of inhaler and shake it. Insert it into end of spacer device. Place the other end of the spacer in the mouth. Press the inhaler canister once to release one dose of the drug. Take one deep breath in and hold, or take 3–4 steady breaths in and out. Repeat as indicated. Valve should rattle. Clean the spacer once a month with mild detergent, rinse, and air-dry. Replace after 6–12 months.
Breath-actuated devices Autohaler® Easibreathe®	Prime the device. If an autohaler, remove the cap and lift the red lever; if an easi-breathe, open the cap. Insert device into mouth. Inhale slowly and deeply. Continue inhaling when the device 'clicks'. Hold breath for up to 10 seconds if possible. Slowly breathe out. To take a second inhaled dose, lower the red lever and lift again. If an autohaler, close the cap and reopen if an easi-breathe and repeat the above sequence.
Dry powder devices Accuhaler® Diskhaler® Turbohaler® Clickhaler® Twisthaler® Cyclohaler® Aerocaps® Spincaps®	Prime the device. Turbohaler: remove the cap, twist the base as far as possible until the click is heard and then twist back again. Clickhaler: shake the device, remove the cap, click the top down and release. Twisthaler: remove the cap by twisting and the dose is then ready. Accuhaler: Open inhaler cover, mouthpiece facing you and push lever down to pierce the blister containing dose. Diskhaler: insert disc into device by opening and pulling out mouthpiece section. To prepare dose, lift up back of lid to 90° until the blister is pierced, then lower the lid. To use all the devices, hold them level, exhale fully, place the mouthpiece into mouth between teeth and inhale steadily. Hold your breath and remove the inhaler. For a second dose, repeat the above actions.
Handihaler®	Flip lid and white mouthpiece open and insert capsule. Close the mouthpiece back down until it clicks. Pierce the capsule by pressing the green button at the side. Exhale as far as is comfortable. Place mouthpiece into mouth and breathe in slowly and deeply. Remove inhaler from your mouth and hold your breath for 10 seconds if possible. Slowly breathe out. Repeat if necessary to ensure all the powder from capsule is gone.

Patient financial entitlements

Patient financial entitlements

Patients with chronic lung disease and their carers may be eligible for financial support. There are a large number of potential benefits that can be claimed for, and the process is often time-consuming and complicated. The best sources of information are

- Benefits Enquiry Line 0800 882200 (0800 220674 in Northern Ireland)
- Website *www.dwp.gov.uk*. Forms can also be completed on line
- The Citizens Advice Bureau *www.nacab.org.uk*
- The ward social worker is usually a good source of information.

Patients who are unable to work may be eligible for:

Statutory sick pay (SSP) A doctor's certificate is usually required for more than one week's sick pay. New rules now make the doctor's certificate the responsibility of the hospital consultant under whom the patient was admitted, and should be completed on discharge, to cover the advised period off work. This also applies to patients needing time off work, and not admitted to hospital. Nursing staff usually complete the forms for the period during which the patient was in hospital.

Incapacity benefit is more complicated and is paid to people not eligible for SSP. It runs for up to a year. After 196 days (the first period is usually covered by a medical certificate) the patient may have to pass a personal capability assessment to show they are incapable of work.

Severe disablement allowance
Income-related benefit
Benefit for the extra cost of disability

Disabled persons tax credit (DPTC). This is not a benefit as such, but a tax credit from the Inland Revenue (paid in addition to benefits).

Severe disablement allowance if a test of 80% disablement is passed.

Disability allowance or attendance allowance are benefits for the extra costs of disability.

Costs for care needs and mobility needs

Industrial diseases disablement benefit. See pneumoconiosis page 480 and asbestosis page 328.

Reduced earning allowance

Constant attendance allowance

Form DS1500, the 'special rules form', is for more urgent benefits for patients with a terminal illness, in whom life expectancy is not expected to exceed 6 months. Patients with a terminal illness can also usually claim attendance allowance, incapacity benefit, and disabled living allowance under 'special rules'. This means that the claim is processed faster, and that higher rates of payment of allowances can be paid from the start.

Further information

There are a number of charities who give grants/aid towards the cost of buying equipment.

www.charitiesdirect.com

www.charity-commission.gov.uk

Part 4

Practical procedures

Airway management

Call for anaesthetic help early.

Patients may require support of their airway and ventilation/oxygenation in situations when they are unable to adequately maintain these. Such situations may be related to a Glasgow Coma Score of <8, which can cause difficulties with airway maintenance, or related to respiratory compromise or arrest in the critically ill patient.

Simple airway adjuncts are used to overcome backward tongue displacement in an unconscious patient.

Oropharyngeal airway (Guedel) A curved plastic tube with a flanged end that is inserted into the mouth. Size is estimated by holding it at the side of the patient's face and estimating required length from angle of the mouth to angle of the jaw. Ensure the mouth is clear, then insert the airway 'upside down', with the curved side towards the tongue. When it is in as far as the soft palate, turn it around by 180 degrees and push it in further, so the flange is at the patient's mouth. If the patient has a gag reflex, remove the airway. Suction can be performed through the airway and oxygen administered via a mask.

Nasopharyngeal airway A soft plastic tube with a bevelled end and a flange at the other end. Better tolerated in the semi-conscious, and should not be used in those with base of skull fractures. Choose a tube size similar to the size of the patient's little finger, and insert a safety pin through the flange. Lubricate it with water-soluble jelly and insert the bevelled end into a nostril and gently push back with a twisting action. Do not force if obstruction is encountered, but remove and try in the other nostril. Nasal bleeding can be caused if the mucosa is damaged. The safety pin ensures the airway is not dislodged into lung. Oxygen can be administered through a mask.

Intubation

Endotracheal tube The optimal method of managing a patient's airway and providing airway protection from aspiration of gastric contents. Requires training in tube insertion. The tube is bevelled at one end with an inflatable cuff and has a connector at the other end. The connector can be removed if the tube needs to be cut, but can be replaced.

- Patient lies flat, with neck flexed and head extended (the 'sniffing the morning air' position). A pillow is placed under the head, not the neck to aid this
- Pre-oxygenate with bag and mask ventilation
- Using the laryngoscope in left hand and standing behind the head, the mouth is opened and the laryngoscope placed over the right side of the tongue and advanced
- It may be necessary to apply suction to clear the mouth of secretions
- When the epiglottis is seen, the laryngoscope is advanced into the vallecula, between the root of the epiglottis and the base of the tongue. Upward pressure in the direction of the laryngoscope handle is applied to lift the jaw slightly and the cords should come into view, taking care not to damage the teeth
- Slide the tube through the cords and then withdraw the laryngoscope
- Inflate the cuff
- Confirm adequate tube position by auscultating for breath sounds over the chest bilaterally
- End tidal CO_2 measurement should be used if available; 5 breaths showing CO_2 confirm an adequate tube position

- If the tube is not in position, usually because it has been passed into the oesophagus or the right main bronchus, deflate the cuff, remove the tube, and reoxygenate with the bag and mask, before trying again. Pull the tube back slightly if the breath sounds are only on the right as this suggests the tube is in the right main bronchus
- Secure the tube
- Administer oxygen with a self-inflating bag with oxygen and reservoir bag
- CXR to confirm correct tube position 2–3 cm above the carina
- Suction can be performed through the tube.

Laryngeal mask airway

An alternative to formal intubation. A wide-bore tube with an inflated cuff at one end, which is positioned over the larynx and inflated, hence forming a seal; thus aspiration of gastric contents and gastric inflation are minimized. It is easy to insert and is used in anaesthetic practice and also used in emergencies. Requires minimal head tilt, so is ideal for use in patients with possible cervical spine injuries. Not suitable for patients with high airway resistance, such as pulmonary oedema, bronchospasm, or COPD. Select a size 4 or 5 tube and, after ensuring the cuff works, deflate it. Put water-soluble lubricating jelly over the cuff. The patient should be lying flat, with head extension if possible. Hold the tube like a pen and insert from behind the patient's head, with the point of the cuff positioned to the back of the mouth. Advance along the roof of the mouth and then press it downwards and backwards until resistance is felt. Inflate the cuff, which will cause the tube to lift out of the mouth a little. Confirm adequate airway position by auscultating for breath sounds over the chest bilaterally. Secure the tube.

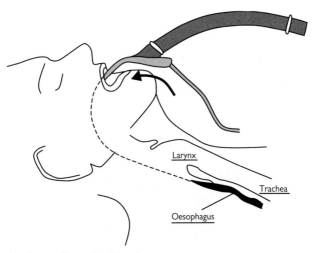

Larynx

Trachea

Oesophagus

Line diagram of laryngeal mask insertion.

Cricothyroidotomy

Call for anaesthetic and ENT help.

In some situations of upper airway obstruction or facial trauma, ventilation and tracheal intubation of a patient is impossible. It may therefore be necessary to create an immediate surgical airway below the level of obstruction.

- Extend the head, with the patient lying flat. Place a pillow under the patient's shoulders, not their head
- Identify cricothyroid membrane: soft triangular area above cricoid ring and below the thyroid cartilage. (Put your fingers on the larynx and move them down to the soft area below, where you are aiming for.) Clean with antiseptic swab
- Puncture the membrane in the midline with a large-bore cannula (18G or larger). Remove the needle, attach a syringe, and aspirate air to confirm correct position. Specific cricothyroidotomy kits are available
- Angle the cannula downwards at 45 degrees and advance. Ensure air can still be aspirated and then connect to high-pressure oxygen supply, with a Y connector if possible
- Occlude one limb of Y connector with a finger until chest rises and then release to allow exhalation, ideally via larynx. Inflate for 1 second and deflate for 4 seconds. Must allow air to be exhaled. If there is no Y connector, a hole is cut in the oxygen tubing, which can be intermittently occluded
- Secure the cannula
- Perform a formal surgical cricothyroidotomy with ENT help, as needle method does not allow adequate ventilation as the tube is too small and the larynx is blocked. Vertical skin incision, press lateral edges outwards to minimize bleeding. Transverse cricothyroid membrane incision, care not to damage cricoid cartilage. Dilate tract with tracheal spreader or scalpel handle and insert a cuffed tube.

Diagram of needle cricothyroidotomy.

Further information

Advanced Life Support Provider Manual, 4th edition 2000. Resuscitation Council UK

Bronchoscopy

Indications and risks

Bronchoscopy is the procedure of passing a telescope or camera into the trachea to inspect the large- and medium-sized airways. It may be performed with a flexible scope using local anaesthetic ± sedation, favoured by physicians, or under a general anaesthetic with a rigid scope, used mostly by surgeons. Airways can be visually inspected and samples taken and therapeutic procedures can be performed. This chapter focuses on flexible bronchoscopy.

Indications for bronchoscopy

- **Suspected lung cancer** Patients who have a central mass <4 cm from the origin of the nearest lobar bronchus, which is likely to be accessible for biopsy at bronchoscopy
- **Suspected pulmonary infection** such as TB in a patient who is unable to produce sputum, or in immunocompromised patients, with fever, cough, hypoxia, or CXR changes (induced sputum with hypertonic saline may be an alternative; see page 701)
- **Suspected interstitial lung disease** if a transbronchial biopsy will provide an adequate sample for diagnostic purposes, such as in sarcoid. Only indicated in a limited number of interstitial lung diseases, as more adequate biopsies are often obtained through open lung biopsy, which may be preferable
- **Foreign body removal** if this is located proximally
- **Therapeutic indications** include diathermy, laser, cryotherapy, argon plasma coagulation, endobronchial brachytherapy, and stenting.

Relative contraindications/take care

- If a patient has saturations below 90% on air at rest, or PaO_2 less than 8 kPa, the risk of significant hypoxia during bronchoscopy is increased
- FEV_1 < 40% predicted
- Blood clotting abnormalities, particularly platelet level < 50,000/mm^3
- Uraemia, pulmonary hypertension, SVCO, liver disease, and immunosuppression predispose to haemorrhage
- Recent myocardial infarction may be associated with cardiac ischaemia during bronchoscopy. Wait until 4–6 weeks after.

Risks associated with bronchoscopy Flexible bronchoscopy is a safe procedure, with reported mortality rates in large series being 0.01–0.04% and major complications of 0.08–0.12%. Complications include respiratory depression, pneumonia, pneumothorax, airway obstruction, laryngospasm, cardiorespiratory arrest, arrhythmias, pulmonary oedema, vasovagal episodes, fever (especially following BAL), septicaemia, haemorrhage, nausea, and vomiting.

Bleeding and bronchoscopy

- Bleeding occurs in approximately 0.7% of patients due to mechanical trauma from the scope, suctioning, brushing, or biopsy, but is more common with transbronchial biopsy (1.6–4.4%). Patients with malignancy, immunocompromise, or uraemia have an increased bleeding tendency
- If bleeding does not stop spontaneously, the bronchoscope should be wedged to tamponade the bleeding in the segmental bronchus. Use minimal suction, to allow clot formation. 1 ml aliquots of 1:10,000 adrenaline solution are administered via the bronchoscope as near to the bleeding point as possible, until it stops. Iced saline may be useful
- If massive haemorrhage occurs, the patient should be turned on to the side of the bleeding to protect the other lung.

Patient preparation and procedure

Patient preparation

- **Information** Patients should be given written information about the procedure ideally more than 24 hours prior to the procedure. Provide an information sheet for the patient to take home following the bronchoscopy, with advice about the effects of any sedation and possible complications, as well as telephone numbers in case help is needed
- **Consent** The physician performing the bronchoscopy should obtain written consent, with a description of the procedure and its associated risks
- **Nil by mouth** Patients should have no food for 4 hours beforehand and clear fluids only until 2 hours beforehand
- **Blood tests** Patients do not need routine pre-procedure blood tests, unless there are specific concerns (uraemia, deranged LFTs, low platelets). Many physicians check platelet counts and clotting times prior to transbronchial biopsy (platelets > 75,000/mm^3, PT and APTT within 1–2 seconds of control)
- **Bedside tests** Consider performing an ECG in patients with a history of cardiac disease. Check blood sugar in patients with diabetes
- **Prophylactic antibiotics** should be given to those at risk of endocarditis. In those with asthma, a nebulized bronchodilator should be given before the bronchoscopy.

Procedure

- Practices vary between centres. Some perform bronchoscopy with the patient sitting up facing the operator; some from behind with the patient lying flat
- **IV access** should be present in all patients
- **Nasal oxygen** should be administered and oximetry measured throughout
- **Pre-medication** may be given in addition for mild sedation, anxiolysis, and anterograde amnesia. A benzodiazepine such as midazolam 2 mg, with 1 mg increments as necessary, may be used with fentanyl. Some patients and operators prefer not to use sedation, due to concerns particularly in elderly patients, those with COPD, or those with cardiac disease. Midazolam can make some patients more agitated. Pre-medication with anticholinergics is not beneficial during bronchoscopy
- **Lidocaine** Local anaesthetic spray or gel is applied to the nostrils and the vocal cords are anaesthetized by spraying local anaesthetic (lidocaine 10 mg/spray) to the back of the throat and allowing time to work. Peak plasma levels occur after 15 minutes
  - Transcricoid injection may be used to administer 4% lidocaine into the trachea, or this may be anaesthetized under direct vision through the bronchoscope, when the vocal cords are open
  - Aliquots of 1–2% lidocaine may be administered to right and left main bronchi via the bronchoscope when it is passed through the vocal cords into the trachea. Use the minimal dose required for

cough suppression. Peak plasma levels occur after 5 minutes via the scope. Airway inflammation increases lidocaine absorption
- Maximum dose of lidocaine is 8 mg/kg (= 29 ml of 2% solution in 70 kg patient); 5 mg/kg if hepatic or cardiac insufficiency. Toxic effects include seizures and arrhythmias
- The half-life of lidocaine is 1.5–2 hours
- Most access the trachea via the nasal route, as this gives increased stability when taking biopsies. If this is not possible, a mouth guard is used and access obtained through the mouth
- All sections of the bronchial tree should be visually inspected, including the cords and trachea. CXR or CT may help localize the area of concern so specimen site can then be targeted. This increases the diagnostic yield of bronchoscopy in cases of suspected lung cancer
- Avoid unnecessary suction, as this can increase hypoxia.

Sampling techniques

Bronchial washings are taken by instilling about 10 ml of saline and then collecting it in a pot/trap to obtain superficial airway cells.

Bronchial brushings are taken by inserting a covered brush into a bronchial segment, uncovering it, rubbing the bronchial wall, covering it, removing it, and wiping it on a slide. The slide is then sprayed with a cell fixing solution.

Bronchial biopsies are taken with biopsy forceps. 5–7 should be taken to optimize yield. These may be taken blindly or from a visibly abnormal area, which gives a higher diagnostic yield than blind biopsies. They can be placed in formalin or saline solution depending on whether they are for histology or microbiology.

Bronchoalveolar lavage (BAL) is performed by inserting 50–100 ml of saline through the bronchoscope when it is wedged well in a small airway. Ideally instil fluid during inspiration and, after allowing the fluid to dwell for 10–30 seconds, aspirate back into the syringe during expiration or collect in a trap. Best performed in the area of abnormality on CXR or CT, or non-dependent lobes such as the right middle lobe or lingula. Poor return if the patient is coughing excessively or if they have emphysema. Can cause hypoxia, proportional to amount of lavage fluid used.

Transbronchial biopsy (TBB) Technique of passing transbronchial biopsy forceps down a terminal bronchus until resistance is first felt and taking a sample of parenchymal tissue. Safe to perform if patient is taking aspirin or on subcutaneous heparin, but omit clopidogrel for 5 days before and if on warfarin, wait until INR < 1.3. Some perform with radiological screening.

Associated with a significant risk of bleeding in 9% and pneumothorax in 3.5%, but up to 14% if patient is mechanically ventilated. Half of all pneumothoraces require chest drains. Therefore perform on one side only and minimize risk by performing TBB in the lower lobes, in dependent segments. Perform CXR one hour after the bronchoscopy. Pneumothorax should be managed according to standard guidelines (page 294). Small pneumothoraces often resolve spontaneously, but the patient may need admission if there are concerns.

When performing bronchoscopy:
- Wear gloves, facemask and eye shields
- Use particulate (duck) masks if there are concerns about TB or HIV.

Interventional bronchoscopy

Transbronchial needle aspirate (TBNA) Technique of inserting a biopsy needle through the bronchial wall into an enlarged lymph node or extrabronchial mass and aspirating cells. Used to give additional staging information in lung cancer. Appropriate lymph nodes should be identified on CT first. Should be performed initially, so the bronchoscope is not contaminated with malignant cells from the airway. Push sheath out through end of bronchoscope until the hub is just visible. Extend the needle and then position over nodal position and insert through bronchial wall. Subcarinal and right hilar nodes are the easiest to sample.

Autofluorescent bronchoscopy (AFB) Emerging technique to differentiate central malignant areas from normal tissue, including pre-invasive tumours *in situ*. However the progression of these abnormalities is not known, so the role of AFB is unclear. Uses blue light to induce tissue autofluorescence, which means normal and abnormal tissues appear different colours when viewed through a specialized bronchoscope. Airway trauma, however, can also cause a different mucosal appearance and the test has low specificity. It is being used in some centres as a screening tool following surgical resection of lung cancer, or in patients with head and neck cancer suspected of having a lung primary, or following positive sputum cytology.

Endobronchial ultrasound (EBUS) Technique of visualizing the bronchial wall and the immediate surrounding structures via an ultrasound probe either incorporated into the tip of the bronchoscope or passed down the scope. A balloon surrounding the probe is inflated with water, in order to achieve close circular contact and view surrounding structures. Useful to assess lymph node involvement in malignancy, to guide TBNA, to identify mediastinal structures or masses next to the airways, to assess the depth of bronchial wall tumour invasion, or to localize masses within the lung for biopsy. Not widely used currently.

Bronchial diathermy, laser resection, argon–plasma coagulation, and cryotherapy These are all procedures that can be used to debulk obstructing endobronchial lesions, or coagulate a bleeding point. Diathermy is the use of an electrical current via a probe to coagulate tissue. Laser achieves the same effect. Argon–plasma coagulation is a non-contact method using argon gas. These are all effective immediately. Cryotherapy is the technique of freezing and then thawing an area with a probe in order to destroy tissue, such as an endobronchial obstructing lesion. It takes hours–days to have its effects. It can also be used to remove a foreign body, as freezing attaches foreign body to the end of the probe.

Bronchial stent insertion via the bronchoscope to re-establish airway patency. Expanding metal stents used in cases of external compression, such as lung cancer, for palliation of breathlessness. Silicone stents are used in mainly benign disease and are inserted via rigid bronchoscopy. They are easily removed and manoeuvred, but can migrate and lead to problems with retained secretions.

Brachytherapy Procedure of endobronchial irradiation using iridium^{192} via bronchoscope for endobronchial and intramural tumours. Delayed effect, requires several sessions. Complementary to other bronchoscopic therapies. Can cause fistulas and haemorrhage.

Rigid bronchoscopy Visualize bronchial tree to level of segmental bronchi. Can remove or core out endobronchial tumours, insert a stent, dilate tracheal or bronchial stenosis, and manage massive haemoptysis. Useful to provide information regarding resectability in lung cancer by measuring airway length. Incidence of serious complications < 5%: hypoxia, laryngospasm, pneumothorax, bleeding.

Further information

Airway stenting for malignant and benign tracheobronchial stenosis. Wood DE et al. Ann Thorac Surg 2003; **76**: 167–74

Therapeutic bronchoscopy in lung cancer. Lee P et al. Clinics in Chest Medicine 2002; **23**: 241–56

BTS Bronchoscopy guidelines. Thorax 2001; **56** (suppl. 1)

ERS/ATS Statement on Interventional Pulmonology. Europ Respir J 2002; **19**: 356–73

An evaluation of CT as an aid to diagnosing patients undergoing bronchoscopy for suspected bronchial carcinoma. Bungay HK et al. Clin Radiol 2000; **55**(7): 554–60

Role of CT scanning of the thorax prior to bronchoscopy in the investigation of suspected lung cancer. Laroche C et al. Thorax 2000; **55**(5): 359–63

Thoracentesis

Thoracentesis ('pleural tap', or pleural fluid aspiration) may be diagnostic or therapeutic.

Diagnostic thoracentesis

Indication Undiagnosed pleural effusion.

There are no absolute *contraindications* to pleural aspiration, although care should be taken if the patient is anticoagulated.

Technique
1. Explain procedure to patient.
2. Position patient sitting forward, leaning on a pillow over a table with their arms folded in front of them.
3. Double-check correct side from chest examination and CXR.
4. Choose aspiration site 1–2 intercostal spaces below upper level of effusion on percussion. Use posterior or lateral approach (although avoid very posterior approaches close to spine, as intercostal artery drops medially to lie in the mid-intercostal space).
5. Sterile skin preparation and aseptic technique.
6. Infiltrate skin, intercostal muscle, and parietal pleura with 10 ml of 1% lidocaine. Aim just above the upper border of the appropriate rib, avoiding the neurovascular bundle that runs below each rib. The parietal pleura is extremely sensitive; use the full 10 ml of lidocaine.
7. Aspirate pleural fluid with a green (21G) needle and 50 ml syringe.
8. Following diagnostic tap:
   • Note pleural fluid *appearance*
   • Send sample in sterile pot to biochemistry for measurement of *protein* and *LDH*
   • Send a fresh, 20 ml sample in sterile pot to cytology for examination for malignant cells and differential cell count. Use of a 3.8% sodium citrate tube may help preserve cells in cytology samples
   • Send samples in sterile pot and blood culture bottles to *microbiology* for Gram stain and microscopy, culture, and AFB stain and culture
   • Process non-purulent, heparinized samples in arterial blood gas analyser for *pH* (consult biochemistry laboratory for local policy of pH analysis beforehand; never put purulent samples in the arterial blood analyser)
   • Consider measurement of cholesterol and triglycerides, haematocrit, glucose (with paired blood sample), and amylase, depending on the clinical circumstances.
9. There is no need for a routine CXR following aspiration.

If unable to aspirate fluid, further attempts should be with ultrasound-guidance. Ultrasound-guidance may also be required for small or loculated effusions, or to distinguish fluid from pleural thickening.

If *mesothelioma* is likely, 'tattoo' the aspiration site with India ink (to guide prophylactic radiotherapy; pierce skin through ink) and perform aspiration in midaxillary line 6th–7th intercostal space (corresponding to the site of thoracoscopy port, to minimize area of radiotherapy required).

Complications of thoracentesis include pneumothorax, cough, bleeding, empyema, spleen or liver puncture, and malignant seeding down aspiration site (particularly in mesothelioma).

Therapeutic thoracentesis

Indication Symptomatic relief of breathlessness due to a pleural effusion, most commonly due to malignancy.

Technique In many cases, can be performed as a day-case procedure.
1. The initial procedure is identical to that of diagnostic thoracentesis (steps 1–7 opposite). It is important to verify that the insertion site is correct by first aspirating pleural fluid with a green (21G) needle. If unable to aspirate fluid, abort the procedure and ultrasound the chest to check the presence and location of fluid.
2. Carefully advance a large-bore intravenous cannula along the anaesthetized track.
3. Remove the inner needle and attach the cannula to a three-way tap.
4. Aspirate fluid from the chest with a 50 ml syringe via the three-way tap, and flush the fluid into a pot through extension tubing. Drain a maximum of 1.5 l of fluid in one sitting (risk of re-expansion pulmonary oedema following sudden removal of very large volumes). Stop the procedure if resistance is felt, or the patient experiences discomfort or severe coughing.
5. Apply dressing to aspiration site.
6. Repeat CXR to document extent of improvement in effusion size and to exclude pneumothorax or trapped lung.

Aspiration of pneumothorax

Indications

- *Primary pneumothorax* Consider aspiration if patient breathless and/or pneumothorax large (rim of air > 2 cm on CXR)
- *Secondary pneumothorax* Consider aspiration if patient aged <50 years, with small pneumothorax (rim of air < 2 cm on CXR) and minimal breathlessness.

Technique Refer to pages 294–5 for treatment algorithms.

1. Discuss procedure with patient and obtain written consent (unless emergency situation).
2. Insert IV cannula.
3. Position patient sitting upright, supported on pillows.
4. Double-check correct side from chest examination and CXR.
5. Choose aspiration site: second intercostal space in midclavicular line on side of pneumothorax.
6. Infiltrate skin, intercostal muscle, and parietal pleura with 10 ml of 1% lidocaine. Aim just above the upper border of the appropriate rib, avoiding the neurovascular bundle that runs below each rib. Parietal pleura is extremely sensitive; use the full 10 ml of lidocaine.
7. Sterile skin preparation. Wear sterile gloves and gown.
8. Whilst waiting for anaesthetic to work, connect 50 ml syringe to 3 way tap, with tap turned 'off' to patient.
9. Confirm presence of pneumothorax by aspirating air with green (21G) needle.
10. Insert large-bore (e.g. 16G) cannula over upper border of rib. Remove inner needle, quickly connect cannula to three-way tap and 50 ml syringe.
11. Aspirate 50 ml air with syringe, turn tap and expel air into atmosphere. Repeat until resistance felt, or 2.5 litres of air aspirated (aspiration of > 2.5 litres suggests a large air-leak, and aspiration is likely to fail). Halt procedure if painful, or patient coughing excessively.
12. Remove cannula; cover insertion site with dressing.
13. Repeat CXR. Ideal timing of CXR following aspiration is unknown; it may be advisable to wait several hours before performing the CXR, in order to detect slow air leaks.
14. Aspiration is successful if lung is fully re-expanded on CXR.
15. If initial aspiration of a primary pneumothorax fails, repeat aspiration should be considered (unless ≥ 2.5 litres has already been aspirated). At least one-third of patients will respond to a second aspiration.

Abrams' pleural biopsy

Indications

- Diagnosis of tuberculous pleural effusion
- Abrams' biopsy is used for the diagnosis of malignant pleural disease in many centres, although a recent randomized-controlled trial has shown that CT-guided cutting-needle biopsy has a greater sensitivity (sensitivity 87% in CT-guided biopsy group vs. 47% in Abrams' group).

Technique An assistant is required.

1. Discuss procedure with patient and obtain written consent.
2. Insert IV cannula.
3. Consider sedation (e.g. midazolam 2–5 mg IV, with oxygen saturations monitoring).
4. Position patient sitting forward, leaning on a pillow over a table with their arms folded in front of them.
5. Double-check correct side from chest examination and CXR.
6. Choose biopsy site: 1–2 intercostal spaces below upper level of effusion on percussion. Use posterior or lateral approach (although avoid very posterior approaches close to spine, as intercostal artery drops medially to lie in mid-intercostal space).
7. Sterile skin preparation. Wear sterile gloves and gown.
8. Infiltrate skin, intercostal muscle, and parietal pleura with 10 ml of 1% lidocaine. Aim just above the upper border of the appropriate rib, avoiding the neurovascular bundle that runs below each rib. Anaesthetize area behind rib below the insertion point.
9. Whilst waiting for anaesthetic to work, assemble Abrams' reverse bevel biopsy needle. The needle consists of an outer sheath with a triangular opening (biopsy port) that can be opened or closed by rotating an inner sheath.
10. Verify that the insertion site is correct by aspirating pleural fluid with a green (21G) needle. If unable to aspirate fluid, do not proceed.
11. Make small (5 mm) skin incision; dissect intercostal muscles with blunt forceps (e.g. Spencer–Wells).
12. Insert biopsy needle gently with biopsy port closed. Do not apply force; the needle should slip into the pleural space without resistance. When in the pleural cavity, fluid can be withdrawn by attaching a syringe to the needle and opening the biopsy port.
13. To take a biopsy, attach a syringe to the needle. Open the biopsy port and angle it downwards, and then pull the biopsy port firmly against the parietal pleura on the rib beneath the entry point (6 o'clock position relative to entry point). Close the biopsy port, thereby pulling a sample of parietal pleura into the needle.
14. Remove the biopsy needle, open the biopsy port, and remove biopsy sample.
15. Repeat procedure four–six times in positions 4–8 o'clock, always sampling below the insertion point (to avoid the neurovascular bundle beneath the rib above).
16. Send biopsy samples in saline for analysis for tuberculosis and in formalin if malignancy is suspected.
17. Apply dressing to biopsy site. May require a single stitch.
18. CXR to exclude pneumothorax.

Complications include pain, pneumothorax, haemothorax, and empyema. Haemorrhage from trauma to an intercostal artery may necessitate emergency thoracotomy. Fatalities are well-documented but rare.

Further information

Standard pleural biopsy versus CT-guided cutting-needle biopsy for diagnosis of malignant disease in pleural effusions: a randomised controlled trial. Maskell NA, *et al. Lancet* 2003; **361**: 1326–31

Chest drains

Indications, drain types, complications

Chest drain insertion is associated with significant morbidity and mortality, and careful consideration should be given to the precise indication for drainage. Ultrasound-guidance may be required for small or loculated effusions (e.g. empyema).

Indications
- Tension pneumothorax (following needle decompression)
- Symptomatic pneumothorax with failed aspiration or underlying lung disease
- Complicated parapneumonic effusion and empyema
- Malignant pleural effusion for symptomatic relief and/or pleurodesis
- Haemothorax
- Traumatic haemopneumothorax
- Rarely, for symptomatic effusions of other aetiology.

Contraindications
- Inexperienced operator
- Lung adherent to chest wall
- Bleeding tendency (a relative contraindication; routine measurement of platelet count and clotting in the absence of risk factors is not required)
- Post-pneumonectomy (not a contraindication, but discuss with cardiothoracic surgical team; imaging may be required for drain placement).

Types of chest drain Traditional *trocar* drains consist of a flexible plastic tube surrounding a metal rod with a blunt tip, and are available in a variety of sizes. When inserted incorrectly, or with excess force by an inexperienced operator, they can cause significant harm and even death. Blue, *portex* drains are inserted over a flexible plastic introducer in a similar manner to trocar drains; they are available in a range of sizes, up to 28F. Newer, *Seldinger*-style drains involve sliding the drain into the pleural cavity over a guide-wire. They are safer than trocar drains, but still require experience and care to be inserted safely and comfortably. Small (10–14F) drains are more comfortable and are adequate for the majority of situations. Large bore chest drains (28–32F) are only rarely required, e.g. secondary pneumothorax with large air-leak and/or surgical emphysema; acute haemothorax.

Complications
- Pain—very common. Opiate analgesia frequently required
- Inadequate drain position—may require withdrawal or insertion of new drain
- Surgical emphysema (in pneumothorax)—air leaks into subcutaneous tissues. May occur if tube blocked or positioned with holes subcutaneously, or with very large air leaks. See page 296 for management

- Infection—empyema rate around 1%, perhaps higher in trauma patients
- Organ damage (e.g. lung, liver, spleen, heart, great vessels, stomach)—particularly if sharp trocar used. Intrapulmonary placement results in significant, continuous bubbling and bleeding; this may occur in up to 6% of all drain insertions. Drainage of gastrointestinal contents suggests bowel perforation (or oesophageal rupture as the cause of the effusion)
- Haemorrhage into drain—bloody pleural fluid is a common finding (e.g. in malignant effusions), but unexpected large volume drainage of frank blood suggests damage to organs or intercostal vessels. Clamp the drain and leave it in place. Urgent imaging and surgical referral
- Re-expansion pulmonary oedema (page 297)
- Vasovagal reaction
- Sudden death due to vagus nerve irritation reported.

Insertion technique

An assistant is required.

1. Discuss procedure with patient and obtain written consent (unless emergency situation).
2. Insert IV cannula.
3. Consider sedation (e.g. midazolam 2–5 mg IV or diamorphine 2.5–5 mg IV) with oxygen saturation monitoring; be cautious in patients with severe underlying lung disease or respiratory failure.
4. Position patient lying with bed head at 30°, with insertion side of trunk rotated about 45° upwards, and arm on insertion side behind their head; stand behind the patient. Alternative position is with patient sitting forward, leaning over a table.
5. Double-check correct side from chest examination and CXR.
6. Choose insertion site: ideally within 'triangle of safety', which avoids major vessels and muscles (boundaries: anteriorly, anterior axillary line and border of pectoralis major; posteriorly, posterior axillary line; inferiorly, horizontal to level of nipple in man or fifth intercostal space in woman). More posterolateral approaches are safe but less comfortable for the patient when lying; avoid posteromedial approaches close to spine, as intercostal artery drops medially to lie in mid-intercostal space.
7. Sterile skin preparation. Wear sterile gloves and gown.
8. Infiltrate skin, intercostal muscle, and parietal pleura with 10 ml of 1% lidocaine. Aim just above the upper border of the appropriate rib, avoiding the neurovascular bundle that runs below each rib. The subcutaneous fat lacks pain receptors and does not require anaesthetic. The parietal pleura however is extremely sensitive; use the full 10 ml of lidocaine.
9. Verify that the site is correct by aspirating pleural fluid or air. Occasionally, a green (21G) needle may be too short in obese patients, and a longer needle is required. If unable to aspirate fluid or air, do not proceed with drain insertion; consider image-guided drainage.
10. Whilst waiting for anaesthetic to work, prepare drain and connections. Assistant should prepare underwater seal.
11. Insert drain:
    - **Trocar drains** Small (1 cm) skin incision parallel to rib. Consider horizontal mattress stitch across incision to facilitate later closure. Dissect intercostal muscles with blunt forceps (e.g. Spencer–Wells)—the fibres can be teased apart by opening and then removing the forceps; do not close forceps within the chest, this may damage underlying structures. This blunt dissection may take some time. Insert trocar and drain smoothly and gently—there should not be any significant resistance. *Never apply force when inserting a chest drain*. Once the chest wall has been entered, withdraw the trocar a few centimetres and insert the drain into the pleural cavity. Never insert the trocar blindly into pleural cavity. An alternative approach is to remove the trocar and grip the end of the chest tube

with blunt forceps, and use these to guide the tube into the chest. Aim towards the apex for a pneumothorax, and the lung base for a pleural effusion.

(Note—in emergencies, or in patients with extreme obesity or subcutaneous emphysema, it may be appropriate to make a larger initial incision and insert an index finger to assist the drain track.)

- *Seldinger drains* Gently insert the introducer needle and check that air or fluid can be easily aspirated through it with a syringe. Remove syringe. Smoothly insert the guide-wire through the introducer needle. Remove introducer needle. Slide plastic dilator around guide-wire to enlarge the entry-track. Remove the dilator and slide the drain into the pleural cavity over the guide-wire. Do not let go of the guide-wire at any time. Remove the wire when the drain is within the chest.

12. Connect the drain to underwater seal bottle via a three-way tap and tubing. If the drain is correctly positioned in the pleural space it should swing in time with respiration, and drain air or fluid.
13. Stitch and tape the drain in place on the chest wall.
14. Ensure adequate analgesia.
15. Warn the patient not to disconnect the tubing or lift the underwater bottle above the level of the insertion site on the chest; supply a 'chest drain information leaflet'.
16. Obtain CXR to check position. The 'ideal' tube position (apex for pneumothorax, base for effusion) is not necessary for effective drainage, so do not reposition functioning drains on this basis. CT may be useful in confirming drain position in certain circumstances. Drains are often positioned in fissures, but in most cases this does not affect their functioning.
17. Small drains may need regular flush to ensure potency; prescribe 10 ml normal saline flush to drain tds.

Further information

BTS guidelines for the insertion of a chest drain. Laws D, *et al. Thorax* 2003; **58** (suppl. II): ii53–ii59

Drain management

General points

- Patients should ideally be managed on a specialist ward by experienced nursing staff. 'Chest drain observations' should be charted regularly, including swinging, bubbling, and volume of fluid output
- If drain water level does not swing with respiration, the drain is kinked (check underneath dressing, as tube enters skin), blocked, clamped, or incorrectly positioned (drainage holes not in pleural space; check CXR). Occluded drains may sometimes be unblocked by a 30 ml saline flush. Non-functioning drains should be removed (risk of introducing infection)
- Suction is sometimes used to encourage drainage, although there is a lack of evidence regarding its use. Consider in cases of pneumothorax with persistent air leak, or following chemical pleurodesis. Suction should be high volume/low pressure, typically starting at a level of 5 cm H_2O and increasing to 10–20 cm H_2O. It is often painful and may not be tolerated by the patient.

To clamp or not to clamp?

Never clamp a bubbling chest drain (risk of tension pneumothorax). Clamping may be considered in two situations:

- To control the rate of drainage of a large pleural effusion. Rapid drainage of large volumes may result in re-expansion pulmonary oedema; clamping, e.g. for one hour after draining 1 litre, may prevent this
- To avoid inappropriate drain removal in cases of pneumothorax with a slow air-leak, when bubbling appears to have ceased. Clamping of a drain for several hours followed by repeat CXR in such situations may detect very slow or intermittent air leaks. This is controversial, however, and should only ever be considered on a specialist ward with experienced nursing staff. If the patient becomes breathless, the drain should be immediately unclamped.

Drain removal Quickly and smoothly remove the drain whilst patient is breath-holding in expiration (although opinions on this differ—some recommend removal in maximal inspiration). Tie previously placed mattress suture, if applicable. Apply dressing. CXR to document lung position.

Pleurodesis

Background

The aim of pleurodesis is to seal the visceral pleura to the parietal pleura with adhesions to prevent pleural fluid or air accumulating. Successful pleurodesis is dependent upon two factors:

- Lung re-expansion following removal of pleural fluid or air, which allows the apposition of visceral and parietal pleura. This may be encouraged by applying suction to an intercostal drain
- Inflammation of the pleural surfaces, which is required to produce pleural fibrosis and adhesions. This may be induced by a chemical sclerosing agent or by pleural abrasion at thoracoscopy.

Indications

- Recurrent and symptomatic pleural effusion (most commonly as a result of malignancy, although pleurodesis is also rarely used in benign recurrent effusions)
- Recurrent pneumothorax (due to concerns regarding the long-term safety of intrapleural talc, surgical abrasion pleurodesis is usually the procedure of choice in younger patients; chemical pleurodesis may be used as a last resort in older patients who are unfit for surgery).

Chemical pleurodesis

Types of sclerosant Choice of sclerosing agents varies. The most commonly used agents are sterile talc, tetracycline, and bleomycin.

- Talc is the most effective (success rate about 90%), and can be administered either as a slurry via a chest drain or as a poudrage at thoracoscopy, but it carries a risk of inducing ARDS (see later)
- Tetracycline is successful in about 65% cases
- Bleomycin has success rates of only 60%, and is expensive.

Other, rarely used agents include doxycycline, minocycline, interferon, interleukins, cisplatin, or the patient's own blood.

Corticosteroids may increase the failure rate of pleurodesis by inhibiting the pleural inflammatory response and development of adhesions, and should be discontinued beforehand. The effect of NSAIDs on the success of pleurodesis is unclear.

Technique Most centres will have a written pleurodesis protocol, usually involving pre-medication and intrapleural local anaesthesia. A typical protocol is set out below:

1. Discuss procedure with patient and obtain written consent.
2. Insert chest drain (page 688): small bore (10–14F) chest tubes are sufficient for fluid drainage and pleurodesis, and are more comfortable than larger drains. Flush drain with 20 ml normal saline 6 hourly.
3. Commence heparin 5000 IU bd as prophylaxis against thromboembolism (increased risk following pleurodesis, especially in patients with malignancy).

4. Drain fluid in a controlled manner. There is a small risk of re-expansion pulmonary oedema if large effusions are drained too quickly; control output by clamping drain; aim to drain a maximum of 1 litre/hour.
5. CXR when drain output slows (<150 ml/day):
   • Consider pleurodesis if fluid removed and lung fully or partially expanded on CXR (although success rates are much lower in the setting of an incompletely expanded lung)
   • Consider trial of suction if lung only partially re-expanded. Aim to gradually increase pressure to −20 cm H_2O. Use of suction may be limited by pain.

For pleurodesis:

6. Insert IV cannula and attach pulse oximeter.
7. Pleurodesis is often extremely painful. Consider pre-medication with opioid (diamorphine 2.5 mg IV), anti-emetic (metoclopramide 10 mg), and benzodiazepine (midazolam 1–2 mg IV, titrate to conscious level, care in elderly and in patients with respiratory failure). The patient should be comfortable but co-operative.
8. Administer intrapleural local anaesthetic (e.g. lidocaine 3 mg/kg, maximum 250 mg) via the chest drain, as intrapleural administration of sclerosants is frequently painful. Clamp drain and wait several minutes.
9. Administer sterile talc slurry (4 grams talc in 30 ml normal saline).
10. Flush drain with 20 ml saline.
11. Further analgesia if required.
12. Clamp drain for one hour after administration of sclerosant. Then unclamp drain and consider applying suction, −20 cm H_2O. Restart drain flushes.
13. Monitor pulse, blood pressure, temperature, respiratory rate, and oxygen saturations half-hourly for two hours and then six hourly.
14. Analgesia and antipyretics as required.
15. Optimal duration of drainage following pleurodesis is unknown; consider drain removal within 12–72 hours if there is adequate drainage of fluid and lung expansion on CXR. Can usually remove tube at 48 hours.
16. In cases of mesothelioma arrange prophylactic radiotherapy for the drain site (total of 21 Gy in 3 fractions over one week). Malignant seeding at drain sites in non-mesothelioma malignant effusions is uncommon and prophylactic radiotherapy is not required.

Complications All sclerosants may cause chest pain and fever as side-effects. Use of sterile talc may rarely (<1%) result in respiratory failure due to adult respiratory distress syndrome, manifest as hypoxia and diffuse pulmonary infiltrates within 48 hours of pleurodesis. The risk appears to be reduced with lower talc doses (<5 grams).

Future developments are likely to focus on more effective and safer sclerosing agents for pleurodesis, for example, transforming growth factor-β, which has been demonstrated to produce an effective pleurodesis in rabbits.

Medical thoracoscopy

Thoracoscopy is the procedure of examining the chest wall, parietal pleura, visceral pleura, and diaphragm with a thoracoscope and taking biopsies. Chemical pleurodesis can also be performed. Performed by chest physicians, using sedation and local anaesthetic.

There needs to be an adequate space into which the thoracoscope is inserted, without damaging the underlying lung. Patients suitable for thoracoscopy are therefore those who have an underlying pleural effusion or a pneumothorax, where the lung is away from the instrument insertion site.

Indications for thoracoscopy

- Undiagnosed pleural effusion—usually an exudate (diagnostic sensitivity of medical thoracoscopy is 95%)
- Suspected mesothelioma
- Staging of pleural effusion in lung cancer
- Treatment of recurrent pleural effusions with pleurodesis
- Pneumothorax requiring chemical pleurodesis, as an alternative to surgery, e.g. the patient unfit for surgical thoracoscopy.

Contraindications/proceed with caution

- Obliterated pleural space
- Pleural adhesions, as these may tear when pneumothorax is induced
- Bleeding disorder
- Hypoxia <92% on air
- Unstable cardiovascular disease
- Persistent uncontrollable cough.

Risks associated with thoracoscopy

Mortality rates are low (<0.01% of cases)
- Haemorrhage—may need diathermy in the pleural space. Rare
- Pulmonary perforations. Rare
- Air or gas embolism during pneumothorax induction. Rare <0.1%
- Local wound infection
- Empyema
- Fever, ARDS with talc poudrage (see page 693).

Preparation of patient and consent

- Patient should have written information >24 hours before the procedure. Written consent taken by doctor performing procedure
- Check recent CXR and any CT scans available
- Check FBC, coagulation, U&E
- Send blood for group and save
- Nil by mouth for 4 hours pre-procedure
- IV cannula in arm on the same side as the thoracoscopy to make repeated sedative administration during the procedure easy
- Pre-medication with analgesia, such as a single dose of oral ibuprofen 800 mg, 1–2 hours before. Also antibiotics, such as cefuroxime 1.5 g IV, for infection prophylaxis
- Baseline oxygen saturations, pulse, BP, temperature. Measure oximetry throughout.

Procedure The patient is placed in the lateral decubitus position, with the side of the pleural effusion uppermost. Sedation is administered and allowed time to work. Oxygen (2–4 l/min) is administered via nasal cannulae. The skin is cleaned and local anaesthetic inserted, in the same way as for a chest drain. The aspiration of fluid or air from the pleural space confirms it is safe to proceed to thoracoscopy. An incision is made and blunt dissection performed through the parietal pleura. The thoracoscope port is then inserted. The pleural effusion is drained via a suction tube through the thoracoscope port. Air is allowed to enter the pleural space through this port so the lung does not reinflate, and effectively a pneumothorax is created. The thoracoscope, with its light source, can then be inserted through the port and the chest cavity inspected. A second smaller incision allows forceps or other instruments to be inserted and biopsies taken.

Thoracoscopic biopsies are usually large and yield good diagnostic results. If the pleural surfaces have appearances consistent with malignancy, pleurodesis can be performed at the end of the procedure, using talc inserted via an insufflator. There is no evidence that pleurodesis performed at thoracoscopy is more efficacious than pleurodesis performed via chest tube, but it may save the patient having a further procedure.

Post thoracoscopy care

- Monitor oxygen saturations, pulse, blood pressure, and temperature
- The patient will have a chest drain *in situ*. This should be on free drainage initially, but continuous suction is required when the drain stops bubbling
- Analgesia as required, such as IV diamorphine 2.5 mg, dihydrocodeine 30–60 mg PO, paracetamol 1 g
- DVT prophylaxis with subcutaneous heparin (increased coagulopathy with talc pleurodesis)
- Mobile CXR on the morning after thoracoscopy
- Remove chest drain when the lung is reinflated on CXR with minimal fluid or air drainage. Trapped lung occurs if the visceral pleura is too thick to allow lung reinflation (see page 304)
- If mesothelioma is diagnosed, refer for radiotherapy to thoracoscopy and chest drain tract sites.

Further information

Diagnostic Thoracoscopy for Pleural Disease. Daniel T. *Ann Thorac Surg* 1993; **56**: 639–40

Thoracoscopy: present diagnostic and therapeutic indications. Loddenkemper R, Boutin C. *Eur Respir J* 1993; **6**: 1544–55

Some diagnostic tests

Skin prick tests

These may be useful in identifying specific allergens causing immediate hypersensitivity reactions. They may influence management and guide allergen avoidance. They are also used to help define atopy. Triggers in contact urticaria, atopic eczema, and suspected food allergy may also be identified. The results are available almost immediately (compared to a RAST test for specific IgE), and correlate well with RAST test results. They should be carried out by staff trained to read the tests and deal with adverse reactions.

The allergens tested should be identified from the history, and usually include common aeroallergens e.g. grass, house dust mite (*D. pteronyssinus*), and cat dander.

Practical points

- Testing should be performed off steroids and anti-histamines
- There is a very small risk of anaphylaxis; adrenaline and resuscitation equipment should be available. Particular care is needed with food and latex testing
- Put a drop of allergen on the skin (usually the inside forearm). A range of allergens are available commercially. Fresh produce should be used for suspected fruit and vegetable hypersensitivity
- Lance the skin through the allergen drop using a needle (do not draw blood). This should be with a calibrated lancet (1 mm), held vertically, or a hypodermic needle held at 45° to the skin
- The positive control is usually histamine, and the negative control the dilutent (usually saline)
- Read the test after 15 minutes
- A positive result is an itchy weal, which should be compared with the controls, as some subjects react to the skin prick alone (dermatographism)
- Test solutions are standardized to give a mean weal diameter of 6 mm
- A weal of 3 mm or more is considered positive (indicating allergen sensitization)
- A positive result does not prove that the clinical symptoms are due to bronchial hyperresponsiveness to the tested allergen, but do raise clinical suspicion. Positive results can occur in those without symptoms, and false negatives do occur.

RAST or radioallergosorbent blood tests are more specific, but less sensitive and more expensive than skin prick tests, but give similar information. There is no risk of anaphylaxis and the patient does not need to stop steroids or antihistamines for the test to be performed.

Unconventional tests Electrodermal allergy testing (using a Vegatest machine) was developed as an aid to homeopathic prescribing, and is widely used in complementary medicine to assess allergic status to food and environmental allergens. It is based on small changes in skin electrical impedance at acupuncture points, in response to allergens placed in an electrical circuit. There is no RCT data to show that this method can identify atopic from non-atopic individuals, as identified from skin prick tests.

Technique of induced sputum

- Used to investigate for infection (e.g. TB, PCP) or airway inflammation
- Patients rinse their mouth and clean their teeth to minimize oral contamination. Give inhaled salbutamol, to minimize bronchconstriction
- Nebulized hypertonic (2.7–5%) saline is administered via a face mask. Afterwards the patient expectorates sputum into a sterile pot
- If infection is likely, perform test in a negative pressure room, with appropriate protection of staff and other patients. Do not perform on the open ward or out-patient department
- Send sputum promptly to microbiology for staining and culture, and direct immunofluorescent testing for PCP (if indicated). Sputum for cell counts is mixed with 0.1% dithiothreitol and diluted with saline and then filtered and centrifuged.

Methacholine challenge testing

- Methacholine induces bronchospasm in people with hyperreactive airways. Helpful if there is diagnostic doubt regarding the diagnosis of asthma
- Should be performed by experienced personnel, with facilities to deal with acute bronchospasm
- Increasing nebulized doses of methacholine are given systematically, with the FEV_1 measured after each dose
- If there is a 20% fall in FEV_1, or if the highest dose of methacholine has been given, the test is stopped
- The concentration of drug causing the 20% fall is known as the PC_{20}
- Asthma is indicated by a PC_{20} of below 8 mg/ml. Normal subjects have a $PC_{20} > 16$ mg/ml.

Appendices

Lung function testing

Flow–volume loop

A good starting point to the understanding of lung function tests is the flow–volume loop. This plots inspiratory and expiratory flow against lung volume during a maximal expiratory and maximal inspiratory manoeuvre.

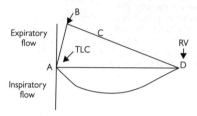

Fig. 1

At the beginning of **expiration** from a full breath in, the expiratory muscles are at their strongest, the lungs at their biggest, and hence the airways are at their most open, (A). Because the lungs are at their largest, the radial attachments to the airways, effectively the alveolar/capillary membranes and their connective tissue, are pulling the hardest and supporting the airways against **dynamic compression** during the exhalation manoeuvre.

This means that the highest flow rates are possible at the beginning of the blow, hence the sudden rise to a **peak expiratory flow rate** in the 100 ms or so of the forced breath out, (B). This is the **peak flow** and is essentially what a peak flow meter measures.

As the lung empties, and the lung volume drops, the dilatory pull on the airways from the radial attachments of the surrounding lung tissue reduces, (C). Hence the airways narrow and become less supported, and are less able to resist dynamic compression. This means that the maximal airflow obtainable, regardless of effort, falls too.

Eventually the expiratory muscles come to the end of their 'travel' and cannot squeeze the chest anymore. Also, increasingly with age, the small airways may actually close off, preventing anymore emptying (D). The volume at which this begins to happen is called the **closing volume**.

As maximal **inspiration** starts, although the inspiratory muscles are at their strongest, the airways are at their smallest. Thus flow rates start low and increase as the airways open up. However, as the airways open up, the inspiratory muscles are approaching the end of their 'travel' and are weakening, this means the flow rates fall again; hence the different, rounded, appearance of the inspiratory limb of the flow volume curve.

Thus normally the inspiratory and expiratory flow rates depend on lung volume and are termed 'volume-dependent'. If there is a **fixed upper airway narrowing**, such as from a fibrous tumour in the trachea, then the size of the airway at this point may become so narrow that it now limits maximal flows. However, its diameter will not vary with lung volumes and hence flow will become 'volume-independent'. Figure 2 shows this.

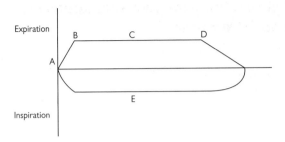

Fig. 2

At A, the rise in flow will initially be normal, but at some point the maximum flow imposed by the upper airway narrowing will cut in, B. From that point onwards the flow rate will be fixed at this maximum (C) until the lower recoil and narrowing small airways again determine the maximum flow (D). The flow volume curve has been severely 'clipped' with a squarish appearance. The same clipped appearance will be present on the inspiratory limb (E), giving rise to the so-called 'square box' appearance.

Sometimes, such upper airways restriction may be *variable* rather than fixed and only present on inspiration (e.g. paralysed and collapsing vocal chords) due to the obstructing elements being sucked in, and then blown open again on expiration.

- Thus a square inspiratory limb, but normal expiratory limb, provides evidence of a mobile, **extrathoracic upper airways obstruction**.

Conversely, a mobile intrathoracic upper airway obstruction (e.g. fleshy tumour at the carina, or retrosternal thyroid) may obstruct more during expiration (when the chest is under compression), compared to inspiration when the chest is being expanded.

- Thus a square expiratory limb, but normal inspiratory limb, is evidence of a **variable intrathoracic upper airways obstruction**.

Sometimes ratios of maximal inspiratory to maximal expiratory flows are used to characterize intra-or extrathoracic airway obstruction.

The other, more common, causes of airway obstruction are due to narrowing of the lower airways (asthma, COPD). In these conditions the airway calibre (and thus flow rates) still remain dependent on lung volume. Hence the flow rates decrease as the lung volume decreases, but particularly so at low lung volumes. This is because resistance to flow is proportional to the airway radius raised to the power of four (r^4) and therefore most significant when airways are already small. Hence increasing airflow obstruction produces expiratory flow volume curves like those in Fig. 3. This greater effect of small airways narrowing at low lung volumes has led some units to report flow rates at, for example, 25% expired lung volume, or averaged between 25 and 75% of the total expired lung volume.

Spirometry, peak flow measurements, and CO transfer

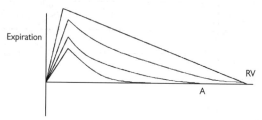

Fig. 3

The airways can be so small such that some begin to close off at lower lung volumes (the *closing volume*); hence a full breath out is not possible, producing air trapping and a raised residual volume (RV) (A). Sensitive tests of small airways narrowing therefore have to concentrate on flows at low lung volumes, and peak flow measurements are relatively insensitive.

- Note that peak flow measurements are the most sensitive to upper airway narrowing and a good way to follow changes in upper airway narrowing during, for example, radiotherapy for a central airway obstructing lung cancer.

Spirometry and peak flow measurements

- The ordinary spirometer (mechanical or electrical) records *volumes against time* rather than *flows against volume*
- The two essential measures are *FEV_1* and *VC*.

The vital capacity (VC) is the maximum amount of air that can be blown out completely. This will be *reduced* if the lungs are *stiff* (preventing a full breath in), the *inspiratory muscles are weak* (preventing a full breath in) or if the *airways are narrowed* such that the small airways collapse during expiration (preventing a full breath out).

The FEV_1 is the amount (forced expiratory volume) that can be blown out in 1 second. Because the value is taken over a second we are capturing much more flow during the breath out than the PEFR measure does, but it is still occurring when the airways are at their largest. It is less effort-dependent and generally more robust. The ratio of the two figures (FEV_1/VC) tells us about the degree of airflow obstruction.

- A ratio of FEV_1/VC of less than about 70–75% indicates airflow obstruction.

This ratio is a very useful figure because it is hardly affected by age, sex, height, ethnic origin, etc.—it is self-normalizing. The individual measures FEV_1 and VC do need corrections for the above factors, however, and are usually quoted as % predicted. It is important to realize that the range of normality is considerable, and it may not be clear if a set of results is simply at the bottom end of normal, or is considerably reduced from the patient's normally much higher figures. Serial measurements indicating continuing deterioration may be the first clue.

If the FEV_1/VC ratio is normal, then the VC can be interpreted as to whether there is a reduced total lung volume, such as from interstitial lung disease. This is called a restrictive pattern, and a low FEV_1/VC ratio an obstructive pattern. The FEV_1/VC ratio may actually be raised in interstitial lung disease as the airways are better supported by the fibrosed radial attachments which therefore reduces dynamic compression. The *slope* of the volume/time plot you get from a spirometer is effectively the *flow rate* at any particular point: because flow is dropping during expiration the slope progressively flattens off. However, if there is any upper airways obstruction (as discussed above) the expiratory flow rate will be constant for a while and hence the spirometer line will be straighter than usual. An interesting index, the ***Empey index***, has been described.

$$\text{Empey index} = \frac{FEV_1 \text{ (in ml)}}{PEFR \text{ (in litre/min)}}$$

Because PEFR is clipped first by the presence of upper airflow obstruction, relative to the FEV_1, the above index gets larger with such a problem. A figure over 10 is indicative of upper airflow obstruction, but it is only a pointer, and there will be false positives and negatives.

Although one-off measures of these flows and volumes can be made, often more interesting information comes from serial measurements. For example in asthma, the measurements will fluctuate with a characteristic morning 'dip' in lung function.

Carbon monoxide (CO) transfer

This test is usually done in the lung function laboratory and measures the amount of **gas exchanging surface area** available. A gas mixture containing CO is inhaled, the breath held for 10 seconds, and then exhaled. The amount that has disappeared (by crossing the alveolar capillary membrane and being taken up by red cells) is calculated. A correction for the haemoglobin concentration is required, as the amount of CO transferred will fall as the available haemoglobin is reduced. The **total amount of CO transferred is the TLCO** (total lung, TL). When divided by the total lung volume during the breath hold, it is called the **kCO, gas transfer per unit lung volume.** The total lung volume 'reached' by the CO is the amount breathed in, *plus* the amount of air already in the lung at the start of the breath in. This is measured by including helium in the inhaled gas mixture that is then diluted by the air already in the lung; thus by comparing inspired helium concentration with the expired, this total lung volume can be calculated.

- The kCO is *reduced* most in emphysema when alveoli have been destroyed
- It is also *reduced* in interstitial lung diseases where the alveolar capillary membrane may be thick enough to reduce CO passage
- It may also be *raised* when lungs are poorly expanded by, say, weak respiratory muscles, because the lung is 'more concentrated' and transfers CO *better* when quoted per unit volume
- kCO may also be *raised* when there has been profuse lung haemorrhage, as can occur in SLE, Wegener's, and Goodpasture's. This is because the free red cells lining the alveoli take up CO directly and 'falsely' elevate the figure.

This test requires more cooperation than simple spirometry, as well as a minimum inspired volume, and therefore cannot always be obtained.

Respiratory muscle function, body plethysmography, and lung volumes

Respiratory muscle function

Respiratory failure and small VCs may be due to weak respiratory muscles. It is therefore useful to be able to assess inspiratory and expiratory muscle power. There may be global weakness or specific inspiratory, usually diaphragm, weakness. In the clinic the simplest test is a **lying and standing VC**. If the diaphragm is paralysed then on lying down the abdominal contents will push up the diaphragm and limit inspiration. On standing the abdominal contents drop and aid inspiration.

- A fall in VC of less than 10% on lying down is probably normal
- A fall of 10–20% is suspicious of diaphragm paralysis
- A fall of more than 20% is abnormal and suggests significant, usually bilateral, diaphragm paralysis.

In the laboratory there are various ways to test respiratory muscle function. The patient blows against a *pressure meter* after a maximum inspiration, and inspires against the meter after a full expiration. This is, of course, highly effort-dependent. A manoeuvre such as a *sniff* is very stereotypic and patients can reproduce this. Measuring the inspiratory pressure produced at the nose during this manoeuvre is a reasonably reliable way of screening for inspiratory muscle weakness. More accurate assessments of inspiratory muscle function, particularly the diaphragm, can be obtained using two oesophageal balloons placed above and below the diaphragm and connected to pressure transducers. The *trans-diaphragmatic pressures* during maximal inspiratory efforts, sniffing, and breathing to TLC all provide reproducible measures of diaphragm function, but depend on good cooperation and effort by the patient. Activating the phrenic nerve directly with a superficial electrical stimulator, or by using high intensity magnetic stimulation over the nerve roots of C3 to C5, provides non-effort-dependent ways to test diaphragm function.

Body plethysmography requires the patient to climb into an airtight cabinet and breathe through a mouthpiece connected to the outside world. It has two particular advantages over simpler lung function tests. It is able to measure the **total lung volume or capacity** (TLC) in the thorax, and it provides a measure of airways obstruction involving little or no effort by the patient.

The other main method of measuring total lung capacity involves helium dilution as described above. However, in the presence of lower airways obstruction, the helium may not 'reach' all parts of the lung during the 10 s breath hold, and the volume of dilution will therefore be lower than the real TLC. The body plethysmograph relies on the pressure changes that occur when all the air in the chest is alternately compressed and expanded by the patient making breathing efforts against a airway closed by a shutter at the mouth. The pressure changes in the oral cavity are then proportional to the volume of air being compressed and rarefied, thus allowing calculation of the volume in the chest at the time. Note that this volume will include any bullae and the *difference between the plethysmographic lung volume and the helium dilution volume will reflect the bullae volume* as well as areas not reached by the helium due to increased airways resistance.

Measurement of *airways resistance* with the body box relies on a similar principle. If there were no airways resistance, then breathing in and out would not compress or rarefy the air in the chest. With increasing resistance, the air in the chest will be compressed during expiration and rarefied on inspiration. It is this phenomenon that allows calculation of the airways resistance during quiet breathing or panting (the latter ensures the vocal chords are fully open and not contributing to the measured resistance).

Lung volumes in normal, obstructive, and restrictive lung conditions.

TLC = total lung capacity
VC = vital capacity
RV = residual volume
FRC = functional residual capacity
FEV_1 = forced expiratory volume in one second

Derivative	Obstructive	Restrictive
FEV_1 (% predicted)	↓↓	↓
VC (% predicted)	↓ or →	↓
FEV_1/VC ratio	↓	→ or ↑ (increased recoil)
TLC (% predicted)	↑ or →	↓
RV (% predicted)	↑	↓
FRC (% predicted)	↑	↓
RV/TLC ratio	↑ (gas trapping)	→ or ↓

Peak flow reference ranges

Wright peak flow meters over-read slightly (approx. 50 l/min) in the mid-range (approx. 300 l/min), compared to gold-standard-measurements. From October 2004, new peak flow meters will have a corrected scale (in yellow to identify them). This will introduce some confusion if old and new meters are mixed indiscriminately. The following page is a conversion chart to be used when rewriting a management plan, based on peak flow measurements, and the patient is converting from an old to a new meter.

Converting peak flow values between Wright and EU scales
Find old peak flow reading on bottom of graph and read off value for a new EU scale meter on the vertical axis.

New EU scale versus Old Wright scale.

Appendix 2

Blood gases and acid–base balance

Interpretation of arterial blood gases: 1

Normal ranges
Breathing air: $PaO_2 > 12$ kPa (>10 in the elderly), $PaCO_2$ 4.7 to 5.9.

How to take
- **Arterial blood gases** Best taken from radial, rather then brachial, artery due to dual radial/ulnar supply to hand. Use a heparinized syringe, analyse immediately, or within 30 minutes if kept in crushed ice. Always record date and time. Record the % inspired O_2
- **Arterialized capillary sample** An under-used technique. Uses small glass pre-heparinized tube to draw up blood from a puncture on the end of the ear lobe. Blood gas machine must take microsamples (most do). $PaCO_2$ levels are accurate enough for clinical practice, but good arterialization, with rubificants (Algipan/Deep Heat) or heat and vigorous rubbing, required for accurate PaO_2: the latter is less important as oxygenation can be assessed by oximetry. Can easily be performed by nursing staff, to monitor response to NIV and O_2 therapy.

The three main things blood gases tell you about gas exchange:
- How much is the patient ventilating their alveoli? This is derived from the $PaCO_2$. $PaCO_2 > 6$ kPa = underventilating, $PaCO_2 < 4$ kPa = overventilating
- Is the PaO_2 high enough to adequately oxygenate tissues and prevent anaerobic metabolism? $PaO_2 > 6$ kPa ($SaO_2 \cong 80\%$) is probably adequate; $PaO_2 > 7$ kPa ($SaO_2 > 87\%$) is adequate
- Is there evidence of V/Q mismatch? Evidence of low V/Q units is derived from the calculated alveolar to arterial (A–a) gradient.

The two main things blood gases tell you about acid/base balance:
(see section below on acid/base balance)
- What is the respiratory component to an abnormal pH? This is derived from the $PaCO_2$
- What is the metabolic component to an abnormal pH? This is derived from the standard base excess/deficit.

The A–a gradient calculator graph sets out the graphical representation of gas exchange.
- Point ① = pO_2 and pCO_2 of *inspired air*. (Point ② = pO_2 and pCO_2 when breathing 24% O_2 via a Ventimask and point ③ = pO_2 and pCO_2 when breathing 28% O_2 via a Ventimask)
- Point ④ = theoretical pO_2/pCO_2 of *alveolar gas* when breathing air, if all the O_2 removed and replaced by CO_2 (equivalent to extreme hypoventilation and impossible!), when the respiratory quotient (RQ=CO_2 produced/O_2 consumed) is 0.8 (usual value)
- The line between ① and ④ with a gradient of 0.8 describes all possible combinations of alveolar gas, moving towards ① if breathing more, and towards ④ if breathing less, called the *alveolar air line*

- Point ⑤ = area in which PaO_2 and $PaCO_2$ of *arterial blood* sit normally. If lungs are perfect gas exchangers, then blood leaving the lungs and entering systemic arterial circulation (⑤) should be perfectly equilibrated with the alveolar gas (A).

pCO_2 versus pO_2, A–a gradient calculator.

Interpretation of arterial blood gases: 2

Point ⑥ = However, the *mixed venous point* (the pulmonary arterial blood) is well to the left of the alveolar air line. This is because capillary PO_2 falls more kPa than the PCO_2 rises during gas exchange in the tissues (CO$_2$ solubility curve is steeper than PaO_2/SaO_2 dissociation curve). Thus if the lungs fail to oxygenate mixed venous blood properly (e.g. area of pneumonia, or low V/Q due to asthma/COPD) then it is as if mixed venous blood has bypassed the lung and leaked into the arterial blood, which therefore moves the eventual arterial $PaO_2/PaCO_2$ point to the left of the alveolar air line, point ⑦. The horizontal distance that the actual arterial point is to the left of the 'ideal' alveolar air line is called the *alveolar to arterial (A–a) gradient* and is a measure of how efficiently mixed venous blood is being equilibrated with alveolar gas, i.e. it is a measure of V/Q mismatch and right-to-left shunts. As well as being read off the graph it can be mathematically calculated as follows.

Calculation of alveolar PO_2 breathing air or 24/28% O_2.

Air, 21% of (100–7) $\cong$ 20 kPa (where 100 kPa is atmospheric pressure, and 7 kPa is water vapour pressure)
24%, 24% of (100–7) $\cong$ 23 kPa
28%, 28% of (100–7) $\cong$ 27 kPa

On the graph the 'alveolar air' line depends on the % inspired O_2, and the two extra lines, for 24% and 28% O_2, are shown. In the calculation the PAO_2 has to be adjusted accordingly, see above.

In normal lung there is not perfect matching of V/Q due to relative under-perfusion of the apices and overperfusion of the bases (gravity effects on pulmonary arterial blood flow). These imperfections in V/Q, and direct drainage of some of the cardiac muscle venous blood into the systemic arterial circulation, lead to a small A–a gradient, 1 to 2 kPa in the young and middle aged, and 2 to 3 in the elderly. Figures in excess of these values are abnormal and indicate areas of low V/Q or increased shunt.

pCO$_2$ versus pO$_2$, A–a gradient calculator.

Use of A–a gradient diagram: examples

Case 1 Consider point (W) in the pO_2/pCO_2 graph, the blood gases on air of a young non-smoker complaining of chest pain 7 days post op. The PaO_2 of 13 is normal; does this reassure you or does it provide supporting evidence for a pulmonary embolus?

- How much is the patient ventilating? $PaCO_2 < 4$ kPa; therefore some hyperventilation
- Is the patient adequately oxygenated? $PaO_2 > 7$ kPa; therefore OK
- Is there an abnormal A–a gradient? Read off graph, horizontal line between W and alveolar line, or calculate:

$$20 - \left(13 + \frac{2}{0.8}\right) = 4.5 \text{ kPa}$$

  >2 kPa, hence yes; therefore the V/Q matching is not normal.
  This provides supporting evidence for a pulmonary embolus, but could just as well be due to a pneumonia, for example
- Remember, PaO_2 cannot be used to assess V/Q matching in the lung without an associated $PaCO_2$ to tell you 'what the PaO_2 ought to be'.

Case 2 Consider point (X) on the pO_2/pCO_2 graph. These are the gases on air from a young man following an overdose of methadone tablets.

- How much is the patient ventilating? $PaCO_2 > 6$ kPa; therefore is hypoventilating
- Is the patient adequately oxygenated? PaO_2 only 6 kPa; therefore not enough and needs added O_2
- Has the patient got an A–a gradient?

$$20 - \left(6 + \frac{11}{0.8}\right) = 0.8 \text{ kPa}$$

  <2 kPa, hence no; therefore there is nothing wrong with the lungs, despite the abnormal gases that represent pure hypoventilation.
  After a messy stomach wash-out he is sent to the ward and 24 h later is febrile. Gases on 24% O_2 are point (Y) on the graph, thus both $PaCO_2$ and PaO_2 are better
- How much is the patient ventilating? $PaCO_2$ just >6 kPa; therefore is still hypoventilating a tiny bit
- Is the patient adequately oxygenated? $PaO_2 > 7$ kPa; therefore adequately oxygenated
- Has the patient got an A–a gradient?

$$23 - \left(11 + \frac{6.5}{0.8}\right) = 4.2 \text{ kPa} \quad \text{(remember, the } PAO_2 \text{ is 23 because he is on 24\% } O_2\text{)}$$

  >2 kPa hence yes; therefore may have developed an aspiration pneumonia.

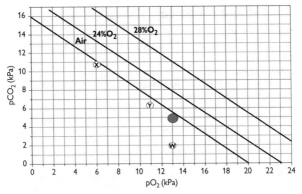

Examples of using A–a gradient.

Acid–base balance

Normal ranges

pH 7.37 to 7.43 (H^+ 37 to 43 nmol/l), $PaCO_2$ 4.7 to 5.9, base excess ±3 mmol/l.

Interpretation Acid/base relationships are best plotted as $PaCO_2$ versus pH graph, as these are the two primary measurements made by a blood gas machine (everything else to do with acid/base balance is calculated). This is shown opposite.

Normal acid/base is the area labelled (N), the pH between 7.37 and 7.43, the $PaCO_2$ between 4 and 6 kPa. As ventilation is decreased or increased ($PaCO_2$ going up or down, respectively), the pH will change depending on the *buffering capacity* of the blood (CO_2 is an acid gas as it combines with water to give $[H^+]$ and $[HCO_3^-]$ ions). Without buffering the pH would fall disastrously with small rises in $PaCO_2$. This buffering capacity depends mainly on *haemoglobin and other proteins*, and results in the normal buffer line running through (N) on the graph.

Therefore *acute hypoventilation and hyperventilation* will move the patient up and down this line, in the direction *b* or *c*, respectively. If the hypoventilation at point *b* persists (e.g. as it may in COPD), then the kidney retains bicarbonate (thus excreting hydrogen ions) to try and correct the pH towards normal, and the patient moves on to a new buffer line displaced to the right, e.g. the one labelled + 10 meq/l (35 meq/l). The degree of displacement represents the *metabolic component to the acid/base status*, and in this case, because the $[HCO_3^-]$ has risen, will be higher than the normal figure of around 25 meq/l. When the raised figure is quoted relative to the normal 25 meq/l (by subtracting 25), this is called the 'base excess'. Thus buffer lines to the right of the normal buffer line represent a metabolic alkalosis or base excess.

These figures are calculated assuming a normal or 'standard' $PaCO_2$, called the 'standard bicarbonate' (SBC on the blood gas machine printout), or 'standard base excess' (usually BE). The other two figures for total bicarbonate on the printout (usually HCO_3^- and TCO_2) are calculated at the patient's actual $PaCO_2$ and are not much use.

Chronic hyperventilation (e.g. at altitude due to the hypoxia) produces the opposite, a resorption of $[H^+]$ by the kidney, and the buffer line shifts to the left giving a negative value for the 'base excess', a 'base deficit'. Thus a metabolic acidosis compensates for a respiratory alkalosis. Note that these corrections rarely bring the pH back to normal as there needs to be an error signal to keep the correction process going.

A *metabolic acidosis* (such as in ketoacidosis) will also move the line to the left (*a*), producing a base deficit (or negative base excess), followed by hyperventilation to try and correct it (i.e. a respiratory alkalosis to correct a metabolic acidosis). This pure ventilatory stimulation in the absence of abnormal lungs often produces deep breathing with little increase in rate and is called Kussmaul's breathing. Thus lines to the left of the normal buffer line represent a metabolic acidosis or base deficit. Such a metabolic acidosis due to anaerobic metabolism can reverse the compensatory metabolic alkalosis secondary to chronic hypercapnia during a severely hypoxic COPD exacerbation, removing the evidence for chronic CO_2 retention.

Finally a *metabolic alkalosis* (e.g. during hypokalaemia when the kidney is forced to use hydrogen ions instead of potassium ions to swap for the sodium that needs resorbing from the tubular fluid). The buffer line will move to the right (*d*), with only limited hypoventilation available to compensate, due to the inevitable attendant hypoxaemia this produces.

Thus the mixture of respiratory and metabolic contributions to a patients acid/base disturbance can be established by plotting the $PaCO_2$ and pH on the graph.

• Remember, there are only two main things to think about when assessing the pH: is the $PaCO_2$ abnormally high or low, and is there a metabolic component evidenced by a shift of the buffer line to the left or right—numerically the base excess (or deficit)?

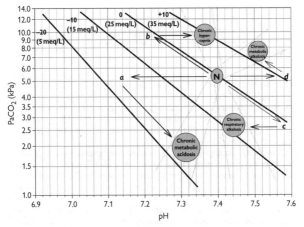

Acid/base balance—$PaCO_2$/pH.

Conversion between arterial oxygen saturation and oxygen tension

A *fall in pH*, or a rise *in body temperature*, will move the dissociation curve to the *right*. This has the effect of making the *PaO₂ higher for any given SaO₂*, e.g. at pH 7.20, a measured saturation (e.g. by oximetry) of 90% is equivalent to a PaO₂ of 9.7 kPa (73 mmHg), rather than 7.7 kPa (58 mmHg): a rise in body temperature to 41°C will do the same, and the effects of pH and temperature are additive.

Conversely, for a given PaO₂, pyrexia and acidosis will lower the SaO₂ and thus oxygen carriage to the tissues. Base deficit/excess has an independent but relatively small effect too. Increasing 2,3-DPG levels shift the curve to the right, but levels fluctuate unpredictably and any changes are small.

Changes in body temperature and acidosis are the usual reasons why measured pulse oximetry saturations apparently 'do not agree' with the measured blood gases (pH *is* taken into account in the *theoretical* calculation of SaO₂ by most analysers, but the patient's body temperature is rarely entered).

Conversion chart*

% saturation	kPa	mmHg
98	15.0	112
97	12.2	92
96	10.8	81
95	9.9	74
94	9.3	70
93	8.8	66
92	8.4	63
91	8.1	60
90	7.7	58
88	7.3	55
86	6.8	51
84	6.5	49
82	6.2	47
80	5.9	45
75	5.4	40
70	4.9	37
65	4.5	34
60	4.2	31
55	3.8	29
50	3.5	27

* kPa and mmHg: conversion factor, 7.5 x kPa = mmHg
assuming normal position of the haemoglobin dissociation curve.

CT anatomy of the thorax

CT anatomy of the thorax: level of C7.

Brachiocephalic vein

Common carotid artery

Subclavian artery

Oesophagus

Upper lobe

Spinal cord

Right brachiocephalic artery

Brachiocephalic vein

Top of inominate artery

Upper lobe

CT anatomy of the thorax: level of T2.

Anterior mediastinal fat and thymic remnants

Aortic arch

Trachea

Oesophagus

Upper lobe

Internal thoracic artery and vein

Superior vena cava

Upper lobe

CT anatomy of the thorax: level of T4.

Pulmonary trunk
Upper lobe
Superior pulmonary vein
Left pulmonary artery
Left main bronchus
Descending aorta
Oblique fissure
Lower lobe

Upper lobe
Descending aorta
Superior vena cava
Upper lobe bronchus
Superior pulmonary vein
Right main bronchus
Oesophagus
Azygos vein
Oblique fissure
Lower lobe

CT anatomy of the thorax: level of T6.

CT anatomy of the thorax: level of T7.

Ascending aorta/ outflow tract

Upper lobe

Left ventricular wall

Left atrium

Inferior left pulmonary vein

Left pulmonary arteries

Descending aorta

Right ventricle

Azygos vein

Middle lobe

Lymph node

Right atrium

Superior vena cava

Oblique fissure

Lower lobe bronchus

Pulmonary artery

Right ventricular wall

Left ventricular cavity

Left ventricular wall

Dome of left diaphragm

Descending aorta

Pericardium

Right ventricular cavity

Right atrium

Liver

Oesophagus

Azygos vein

CT anatomy of the thorax: level of T9.

3

CT patterns of lung disease

Term	Process	Causes
Air space consolidation	Fluid/secretion accumulation in alveoli	Pneumonia, pulmonary oedema or haemorrhage, ARDS, COP, lymphoma
Air trapping	Partial small airway obstruction	Asthma, obliterative bronchiolitis
Cystic air spaces	Clearly defined air-containing space with definable wall	LAM, LCH, end-stage UIP, PCP, LIP
Fissural nodularity	Nodules seen along the pulmonary fissures	Sarcoidosis. Also described in Kaposi's sarcoma
Ground-glass shadowing	Grey appearance to lung interstitium; air in bronchus looks blacker	Parenchymal inflammatory conditions, such as sarcoidosis, alveolitis, hyper-sensitivity pneumonitis, pulmonary oedema or haemorrhage, PCP, drug/radiation injury
Honeycomb lung	End-stage fibrotic lung	UIP
Mosaic attenuation pattern	Well-defined areas of normal lung abutting abnormal lung, giving a mosaic pattern. Seen particularly in expiration	Indicates small airways disease such as asthma, vascular disease such as PE, or infiltrative disease such as obliterative bronchiolitis, hypersensitivity pneumonitis
Nodularity	Small discrete dots 2–10 mm, may be in air spaces or interstitium	Metastases, sarcoidosis, pneumoconiosis, hypersensitivity pneumonitis, miliary TB, fungal infection, idiopathic pulmonary haemorrhage, alveolar microlithiasis, varicella pneumonitis
Poorly defined centrilobular nodules	Peribronchiolar inflammation in the absence of intraluminal secretion	Hypersensitivity pneumonitis, RB-ILD
Reticular pattern	Linear fine lines, indicating thickened interlobular septa. Sub-pleural reticulation	ILD, pulmonary oedema, pulmonary haemorrhage, lymphangitis, UIP
Tree-in-bud	Mucus/pus/secretions filling bronchioles and causing dilatation	Small airways disease, particularly infection including MTB, haemophilus, diffuse pan-bronchiolitis, CF, yellow nail syndrome, primary pulmonary lymphoma

BMI calculator and height converter

Height in metres

Weight in kilograms	1.36	1.40	1.44	1.48	1.52	1.56	1.60	1.64	1.68	1.72	1.76	1.80	1.84	1.88	1.92	1.96	2.00
125	68	64	60	57	54	51	49	46	44	42	40	39	37	35	34	33	31
123	67	63	59	56	53	51	48	46	44	42	40	38	36	35	33	32	31
121	65	62	58	55	52	50	47	45	43	41	39	37	36	34	33	31	30
119	64	61	57	54	52	49	46	44	42	40	38	37	35	34	32	31	30
117	63	60	56	53	51	48	46	44	41	40	38	36	35	33	32	30	29
115	62	59	55	53	50	47	45	43	41	39	37	35	34	33	31	30	29
113	61	58	54	52	49	46	44	42	40	38	36	35	33	32	31	29	28
111	60	57	54	51	48	46	43	41	39	38	36	34	33	31	30	29	28
109	59	56	53	50	47	45	43	41	39	37	35	34	32	31	30	28	27
107	58	55	52	49	46	44	42	40	38	36	35	33	32	30	29	28	27
105	57	54	51	48	45	43	41	39	37	35	34	32	31	30	28	27	26
103	56	53	50	47	45	42	40	38	36	35	33	32	30	29	28	27	26
101	55	52	49	46	44	42	39	38	36	34	33	31	30	29	27	26	25
99	54	51	48	45	43	41	39	37	35	33	32	31	29	28	27	26	25
97	52	49	47	44	42	40	38	36	34	33	31	30	28	27	26	25	24
95	51	48	46	43	41	39	37	35	34	32	31	29	28	27	26	25	24
93	50	47	45	42	40	38	36	34	32	31	30	29	27	26	25	24	23
91	49	46	44	42	39	37	36	34	32	31	29	28	27	26	25	24	23
89	48	45	43	41	39	37	35	33	32	30	29	27	26	25	24	23	22
87	47	44	42	40	38	36	34	32	31	29	28	27	26	25	24	23	22
85	46	43	41	39	37	35	33	32	30	29	27	26	25	24	23	22	21
83	45	42	40	38	36	34	32	31	29	28	27	26	25	23	22	22	21
81	44	41	39	37	35	33	32	30	29	27	26	25	24	23	22	21	20
79	43	40	38	36	34	32	31	29	28	27	26	24	23	22	21	21	20
77	42	39	37	35	33	32	30	29	27	26	25	24	23	22	21	20	19
75	41	38	36	34	32	31	29	28	27	25	24	23	22	21	20	20	19
73	39	37	35	33	32	30	29	27	26	25	24	23	22	21	20	19	18
71	38	36	34	32	31	29	28	26	25	24	23	22	21	20	19	18	18
69	37	35	33	32	30	28	27	26	24	23	22	21	20	20	19	18	17
67	36	34	32	31	29	28	26	25	24	23	22	21	20	19	18	17	17
65	35	33	31	30	28	27	25	24	23	22	21	20	19	18	18	17	16
63	34	32	30	29	27	26	25	23	22	21	20	19	19	18	17	16	16
61	33	31	29	28	26	25	24	23	22	21	20	19	18	17	17	16	15
59	32	30	28	27	26	24	23	22	21	20	19	18	17	17	16	15	15
57	31	29	27	26	25	23	22	21	20	19	18	18	17	16	15	15	14
55	30	28	27	25	24	23	21	20	19	19	18	17	16	16	15	14	14
53	29	27	26	24	23	22	21	20	19	18	17	16	16	15	14	14	13
51	28	26	25	23	22	21	20	19	18	17	16	16	15	14	14	13	13
49	26	25	24	22	21	20	19	18	17	17	16	15	14	14	13	13	12
47	25	24	23	21	20	19	18	17	17	16	15	15	14	13	13	12	12
45	24	23	22	21	19	18	18	17	16	15	15	14	13	13	12	12	11
43	23	22	21	20	19	18	17	16	15	15	14	13	13	12	12	11	11

BMI <18.5 – underweight

BMI 18.5–24.9 – acceptable weight

BMI 25–29.9 – overweight

BMI 30–39.9 – obese

BMI >= 40 – morbid obesity

BMI calculator

Height Converter

Height (ft and in)	Height (m)
5'0"	1.52
5'1"	1.55
5'2"	1.58
5'3"	1.60
5'4"	1.63
5'5"	1.65
5'6"	1.68
5'7"	1.70
5'8"	1.73
5'9"	1.75
5'10"	1.78
5'11"	1.80
6'0"	1.83
6'1"	1.85
6'2"	1.88
6'3"	1.90
6'4"	1.93
6'5"	1.96
6'6"	1.98

Useful websites

Thoracic societies
American College of Chest Physicians *www.chestnet.org*
American Thoracic Society *www.thoracic.org*
British Society for Allergy and Clinical Immunology *www.bsaci.org*
British Thoracic Society *www.brit-thoracic.org.uk*
Canadian Thoracic Society *www.lung.ca*
European Respiratory Society *www.ersnet.org*
Society of Thoracic Surgeons *www.sts.org*
Thoracic Society of Australia and New Zealand *www.thoracic.org.au*

Thoracic journals
American Journal of Respiratory and Critical Care Medicine ('Blue journal') *ajrccm.atsjournals.org*
American Journal of Respiratory Cell and Molecular Biology *www.ajrcmb.org*
Chest *www.chestjournal.org*
European Respiratory Journal access via *www.ersnet.org*
Thorax *thorax.bmjjournals.com*

General journals
British Medical Journal *bmj.bmjjournals.com*
Free medical journals site *www.freemedicaljournals.com*
Journal of the American Medical Association *jama.ama-assn.org*
The Lancet *www.thelancet.com*
National Library of Medicine (Pub Med) *www.ncbi.nlm.nih.gov/entrez/query.fcgi*
New England Journal of Medicine *content.nejm.org*

Teaching resources
BTS training site *www.chestnet.net*
Drugs that cause lung disease *www.pneumotox.com*
Evidence-based medicine site *www.bestbets.org*
Simple thoracic and other anatomy site *anatomy.uams.edu*
Supercourse lectures on public health *www.pitt.edu/~super1*
University of New South Wales teaching/pathology site *www.med.unsw.edu.au/pathology/pathmus*

Fitness to drive
www.dvla.gov.uk

Charities
British Lung Foundation *www.lunguk.org*

Index